Principles of Computerized Tomographic Imaging

SIAM's Classics in Applied Mathematics series consists of books that were previously allowed to go out of print. These books are republished by SIAM as a professional service because they continue to be important resources for mathematical scientists.

Editor-in-Chief

Robert E. O'Malley, Jr., *University of Washington*

Editorial Board

Richard A. Brualdi, *University of Wisconsin-Madison*

Herbert B. Keller, *California Institute of Technology*

Andrzej Z. Manitius, *George Mason University*

Ingram Olkin, *Stanford University*

Stanley Richardson, *University of Edinburgh*

Ferdinand Verhulst, *Mathematisch Instituut, University of Utrecht*

Classics in Applied Mathematics

C. C. Lin and L. A. Segel, *Mathematics Applied to Deterministic Problems in the Natural Sciences*

Johan G. F. Belinfante and Bernard Kolman, *A Survey of Lie Groups and Lie Algebras with Applications and Computational Methods*

James M. Ortega, *Numerical Analysis: A Second Course*

Anthony V. Fiacco and Garth P. McCormick, *Nonlinear Programming: Sequential Unconstrained Minimization Techniques*

F. H. Clarke, *Optimization and Nonsmooth Analysis*

George F. Carrier and Carl E. Pearson, *Ordinary Differential Equations*

Leo Breiman, *Probability*

R. Bellman and G. M. Wing, *An Introduction to Invariant Imbedding*

Abraham Berman and Robert J. Plemmons, *Nonnegative Matrices in the Mathematical Sciences*

Olvi L. Mangasarian, *Nonlinear Programming*

*Carl Friedrich Gauss, *Theory of the Combination of Observations Least Subject to Errors: Part One, Part Two, Supplement.* Translated by G. W. Stewart

Richard Bellman, *Introduction to Matrix Analysis*

U. M. Ascher, R. M. M. Mattheij, and R. D. Russell, *Numerical Solution of Boundary Value Problems for Ordinary Differential Equations*

K. E. Brenan, S. L. Campbell, and L. R. Petzold, *Numerical Solution of Initial-Value Problems in Differential-Algebraic Equations*

Charles L. Lawson and Richard J. Hanson, *Solving Least Squares Problems*

J. E. Dennis, Jr. and Robert B. Schnabel, *Numerical Methods for Unconstrained Optimization and Nonlinear Equations*

Richard E. Barlow and Frank Proschan, *Mathematical Theory of Reliability*

*First time in print.

Classics in Applied Mathematics (continued)

Cornelius Lanczos, *Linear Differential Operators*

Richard Bellman, *Introduction to Matrix Analysis, Second Edition*

Beresford N. Parlett, *The Symmetric Eigenvalue Problem*

Richard Haberman, *Mathematical Models: Mechanical Vibrations, Population Dynamics, and Traffic Flow*

Peter W. M. John, *Statistical Design and Analysis of Experiments*

Tamer Başar and Geert Jan Olsder, *Dynamic Noncooperative Game Theory, Second Edition*

Emanuel Parzen, *Stochastic Processes*

Petar Kokotović, Hassan K. Khalil, and John O'Reilly, *Singular Perturbation Methods in Control: Analysis and Design*

Jean Dickinson Gibbons, Ingram Olkin, and Milton Sobel, *Selecting and Ordering Populations: A New Statistical Methodology*

James A. Murdock, *Perturbations: Theory and Methods*

Ivar Ekeland and Roger Témam, *Convex Analysis and Variational Problems*

Ivar Stakgold, *Boundary Value Problems of Mathematical Physics, Volumes I and II*

J. M. Ortega and W. C. Rheinboldt, *Iterative Solution of Nonlinear Equations in Several Variables*

David Kinderlehrer and Guido Stampacchia, *An Introduction to Variational Inequalities and Their Applications*

F. Natterer, *The Mathematics of Computerized Tomography*

Avinash C. Kak and Malcolm Slaney, *Principles of Computerized Tomographic Imaging*

R. Wong, *Asymptotic Approximations of Integrals*

O. Axelsson and V. A. Barker, *Finite Element Solution of Boundary Value Problems: Theory and Computation*

David R. Brillinger, *Time Series: Data Analysis and Theory*

Joel N. Franklin, *Methods of Mathematical Economics: Linear and Nonlinear Programming, Fixed-Point Theorems*

Philip Hartman, *Ordinary Differential Equations, Second Edition*

Michael D. Intriligator, *Mathematical Optimization and Economic Theory*

Philippe G. Ciarlet, *The Finite Element Method for Elliptic Problems*

Jane K. Cullum and Ralph A. Willoughby, *Lanczos Algorithms for Large Symmetric Eigenvalue Computations, Vol. I: Theory*

M. Vidyasagar, *Nonlinear Systems Analysis, Second Edition*

Robert Mattheij and Jaap Molenaar, *Ordinary Differential Equations in Theory and Practice*

Shanti S. Gupta and S. Panchapakesan, *Multiple Decision Procedures: Theory and Methodology of Selecting and Ranking Populations*

Eugene L. Allgower and Kurt Georg, *Introduction to Numerical Continuation Methods*

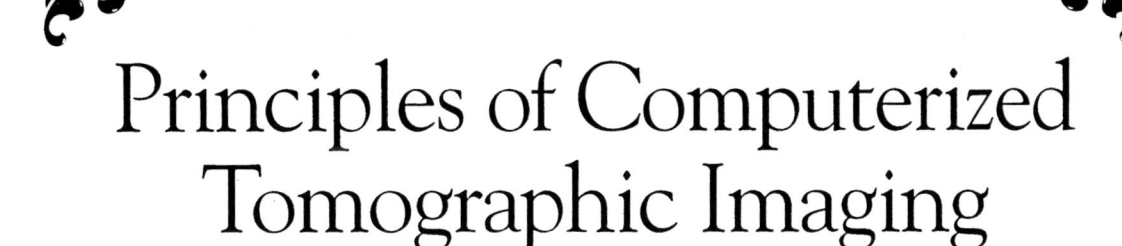

Principles of Computerized Tomographic Imaging

Avinash C. Kak
Purdue University
West Lafayette, Indiana

Malcolm Slaney
IBM Almaden Research Center
San Jose, California

siam.
Society for Industrial and Applied Mathematics
Philadelphia

Copyright © 2001 by the Society for Industrial and Applied Mathematics.

This SIAM edition is an unabridged republication of the work first published by IEEE Press, New York, 1988.

10 9 8 7 6 5 4 3 2

All rights reserved. Printed in the United States of America. No part of this book may be reproduced, stored, or transmitted in any manner without the written permission of the publisher. For information, write to the Society for Industrial and Applied Mathematics, 3600 University City Science Center, Philadelphia, PA 19104-2688.

Library of Congress Cataloging-in-Publication Data

Kak, Avinash C.
    Principles of computerized tomographic imaging / Avinash C. Kak, Malcolm Slaney.
      p. cm. -- (Classics in applied mathematics ; 33)
    "This SIAM edition is an abridged republication of the work first published
  by IEEE Press, New York, 1988."
    Includes bibliographical references and index.
    ISBN 0-89871-494-X (pbk.)
      1. Tomography. I. Slaney, Malcolm. II. Title. III. Series.

RC78.7.T6 K35 2001
616.07'57--dc21

                                                               2001020475

siam is a registered trademark.

Contents

Preface to the Classics Edition   xi

Preface   xiii

1 *Introduction*   1
       References   3

2 *Signal Processing Fundamentals*   5
    2.1   One-Dimensional Signal Processing   5

         Continuous and Discrete One-Dimensional Functions • Linear Operations • Fourier Representation • Discrete Fourier Transform (DFT) • Finite Fourier Transform • Just How Much Data Is Needed? • Interpretation of the FFT Output • How to Increase the Display Resolution in the Frequency Domain • How to Deal with Data Defined for Negative Time • How to Increase Frequency Domain Display Resolution of Signals Defined for Negative Time • Data Truncation Effects

    2.2   Image Processing   28

         Point Sources and Delta Functions • Linear Shift Invariant Operations • Fourier Analysis • Properties of Fourier Transforms • The Two-Dimensional Finite Fourier Transform • Numerical Implementation of the Two-Dimensional FFT

    2.3   References   47

3 *Algorithms for Reconstruction with Nondiffracting Sources*   49
    3.1   Line Integrals and Projections   49
    3.2   The Fourier Slice Theorem   56
    3.3   Reconstruction Algorithms for Parallel Projections   60

         The Idea • Theory • Computer Implementation of the Algorithm

    3.4   Reconstruction from Fan Projections   75

         Equiangular Rays • Equally Spaced Collinear Detectors • A Re-sorting Algorithm

    3.5   Fan Beam Reconstruction from a Limited Number of Views   93
    3.6   Three-Dimensional Reconstructions   99

         Three-Dimensional Projections • Three-Dimensional Filtered Backprojection

3.7 Bibliographic Notes   107
3.8 References   110

4 Measurement of Projection Data—The Nondiffracting Case   113

4.1 X-Ray Tomography   114

Monochromatic X-Ray Projections • Measurement of Projection Data with Polychromatic Sources • Polychromaticity Artifacts in X-Ray CT • Scatter • Different Methods for Scanning • Applications

4.2 Emission Computed Tomography   134

Single Photon Emission Tomography • Attenuation Compensation for Single Photon Emission CT • Positron Emission Tomography • Attenuation Compensation for Positron Tomography

4.3 Ultrasonic Computed Tomography   147

Fundamental Considerations • Ultrasonic Refractive Index Tomography • Ultrasonic Attenuation Tomography • Applications

4.4 Magnetic Resonance Imaging   158
4.5 Bibliographic Notes   168
4.6 References   169

5 Aliasing Artifacts and Noise in CT Images   177

5.1 Aliasing Artifacts   177

What Does Aliasing Look Like? • Sampling in a Real System

5.2 Noise in Reconstructed Images   190

The Continuous Case • The Discrete Case

5.3 Bibliographic Notes   200
5.4 References   200

6 Tomographic Imaging with Diffracting Sources   203

6.1 Diffracted Projections   204

Homogeneous Wave Equation • Inhomogeneous Wave Equation

6.2 Approximations to the Wave Equation   211

The First Born Approximation • The First Rytov Approximation

6.3 The Fourier Diffraction Theorem   218

Decomposing the Green's Function • Fourier Transform Approach • Short Wavelength Limit of the Fourier Diffraction Theorem • The Data Collection Process

6.4 Interpolation and a Filtered Backpropagation Algorithm for Diffracting Sources   234

Frequency Domain Interpolation • Backpropagation Algorithms

6.5 Limitations 247

    Mathematical Limitations • Evaluation of the Born Approximation • Evaluation of the Rytov Approximation • Comparison of the Born and Rytov Approximations

6.6 Evaluation of Reconstruction Algorithms 252
6.7 Experimental Limitations 261

    Evanescent Waves • Sampling the Received Wave • The Effects of a Finite Receiver Length • Evaluation of the Experimental Effects • Optimization • Limited Views

6.8 Bibliographic Notes 268
6.9 References 270

7 Algebraic Reconstruction Algorithms 275

7.1 Image and Projection Representation 276
7.2 ART (Algebraic Reconstruction Techniques) 283
7.3 SIRT (Simultaneous Iterative Reconstructive Technique) 284
7.4 SART (Simultaneous Algebraic Reconstruction Technique) 285

    Modeling the Forward Projection Process • Implementation of the Reconstruction Algorithm

7.5 Bibliographic Notes 292
7.6 References 295

8 Reflection Tomography 297

8.1 Introduction 297
8.2 B-Scan Imaging 298
8.3 Reflection Tomography 303

    Plane Wave Reflection Transducers • Reflection Tomography vs. Diffraction Tomography • Reflection Tomography Limits

8.4 Reflection Tomography with Point Transmitter/Receivers 313

    Reconstruction Algorithms • Experimental Results

8.5 Bibliographic Notes 321
8.6 References 321

Index 323

Preface to the Classics Edition

We are pleased that SIAM is republishing this book on the principles of computerized tomography. We enjoyed writing it and have heard from many people who found the book valuable. We're glad that the book is now back in print.

The worlds of tomography and medical imaging have not stood still in the twelve years since this book was first published, yet the basic algorithms presented in this book are just as important today as when they were first applied to tomographic imaging. The reconstruction formalism that underlies these algorithms helps us create efficient implementations for medical scanners and provides us with a theoretical framework to think about issues such as noise, sampling, resolution and artifacts. We hope that the new readers of our book will also appreciate the beauty of these algorithms.

The primary strength of this book consists of derivations that are appropriate for engineers and scientists who want to understand the principles of computerized tomographic imaging. We hope that these derivations will provide readers with insights to create their own implementations. For our readers more interested in the medical applications of computerized tomography we suggest they also consult Lee's [Lee98] or Haaga's [Haa94] books. For readers interested in more mathematical rigor or a discussion of the mathematical foundations of cross-sectional imaging we suggest they supplement our book with the book by Natterer and Wübbeling [Nat01].

The years since our book was first published have witnessed an increased interest in helical acquisition and reconstruction methods. We cover the basics of this topic in Section 3.6. Interested readers should also consult the paper by Crawford and King [Cra90] and the special issue of *Transactions on Medical Imaging* [Wan00] for an overview of current approaches.

Perhaps the most surprising development in the tomography field has been the application of these algorithms to geophysical phenomena. Researchers have used tomography to study the ocean [Mun95] at scales we are sure were not imagined by Hounsfield when he created his first scans. Likewise, tomographic algorithms have been used for whole-earth imaging [Iye93].

Lately, much work has used tomographic data (and MRI data) to generate volume renderings of internal organs. This work can allow physicians to "fly" through internal organs and provide interesting ways for radiologists to understand the state of a human body.

Before we wrote this book, it taxed our laboratory's abilities to collect the data and create 64 × 64 reconstructions. Today, high-end medical scanners do helical cone-beam tomography, collect four rows of data (1000 detectors per row and 1000 views per rotation) in one-half second, and produce 512 × 512 images in near-real time. We hope our book will help people understand both ends of this spectrum.

The authors would like to thank the IEEE for their many years of support and for allowing us to republish our book. We would also like to thank our colleague Carl Crawford for his support over the years and his creative means of encouraging us to publish a new edition. One of the authors (MS) would like to publicly thank Barb Booth, Jim Ziegler, Gordon Speer, and Anne (Atkins) Burch for their early encouragement in the areas of mathematics, science, and publishing.

A number of corrections and some sample codes are available on the Web at *http://www.slaney.org/pct*.

[Cra90] C. R. Crawford, K. F. King, *Computed tomography scanning with simultaneous patient translation*, Medical Physics, Vol. 17, No. 6, pp. 967–982, November/December 1990.

[Haa94] J. R. Haaga, C. F. Lanzieri, D. J. Sartoris (Eds.), *Computed Tomography and Magnetic Resonance Imaging of the Whole Body*. 3rd edition, St. Louis, MO: Mosby, 1994.

[Iye93] H.M. Iyer, K. Hirahara (Eds.), *Seismic Tomography: Theory and Practice*. London; New York: Chapman & Hall, 1993.

[Lee98] J. K. T. Lee, S. S. Sagel, R. J. Stanley, J. P. Heiken (Eds.), *Computed Body Tomography with MRI Correlation*. 3rd edition, Philadelphia, PA: Lippincott Williams & Wilkins, 1998.

[Mun95] W. H. Munk, P. Worchester, C. Wunsch, *Ocean Acoustic Tomography*. Cambridge: Cambridge University Press, 1995.

[Nat01] F. Natterer, F. Wübbeling, *Mathematical Methods in Image Reconstruction*. Philadelphia, PA: SIAM, 2001.

[Wan00] G. Wang, C. Crawford, W. Kalender (Eds.), *Special Issue on Multirow Detector and Cone-Beam Spiral/Helical Computed Tomography*, IEEE Transactions on Medical Imaging, Vol. 19, No. 9, September 2000.

Preface

The purpose of this book is to provide a tutorial overview on the subject of computerized tomographic imaging. We expect the book to be useful for practicing engineers and scientists for gaining an understanding of what can and cannot be done with tomographic imaging. Toward this end, we have tried to strike a balance among purely algorithmic issues, topics dealing with how to generate data for reconstruction in different domains, and artifacts inherent to different data collection strategies.

Our hope is that the style of presentation used will also make the book useful for a beginning graduate course on the subject. The desired prerequisites for taking such a course will depend upon the aims of the instructor. If the instructor wishes to teach the course primarily at a theoretical level, with not much emphasis on computer implementations of the reconstruction algorithms, the book is mostly self-contained for graduate students in engineering, the sciences, and mathematics. On the other hand, if the instructor wishes to impart proficiency in the implementations, it would be desirable for the students to have had some prior experience with writing computer programs for digital signal or image processing. The introductory material we have included in Chapter 2 should help the reader review the relevant practical details in digital signal and image processing. There are no homework problems in the book, the reason being that in our own lecturing on the subject, we have tended to emphasize the implementation aspects and, therefore, the homework has consisted of writing computer programs for reconstruction algorithms.

The lists of references by no means constitute a complete bibliography on the subject. Basically, we have included those references that we have found useful in our own research over the years. Whenever possible, we have referenced books and review articles to provide the reader with entry points for more exhaustive literature citations. Except in isolated cases, we have not made any attempts to establish historical priorities. No value judgments should be implied by our including or excluding a particular work.

Many of our friends and colleagues deserve much credit for helping bring this book to fruition. This book draws heavily from research done at Purdue by our past and present colleagues and collaborators: Carl Crawford, Mani Azimi, David Nahamoo, Anders Andersen, S. X. Pan, Kris Dines, and Barry Roberts. A number of people, Carl Crawford, Rich Kulawiec, Gary S. Peterson, and the anonymous reviewers, helped us proofread the manuscript;

we are grateful for the errors they caught and we acknowledge that any errors that remain are our own fault. We are also grateful to Carl Crawford and Kevin King at GE Medical Systems Division, Greg Kirk at Resonex, Dennis Parker at the University of Utah, and Kris Dines of XDATA, for sharing their knowledge with us about many newly emerging aspects of medical imaging.

Our editor, Randi Scholnick, at the IEEE PRESS was most patient with us; her critical eye did much to improve the quality of this work.

Sharon Katz, technical illustrator for the School of Electrical Engineering at Purdue University, was absolutely wonderful. She produced most of the illustrations in this book and always did it with the utmost professionalism and a smile. Also, Pat Kerkhoff (Purdue), and Tammy Duarte, Amy Atkinson, and Robin Wallace (SPAR) provided excellent secretarial support, even in the face of deadlines and garbled instructions.

Finally, one of the authors (M.S.) would like to acknowledge the support of his friend Kris Meade during the long time it took to finish this project.

AVINASH C. KAK
MALCOLM SLANEY

1 Introduction

Tomography refers to the cross-sectional imaging of an object from either transmission or reflection data collected by illuminating the object from many different directions. The impact of this technique in diagnostic medicine has been revolutionary, since it has enabled doctors to view internal organs with unprecedented precision and safety to the patient. The first medical application utilized x-rays for forming images of tissues based on their x-ray attenuation coefficient. More recently, however, medical imaging has also been successfully accomplished with radioisotopes, ultrasound, and magnetic resonance; the imaged parameter being different in each case.

There are numerous nonmedical imaging applications which lend themselves to the methods of computerized tomography. Researchers have already applied this methodology to the mapping of underground resources via cross-borehole imaging, some specialized cases of cross-sectional imaging for nondestructive testing, the determination of the brightness distribution over a celestial sphere, and three-dimensional imaging with electron microscopy.

Fundamentally, tomographic imaging deals with reconstructing an image from its projections. In the strict sense of the word, a projection at a given angle is the integral of the image in the direction specified by that angle, as illustrated in Fig. 1.1. However, in a loose sense, projection means the information derived from the transmitted energies, when an object is illuminated from a particular angle; the phrase "diffracted projection" may be used when energy sources are diffracting, as is the case with ultrasound and microwaves.

Although, from a purely mathematical standpoint, the solution to the problem of how to reconstruct a function from its projections dates back to the paper by Radon in 1917, the current excitement in tomographic imaging originated with Hounsfield's invention of the x-ray computed tomographic scanner for which he received a Nobel prize in 1972. He shared the prize with Allan Cormack who independently discovered some of the algorithms. His invention showed that it is possible to compute high-quality cross-sectional images with an accuracy now reaching one part in a thousand in spite of the fact that the projection data do not strictly satisfy the theoretical models underlying the efficiently implementable reconstruction algorithms. His invention also showed that it is possible to process a very large number of measurements (now approaching a million for the case of x-ray tomography) with fairly complex mathematical operations, and still get an image that is incredibly accurate.

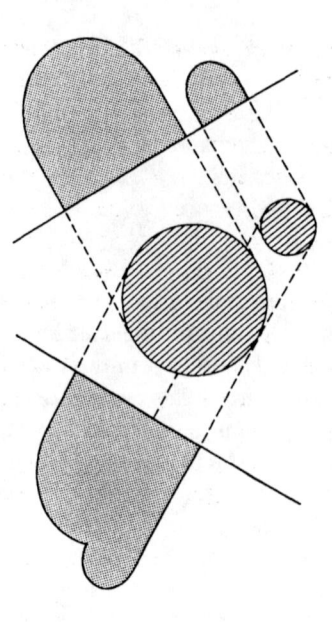

Fig. 1.1: *Two projections are shown of an object consisting of a pair of cylinders.*

It is perhaps fair to say that the breakneck pace at which x-ray computed tomography images improved after Hounsfield's invention was in large measure owing to the developments that were made in reconstruction algorithms. Hounsfield used algebraic techniques, described in Chapter 7, and was able to reconstruct noisy looking 80 × 80 images with an accuracy of one part in a hundred. This was followed by the application of convolution-backprojection algorithms, first developed by Ramachandran and Lakshminarayanan [Ram71] and later popularized by Shepp and Logan [She74], to this type of imaging. These later algorithms considerably reduced the processing time for reconstruction, and the image produced was numerically more accurate. As a result, commercial manufacturers of x-ray tomographic scanners started building systems capable of reconstructing 256 × 256 and 512 × 512 images that were almost photographically perfect (in the sense that the morphological detail produced was unambiguous and in perfect agreement with the anatomical features). The convolution-backprojection algorithms are discussed in Chapter 3.

Given the enormous success of x-ray computed tomography, it is not surprising that in recent years much attention has been focused on extending this image formation technique to nuclear medicine and magnetic resonance on the one hand; and ultrasound and microwaves on the other. In nuclear medicine, our interest is in reconstructing a cross-sectional image of radioactive isotope distributions within the human body; and in imaging with magnetic resonance we wish to reconstruct the magnetic properties of the object. In both these areas, the problem can be set up as reconstructing an image from its projections of the type shown in Fig. 1.1. This is not the case when ultrasound and microwaves are used as energy sources; although the aim is the same as with x-rays, viz., to reconstruct the cross-sectional image of, say, the attenuation coefficient. X-rays are nondiffracting, i.e., they travel in straight lines, whereas microwaves and ultrasound are diffracting. When an object is illuminated with a diffracting source, the wave field is scattered in practically all directions, although under certain conditions one might be able to get away with the assumption of straight line propagation; these conditions being satisfied when the inhomogeneities are much larger than the wavelength and when the imaging parameter is the refractive index. For situations when one must take diffraction effects (inhomogeneity caused scattering of the wave field) into account, tomographic imaging can in principle be accomplished with the algorithms described in Chapter 6.

This book covers three aspects of tomography: Chapters 2 and 3 describe the mathematical principles and the theory. Chapters 4 and 5 describe how to apply the theory to actual problems in medical imaging and other fields. Finally, Chapters 6, 7, and 8 introduce several variations of tomography that are currently being researched.

During the last decade, there has been an avalanche of publications on different aspects of computed tomography. No attempt will be made to present a comprehensive bibliography on the subject, since that was recently accomplished in a book by Dean [Dea83]. We will only give selected references at the end of each chapter, their purpose only being to cite material that provides further details on the main ideas discussed in the chapter.

The principal textbooks that have appeared on the subject of tomographic imaging are [Her80], [Dea83], [Mac83], [Bar81]. The reader is also referred to the review articles in the field [Gor74], [Bro76], [Kak79] and the two special issues of IEEE journals [Kak81], [Her83]. Reviews of the more popular algorithms also appeared in [Ros82], [Kak84], [Kak85], [Kak86].

References

[Bar81]   H. H. Barrett and W. Swindell, *Radiological Imaging: The Theory of Image Formation, Detection and Processing*. New York, NY: Academic Press, 1981.

[Bro76]   R. A. Brooks and G. DiChiro, "Principles of computer assisted tomography (CAT) in radiographic and radioisotopic imaging," *Phys. Med. Biol.*, vol. 21, pp. 689-732, 1976.

[Dea83]   S. R. Dean, *The Radon Transform and Some of Its Applications*. New York, NY: John Wiley and Sons, 1983.

[Gor74]   R. Gordon and G. T. Herman, "Three-dimensional reconstructions from projections: A review of algorithms," in *International Review of Cytology*, G. H. Bourne and J. F. Danielli, Eds. New York, NY: Academic Press, 1974, pp. 111-151.

[Her80]   G. T. Herman, *Image Reconstructions from Projections*. New York, NY: Academic Press, 1980.

[Her83]   ——, Guest Editor, Special Issue on Computerized Tomography, *Proceedings of the IEEE*, vol. 71, Mar. 1983.

[Kak79]   A. C. Kak, "Computerized tomography with x-ray emission and ultrasound sources," *Proc. IEEE*, vol. 67, pp. 1245-1272, 1979.

[Kak81]   ——, Guest Editor, Special Issue on Computerized Medical Imaging, *IEEE Transactions on Biomedical Engineering*, vol. BME-28, Feb. 1981.

[Kak84] ——, "Image reconstructions from projections," in *Digital Image Processing Techniques,* M. P. Ekstrom, Ed. New York, NY: Academic Press, 1984.

[Kak85] ——, "Tomographic imaging with diffracting and non-diffracting sources," in *Array Signal Processing,* S. Haykin, Ed. Englewood Cliffs, NJ: Prentice-Hall, 1985.

[Kak86] A. C. Kak and B. Roberts, "Image reconstruction from projections," in *Handbook of Pattern Recognition and Image Processing,* T. Y. Young and K. S. Fu, Eds. New York, NY: Academic Press, 1986.

[Mac83] A. Macovski, *Medical Imaging Systems*. Englewood Cliffs, NJ: Prentice-Hall, 1983.

[Ram71] G. N. Ramachandran and A. V. Lakshminarayanan, "Three dimensional reconstructions from radiographs and electron micrographs: Application of convolution instead of Fourier transforms," *Proc. Nat. Acad. Sci.,* vol. 68, pp. 2236–2240, 1971.

[Ros82] A. Rosenfeld and A. C. Kak, *Digital Picture Processing,* 2nd ed. New York, NY: Academic Press, 1982.

[She74] L. A. Shepp and B. F. Logan, "The Fourier reconstruction of a head section," *IEEE Trans. Nucl. Sci.,* vol. NS-21, pp. 21–43, 1974.

2 Signal Processing Fundamentals

We can't hope to cover all the important details of one- and two-dimensional signal processing in one chapter. For those who have already seen this material, we hope this chapter will serve as a refresher. For those readers who haven't had prior exposure to signal and image processing, we hope that this chapter will provide enough of an introduction so that the rest of the book will make sense.

All readers are referred to a number of excellent textbooks that cover one- and two-dimensional signal processing in more detail. For information on 1-D processing the reader is referred to [McG74], [Sch75], [Opp75], [Rab75]. The theory and practice of image processing have been described in [Ros82], [Gon77], [Pra78]. The more general case of multidimensional signal processing has been described in [Dud84].

2.1 One-Dimensional Signal Processing

2.1.1 Continuous and Discrete One-Dimensional Functions

One-dimensional continuous functions, such as in Fig. 2.1(a), will be represented in this book by the notation

$$x(t) \tag{1}$$

where $x(t)$ denotes the value as a function at t. This function may be given a discrete representation by sampling its value over a set of points as illustrated in Fig. 2.1(b). Thus the discrete representation can be expressed as the list

$$\cdots x(-\tau),\ x(0),\ x(\tau),\ x(2\tau),\ \cdots,\ x(n\tau),\ \cdots. \tag{2}$$

As an example of this, the discrete representation of the data in Fig. 2.1(c) is

$$1,\ 3,\ 4,\ 5,\ 4,\ 3,\ 1. \tag{3}$$

It is also possible to represent the samples as a single vector in a multidimensional space. For example, the set of seven samples could also be represented as a vector in a 7-dimensional space, with the first element of the vector equal to 1, the second equal to 3, and so on.

There is a special function that is often useful for explaining operations on functions. It is called the Dirac delta or impulse function. It can't be defined

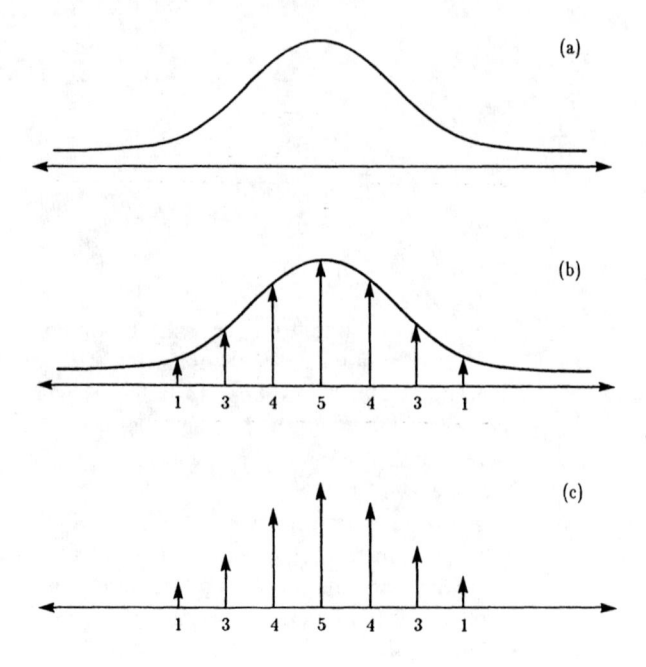

Fig. 2.1: *A one-dimensional signal is shown in (a) with its sampled version in (b). The discrete version of the signal is illustrated in (c).*

directly; instead it must be expressed as the limit of a sequence of functions. First we define a new function called rect (short for rectangle) as follows

$$\text{rect }(t) = \begin{cases} 1 & |t| < \frac{1}{2} \\ 0 & \text{elsewhere.} \end{cases} \quad (4)$$

This is illustrated in Fig. 2.2(a). Consider a sequence of functions of ever decreasing support on the t-axis as described by

$$\delta_n(t) = n \text{ rect }(nt) \quad (5)$$

and illustrated in Fig. 2.2(b). Each function in this sequence has the same area but is of ever increasing height, which tends to infinity as $n \to \infty$. The limit of this sequence of functions is of infinite height but zero width in such a manner that the area is still unity. This limit is often pictorially represented as shown in Fig. 2.2(c) and denoted by $\delta(t)$. Our explanation leads to the definition of the Dirac delta function that follows

$$\int_{-\infty}^{\infty} \delta(t) \, dt = 1. \quad (6)$$

The delta function has the following "sampling" property

$$\int_{-\infty}^{\infty} x(t)\delta(t-t') \, dt = x(t') \quad (7)$$

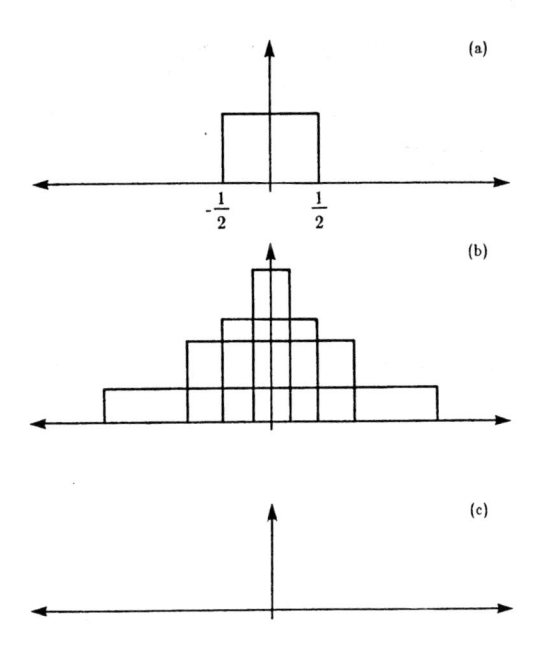

Fig. 2.2: *A rectangle function as shown in (a) is scaled in both width and height (b). In the limit the result is the delta function illustrated in (c).*

where $\delta(t - t')$ is an impulse shifted to the location $t = t'$. When an impulse enters into a product with an arbitrary $x(t)$, all the values of $x(t)$ outside the location $t = t'$ are disregarded. Then by the integral property of the delta function we obtain (7); so we can say that $\delta(t - t')$ samples the function $x(t)$ at t'.

2.1.2 Linear Operations

Functions may be operated on for purposes such as filtering, smoothing, etc. The application of an operator O to a function $x(t)$ will be denoted by

$$O[x(t)]. \tag{8}$$

The operator is linear provided

$$O[\alpha x(t) + \beta y(t)] = \alpha O[x(t)] + \beta O[y(t)] \tag{9}$$

for any pair of constants α and β and for any pair of functions $x(t)$ and $y(t)$.

An interesting class of linear operations is defined by the following integral form

$$z(t) = \int_{-\infty}^{\infty} x(t')h(t, t') \, dt' \tag{10}$$

where h is called the impulse response. It is easily shown that h is the system response of the operator applied to a delta function. Assume that the input function is an impulse at $t = t_0$ or

$$x(t) = \delta(t - t_0). \tag{11}$$

Substituting into (10), we obtain

$$z(t) = \int_{-\infty}^{\infty} \delta(t' - t_0) h(t, t') \, dt' \tag{12}$$

$$= h(t, t_0). \tag{13}$$

Therefore $h(t, t')$ can be called the impulse response for the impulse applied at t'.

A linear operation is called shift invariant when

$$y(t) = O[x(t)] \tag{14}$$

implies

$$y(t - \tau) = O[x(t - \tau)] \tag{15}$$

or equivalently

$$h(t, t') = h(t - t'). \tag{16}$$

This implies that when the impulse is shifted by t', so is the response, as is further illustrated in Fig. 2.3. In other words, the response produced by the linear operation does not vary with the location of the impulse; it is merely shifted by the same amount.

For shift invariant operations, the integral form in (10) becomes

$$z(t) = \int_{-\infty}^{\infty} x(t') h(t - t') \, dt'. \tag{17}$$

This is now called a convolution and is represented by

$$z(t) = x(t) * h(t). \tag{18}$$

Fig. 2.3: *The impulse response of a shift invariant filter is shown convolved with three impulses.*

The process of convolution can be viewed as flipping one of the two functions, shifting one with respect to the other, multiplying the two and integrating the product for every shift as illustrated by Fig. 2.4.

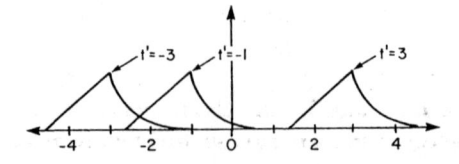

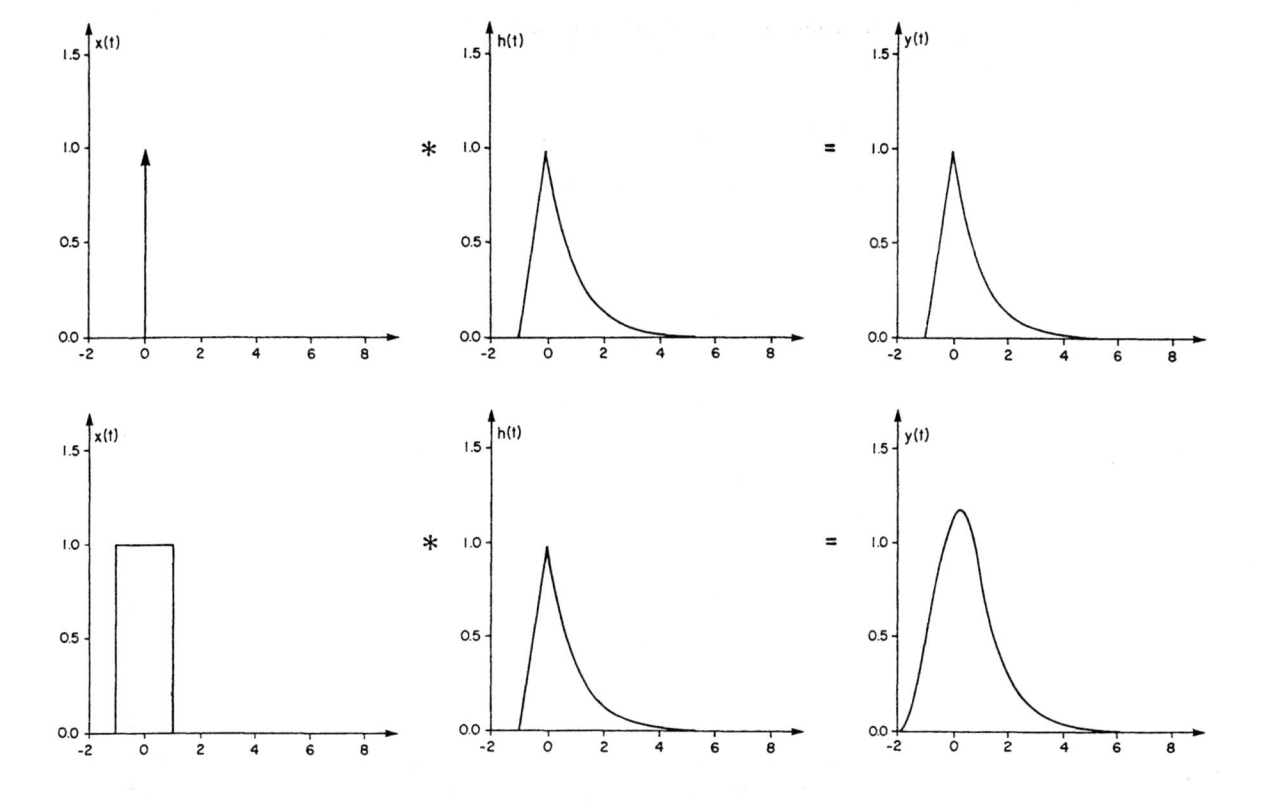

Fig. 2.4: *The results of convolving an impulse response with an impulse (top) and a square pulse (bottom) are shown here.*

Convolution can also be defined for discrete sequences. If

$$x_i = x(i\tau) \tag{19}$$

and

$$y_i = y(i\tau) \tag{20}$$

then the convolution of x_i with y_i can be written as

$$y_i = \tau \sum_{j=-\infty}^{\infty} x_j h_{i-j}. \tag{21}$$

This is a discrete approximation to the integral of (17).

2.1.3 Fourier Representation

For many purposes it is useful to represent functions in the frequency domain. Certainly the most common reason is because it gives a new perspective to an otherwise difficult problem. This is certainly true with the

SIGNAL PROCESSING FUNDAMENTALS 9

convolution integral; in the time domain convolution is an integral while in the frequency domain it is expressed as a simple multiplication.

In the sections to follow we will describe four different varieties of the Fourier transform. The continuous Fourier transform is mostly used in theoretical analysis. Given that with real world signals it is necessary to periodically sample the data, we are led to three other Fourier transforms that approximate either the time or frequency data as samples of the continuous functions. The four types of Fourier transforms are summarized in Table 2.1.

Assume that we have a continuous function $x(t)$ defined for $T_1 \leq t \leq T_2$. This function can be expressed in the following form:

$$x(t) = \sum_{k=-\infty}^{\infty} z_k e^{jk\omega_0 t} \qquad (22)$$

where $j = \sqrt{-1}$ and $\omega_0 = 2\pi f_0 = 2\pi/T$, $T = T_2 - T_1$ and z_k are complex coefficients to be discussed shortly. What is being said here is that $x(t)$ is the sum of a number of functions of the form

$$e^{jk\omega_0 t}. \qquad (23)$$

This function represents

$$e^{jk\omega_0 t} = \cos k\omega_0 t + j \sin k\omega_0 t. \qquad (24)$$

The two functions on the right-hand side, commonly referred to as sinusoids, are oscillatory with kf_0 cycles per unit of t as illustrated by Fig. 2.5. kf_0 is

Table 2.1: Four different Fourier transforms can be defined by sampling the time and frequency domains.*

	Continuous Time	Discrete Time
Continuous Frequency	Name: Fourier Transform Forward: $X(\omega) = \int_{-\infty}^{\infty} x(t) e^{-j\omega t} dt$ Inverse: $x(t) = 1/2\pi \int_{-\infty}^{\infty} X(\omega) e^{j\omega t} d\omega$ Periodicity: None	Name: Discrete Fourier Transform Forward: $X(\omega) = \sum_{n=-\infty}^{\infty} x(n\tau) e^{-j\omega n\tau}$ Inverse: $x(n\tau) = \tau/2\pi \int_{-\pi/\tau}^{\pi/\tau} X(\omega) e^{j\omega n\tau} d\omega$ Periodicity: $X(\omega) = X(\omega + i(2\pi/\tau))$
Discrete Frequency	Name: Fourier Series Forward: $X_n = 1/T \int_0^T x(t) e^{-jn(2\pi/T)t}$ Inverse: $x(t) = \sum_{n=-\infty}^{\infty} X_n e^{jn(2\pi/T)t}$ Periodicity: $x(t) = x(t + iT)$	Name: Finite Fourier Transform Forward: $X_k = 1/N \sum_{n=0}^{N} x_n e^{-j(2\pi/N)kn}$ Inverse: $x_k = \sum_{n=0}^{N} X_n e^{j(2\pi/N)kn}$ Periodicity: $x_k = x_{k+iN}$ and $X_k = X_{k+iN}$

* In the above table time domain functions are indicated by x and frequency domain functions are X. The time domain sampling interval is indicated by τ.

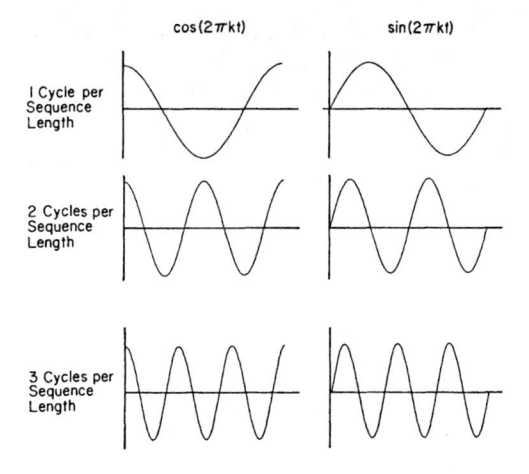

Fig. 2.5: *The first three components of a Fourier series are shown. The cosine waves represent the real part of the signal while the sine waves represent the imaginary.*

called the frequency of the sinusoids. Note that the sinusoids in (24) are at multiples of the frequency f_0, which is called the fundamental frequency.

The coefficients z_k in (22) are called the complex amplitude of the kth component, and can be obtained by using the following formula

$$z_k = \frac{1}{T} \int_{T_1}^{T_2} x(t) e^{-jk\omega_0 T}. \tag{25}$$

The representation in (22) is called the Fourier Series. To illustrate pictorially the representation in (22), we have shown in Fig. 2.6, a triangular function and some of the components from the expansion.

A continuous signal $x(t)$ defined for t between $-\infty$ and ∞ also possesses another Fourier representation called the continuous Fourier transform and defined by

$$X(\omega) = \int_{-\infty}^{\infty} x(t) e^{-j\omega t} \, dt. \tag{26}$$

One can show that this relationship may be inverted to yield

$$x(t) = \frac{1}{2\pi} \int_{-\infty}^{\infty} X(\omega) e^{j\omega t} \, d\omega. \tag{27}$$

Comparing (22) and (27), we see that in both representations, $x(t)$ has been expressed as a sum of sinusoids, $e^{j\omega t}$; the difference being that in the former, the frequencies of the sinusoids are at multiples of ω_0, whereas in the latter we have all frequencies between $-\infty$ to ∞. The two representations are not independent of each other. In fact, the series representation is contained in the continuous transform representation since z_k's in (25) are similar to $X(\omega)$ in (26) for $\omega = k\omega_0 = k(2\pi/T)$, especially if we assume that $x(t)$ is zero outside $[T_1, T_2]$, in which case the range of integration in (27) can be cut

SIGNAL PROCESSING FUNDAMENTALS 11

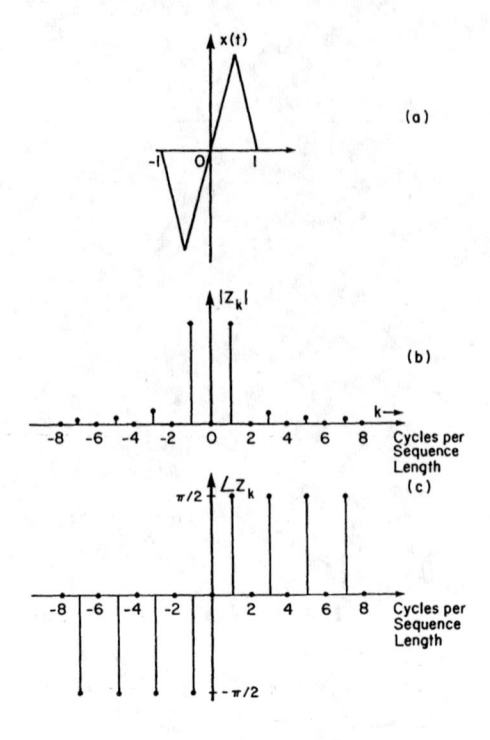

Fig. 2.6: *This illustrates the Fourier series for a simple waveform. A triangle wave is shown in (a) with the magnitude (b) and phase (c) of the first few terms of the Fourier series.*

down to $[T_1, T_2]$. For the case when $x(t)$ is zero outside $[T_1, T_2]$, the reader might ask that since one can recover $x(t)$ from z_k using (22), why use (27) since we require $X(\omega)$ at frequencies in addition to $k\omega_0$'s. The information in $X(\omega)$ for $\omega \neq k\omega_0$ is necessary to constrain the values of $x(t)$ *outside* the interval $[T_1, T_2]$.

If we compute z_k's using (25), and then reconstruct $x(t)$ from z_k's using (22), we will of course obtain the correct values of $x(t)$ within $[T_1, T_2]$; however, if we insist on carrying out this reconstruction outside $[T_1, T_2]$, we will obtain *periodic replications* of the original $x(t)$ (see Fig. 2.7). On the other hand, if $X(\omega)$ is used for reconstructing the signal, we will obtain $x(t)$ within $[T_1, T_2]$ and zero everywhere outside.

The continuous Fourier transform defined in (26) may not exist unless $x(t)$ satisfies certain conditions, of which the following are typical [Goo68]:

1) $\int_{-\infty}^{\infty} |x(t)| \, dt < \infty$.
2) $g(t)$ must have only a finite number of discontinuities and a finite number of maxima and minima in any finite interval.
3) $g(t)$ must have no infinite discontinuities.

Some useful mathematical functions, like the Dirac δ function, do not obey the preceding conditions. But if it is possible to represent these functions as limits of a sequence of well-behaved functions that do obey these conditions then the Fourier transforms of the members of this sequence will also form a

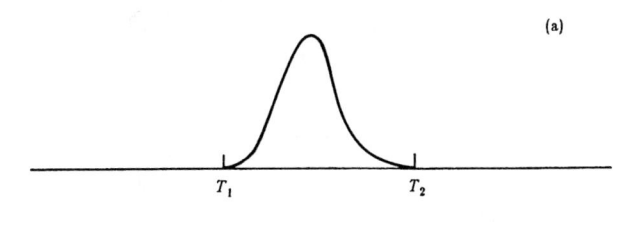

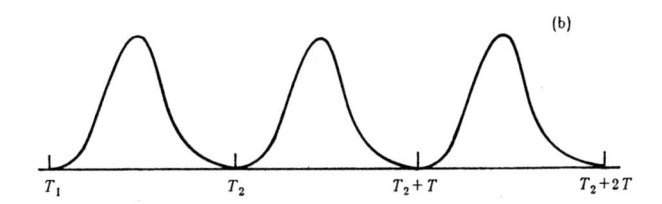

Fig. 2.7: *The signal represented by a Fourier series is actually a periodic version of the original signal defined between T_1 and T_2. Here the original function is shown in (a) and the replications caused by the Fourier series representation are shown in (b).*

sequence. Now if this sequence of Fourier transforms possesses a limit, then this limit is called the "generalized Fourier transform" of the original function. Generalized transforms can be manipulated in the same manner as the conventional transforms, and the distinction between the two is generally ignored; it being understood that when a function fails to satisfy the existence conditions and yet is said to have a transform, then the generalized transform is actually meant [Goo68], [Lig60].

Various transforms described in this section obey many useful properties; these will be shown for the two-dimensional case in Section 2.2.4. Given a relationship for a function of two variables, it is rather easy to suppress one and visualize the one-dimensional case; the opposite is usually not the case.

2.1.4 Discrete Fourier Transform (DFT)

As in the continuous case, a discrete function may also be given a frequency domain representation:

$$X(\omega) = \sum_{n=-\infty}^{\infty} x(n\tau) e^{-j\omega n\tau} \tag{28}$$

where $x(n\tau)$ are the samples of some continuous function $x(t)$, and $X(\omega)$ the frequency domain representation for the sampled data. (*In this book we will generally use lowercase letters to represent functions of time or space and the uppercase letters for functions in the frequency domain.*)

Note that our strategy for introducing the frequency domain representation is opposite of that in the preceding subsection. In describing Fourier series we defined the inverse transform (22), and then described how to compute its coefficients. Now for the DFT we have first described the transform from time into the frequency domain. Later in this section we will describe the inverse transform.

As will be evident shortly, $X(\omega)$ represents the complex amplitude of the sinusoidal component $e^{j\omega\tau n}$ of the discrete signal. Therefore, with one important difference, $X(\omega)$ plays the same role here as z_k in the preceding subsection; the difference being that in the preceding subsection the frequency domain representation was discrete (since it only existed at multiples of the fundamental frequency), while the representation here is continuous as $X(\omega)$ is defined for all ω.

For example, assume that

$$x(n\tau) = \begin{cases} 1 & n=0 \\ -1 & n=1 \\ 0 & \text{elsewhere.} \end{cases} \qquad (29)$$

For this signal

$$X(\omega) = 1 - e^{-j\omega\tau}. \qquad (30)$$

Note that $X(\omega)$ obeys the following periodicity

$$X(\omega) = X\left(\omega + \frac{2\pi}{\tau}\right) \qquad (31)$$

which follows from (28) by simple substitution. In Fig. 2.8 we have shown several periods of this $X(\omega)$.

$X(\omega)$ is called the discrete Fourier transform of the function $x(n\tau)$. From the DFT, the function $x(n\tau)$ can be recovered by using

$$x(n\tau) = \frac{\tau}{2\pi} \int_{-\pi/\tau}^{\pi/\tau} X(\omega) e^{j\omega n\tau} \, d\omega \qquad (32)$$

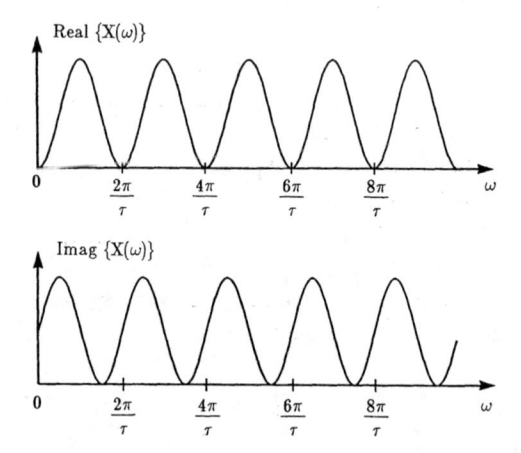

Fig. 2.8: *The discrete Fourier transform (DFT) of a two element sequence is shown here.*

which points to the discrete function $x(n\tau)$ being a sum (an integral sum, to be more specific) of sinusoidal components like $e^{j\omega n\tau}$.

An important property of the DFT is that it provides an alternate method for calculating the convolution in (21). Given a pair of sequences $x_i = x(i\tau)$ and $h_i = h(i\tau)$, their convolution as defined by

$$y_i = \sum_{j=-\infty}^{\infty} x_j h_{i-j}, \tag{33}$$

can be calculated from

$$Y(\omega) = X(\omega) H(\omega). \tag{34}$$

This can be derived by noting that the DFT of the convolution is written as

$$Y(\omega) = \sum_{i=-\infty}^{\infty} \left[\sum_{k=-\infty}^{\infty} x_k h_{i-k} \right] e^{-j\omega i\tau}. \tag{35}$$

Rewriting the exponential we find

$$Y(\omega) = \sum_{i=-\infty}^{\infty} \left[\sum_{k=-\infty}^{\infty} x_k h_{i-k} \right] e^{-j\omega(i-k+k)\tau}. \tag{36}$$

The second summation now can be written as

$$Y(\omega) = \sum_{i=-\infty}^{\infty} x_k e^{-j\omega k\tau} \sum_{m=-\infty}^{\infty} h_m e^{-j\omega m\tau}. \tag{37}$$

Note that the limits of the summation remain from $-\infty$ to ∞. At this point it is easy to see that

$$Y(\omega) = X(\omega) H(\omega). \tag{38}$$

A dual to the above relationship can be stated as follows. Let's multiply two discrete functions, x_n and y_n, each obtained by sampling the corresponding continuous function with a sampling interval of τ and call the resulting sequence z_n

$$z_n = x_n y_n. \tag{39}$$

Then the DFT of the new sequence is given by the following convolution in the frequency domain

$$Z(\omega) = \frac{\tau}{2\pi} \int_{-\pi/\tau}^{\pi/\tau} X(\alpha) Y(\omega - \alpha) \, d\alpha. \tag{40}$$

2.1.5 Finite Fourier Transform

Consider a discrete function

$$x(0), x(\tau), x(2\tau), \cdots, x((N-1)\tau) \qquad (41)$$

that is N elements long. Let's represent this sequence with the following subscripted notation

$$x_0, x_1, x_2, \cdots x_{N-1}. \qquad (42)$$

Although the DFT defined in Section 2.1.4 is useful for many theoretical discussions, for practical purposes it is the following transformation, called the finite Fourier transform (FFT),[1] that is actually calculated with a computer:

$$X_u = \frac{1}{N} \sum_{n=0}^{N-1} x_n e^{-j(2\pi/N)un} \qquad (43)$$

for $u = 0, 1, 2, \cdots, N-1$. To explain the meaning of the values X_u, rewrite (43) as

$$X\left(u\frac{1}{N\tau}\right) = \frac{1}{N} \sum_{n=0}^{N-1} x(n\tau)e^{-j2\pi(u(1/N\tau))(n\tau)}. \qquad (44)$$

Comparing (44) and (28), we see that the X_u's are the samples of the continuous function $X(\omega)$ for

$$\omega = u\frac{1}{N\tau} \quad \text{with } u = 0, 1, 2, \cdots, N-1. \qquad (45)$$

Therefore, we see that if (43) is used to compute the frequency domain representation of a discrete function, a sampling interval of τ in the t-domain implies a sampling interval of $1/N\tau$ in the frequency domain. The inverse of the relationship shown in (43) is

$$x_n = \sum_{u=0}^{N-1} X_u e^{j(2\pi/N)un}, \quad n = 0, 1, 2, \cdots, N-1. \qquad (46)$$

Both (43) and (46) define sequences that are periodically replicated. First consider (43). If the $u = Nm + i$ term is calculated then by noting that $e^{j(2\pi/N)Nm} = 1$ for all integer values of m, it is easy to see that

$$X_{Nm+i} = X_i. \qquad (47)$$

---

[1] The acronym FFT also stands for fast Fourier transform, which is an efficient algorithm for the implementation of the finite Fourier transform.

A similar analysis can be made for the inverse case so that

$$x_{Nm+i} = x_i. \tag{48}$$

When the finite Fourier transforms of two sequences are multiplied the result is still a convolution, as it was for the discrete Fourier transform defined in Section 2.1.4, but now the convolution is with respect to replicated sequences. This is often known as circular convolution because of the effect discussed below.

To see this effect consider the product of two finite Fourier transforms. First write the product of two finite Fourier transforms

$$Z_u = X_u Y_u \tag{49}$$

and then take the inverse finite Fourier transform to find

$$z_n = \sum_{u=0}^{N-1} e^{j(2\pi/N)un} X_u Y_u. \tag{50}$$

Substituting the definition of X_u and Y_u as given by (43) the product can now be written

$$z_n = \frac{1}{N^2} \sum_{u=0}^{N-1} e^{j(2\pi/N)un} \sum_{i=0}^{N-1} x_i e^{j(2\pi/N)iu} \sum_{k=0}^{N-1} y_k e^{j(2\pi/N)ku}. \tag{51}$$

The order of summation can be rearranged and the exponential terms combined to find

$$z_n = \frac{1}{N^2} \sum_{i=0}^{N-1} \sum_{k=0}^{N-1} x_i y_k \sum_{u=0}^{N-1} e^{j(2\pi/N)un - ui - uk}. \tag{52}$$

There are two cases to consider. When $n - i - k \neq 0$ then as a function of u the samples of the exponential $e^{j(2\pi/N)un - ui - uk}$ represent an integral number of cycles of a complex sinusoid and their sum is equal to zero. On the other hand, when $i = n - k$ then each sample of the exponential is equal to one and thus the summation is equal to N. The summation in (52) over i and k represents a sum of all the possible combinations of x_i and y_k. When $i = n - k$ then the combination is multiplied by a factor of N while when $i \neq n - k$ then the term is ignored. This means that the original product of two finite Fourier transforms can be simplified to

$$z_n = \frac{1}{N} \sum_{k=0}^{N-1} x_{n-k} y_k. \tag{53}$$

This expression is very similar to (21) except for the definition of x_{n-k} and y_k for negative indices. Consider the case when $n = 0$. The first term of the summation is equal to $x_0 y_0$ but the second term is equal to $x_{-1} y_1$. Although in the original formulation of the finite Fourier transform, the x sequence was only specified for indices from 0 through $N - 1$, the periodicity property in (48) implies that x_{-1} be equal to x_{N-1}. This leads to the name circular convolution since the undefined portions of the original sequence are replaced by a circular replication of the original data.

The effect of circular convolution is shown in Fig. 2.9(a). Here we have shown an exponential sequence convolved with an impulse. The result represents a circular convolution and not samples of the continuous convolution.

A circular convolution can be turned into an aperiodic convolution by zero-padding the data. As shown in Fig. 2.9(b) if the original sequences are doubled in length by adding zeros then the original N samples of the product sequence will represent an aperiodic convolution of the two sequences.

Efficient procedures for computing the finite Fourier transform are known as fast Fourier transform (FFT) algorithms. To calculate each of the N points of the summation shown in (43) requires on the order of N^2 operations. In a fast Fourier transform algorithm the summation is rearranged to take advantage of common subexpressions and the computational expense is reduced to $N \log N$. For a 1024 point signal this represents an improvement by a factor of approximately 100. The fast Fourier transform algorithm has revolutionized digital signal processing and is described in more detail in [Bri74].

Fig. 2.9: *The effect of circular convolution is shown in (a). (b) shows how the data can be zero-padded so that when an FFT convolution is performed the result represents samples of an aperiodic convolution.*

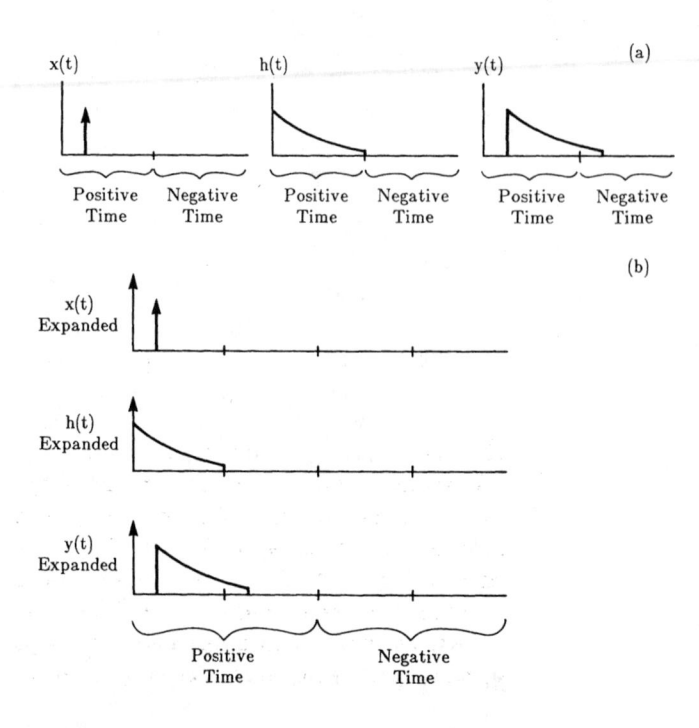

18   COMPUTERIZED TOMOGRAPHIC IMAGING

2.1.6 Just How Much Data Is Needed?

In Section 2.1.1 we used a sequence of numbers x_i to approximate a continuous function $x(t)$. An important question is, how finely must the data be sampled for x_i to accurately represent the original signal? This question was answered by Nyquist who observed that a signal must be sampled at least twice during each cycle of the highest frequency of the signal. More rigorously, if a signal $x(t)$ has a Fourier transform such that

$$X(\omega) = 0 \quad \text{for } \omega \geq \frac{\omega_N}{2} \tag{54}$$

then samples of x must be measured at a rate greater than ω_N. In other words, if T is the interval between consecutive samples, we want $2\pi/T \geq \omega_N$. The frequency ω_N is known as the Nyquist rate and represents the minimum frequency at which the data can be sampled without introducing errors.

Since most real world signals aren't limited to a small range of frequencies, it is important to know the consequences of sampling at below the Nyquist rate. We can consider the process of sampling to be equivalent to multiplication of the original continuous signal $x(t)$ by a sampling function given by

$$h(t) = \sum_{-\infty}^{\infty} \delta(t - iT). \tag{55}$$

The Fourier transform of $h(t)$ can be computed from (26) to be

$$H(\omega) = \left(\frac{2\pi}{T}\right) \sum_{-\infty}^{\infty} \delta\left(\omega - \frac{2\pi i}{T}\right). \tag{56}$$

By (40) we can convert the multiplication to a convolution in the frequency domain. Thus the result of the sampling can be written

$$Z(\omega) = \left(\frac{2\pi}{T}\right) \sum_{i=-\infty}^{\infty} X\left(\omega - \frac{2i\pi}{T}\right). \tag{57}$$

This result is diagrammed in Fig. 2.10.

It is important to realize that when sampling the original data (Fig. 2.10(a)) at a rate faster than that defined by the Nyquist rate, the sampled data are an exact replica of the original signal. This is shown in Fig. 2.10(b). If the sampled signal is filtered such that all frequencies above the Nyquist rate are removed, then the original signal will be recovered.

On the other hand, as the sampling interval is increased the replicas of the signal in Fig. 2.10(c) move closer together. With a sampling interval greater than that predicted by the Nyquist rate some of the information in the original data has been smeared by replications of the signal at other frequencies and the original signal is unrecoverable. (See Fig. 2.10(d).) The error caused by the sampling process is given by the inverse Fourier transform of the frequency information in the overlap as shown in Fig. 2.10(d). These errors are also known as aliasing.

2.1.7 Interpretation of the FFT Output

Correct interpretation of the X_u's in (43) is obviously important. Toward that goal, it is immediately apparent that X_0 stands for the average (or, what is more frequently called the dc) component of the discrete function, since from (43)

$$X_0 = \frac{1}{N} \sum_{n=0}^{N-1} x_n. \qquad (58)$$

Interpretation of X_1 requires, perhaps, a bit more effort; it stands for 1 cycle per sequence length. This can be made obvious by setting $X_1 = 1$, while all

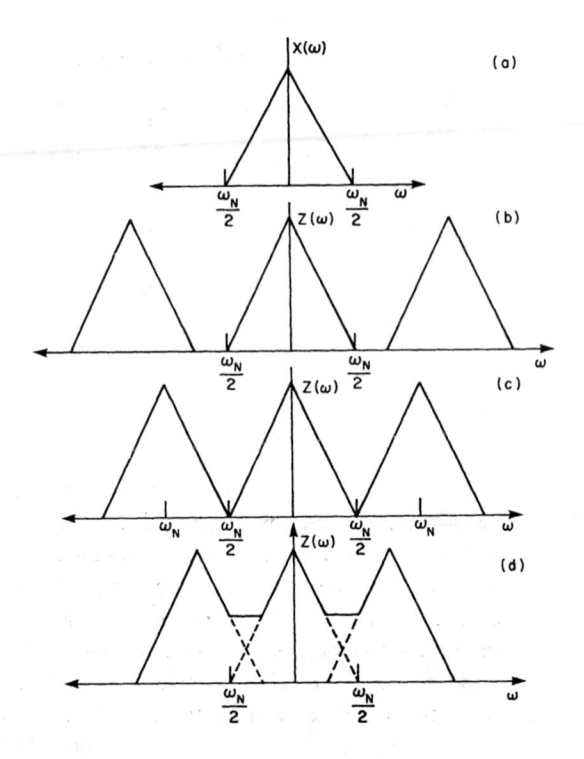

Fig. 2.10: *Sampling a waveform generates replications of the original Fourier transform of the object at periodic intervals. If the signal is sampled at a frequency of ω then the Fourier transform of the object will be replicated at intervals of 2ω. (a) shows the Fourier transform of the original signal, (b) shows the Fourier transform when x(t) is sampled at a rate faster than the Nyquist rate, (c) when sampled at the Nyquist rate and finally (d) when the data are sampled at a rate less than the Nyquist rate.*

other X_i's are set equal to 0 in (46). We obtain

$$x_n = e^{j2(\pi/N)n} \tag{59}$$

$$= \cos\left(\frac{2\pi}{N}n\right) + j\,\sin\left(\frac{2\pi}{N}n\right) \tag{60}$$

for $n = 0, 1, 2, \cdots, N - 1$. A plot of either the cosine or the sine part of this expression will show just one cycle of the discrete function x_n, which is why we consider X_1 as representing one cycle per sequence length. One may similarly show that X_2 represents two cycles per sequence length. Unfortunately, this straightforward approach for interpreting X_u breaks down for $u > N/2$. For these high values of the index u, we make use of the following periodicity property

$$X_{-u} = X_{N-u} \tag{61}$$

which is easily proved by substitution in (43). For further explanation, consider now a particular value for N, say 8. We already know that

X_0 represents dc
X_1 represents 1 cycle per sequence length
X_2 represents 2 cycles per sequence length
X_3 represents 3 cycles per sequence length
X_4 represents 4 cycles per sequence length.

From the periodicity property we can now add the following

X_5 represents -3 cycles per sequence length
X_6 represents -2 cycles per sequence length
X_7 represents -1 cycle per sequence length.

Note that we could also have added "X_4 represents -4 cycles per sequence length." The fact is that for any N element sequence, $X_{N/2}$ will always be equal to $X_{-N/2}$, since from (43)

$$X_{N/2} = X_{-N/2} = \sum_{0}^{N-1} x_n(-1)^n. \tag{62}$$

The discussion is diagrammatically represented by Fig. 2.11, which shows that when an N element data sequence is fed into an FFT program, the output sequence, also N elements long, consists of the dc frequency term, followed by positive frequencies and then by negative frequencies. This type of an output where the negative axis information follows the positive axis information is somewhat unnatural to look at.

To display the FFT output with a more natural progression of frequencies, we can, of course, rearrange the output sequence, although if the aim is

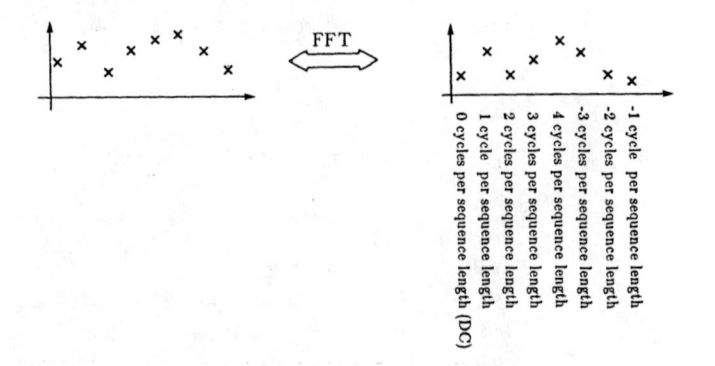

Fig. 2.11: *The output of an 8 element FFT is shown here.*

merely to filter the data, it may not be necessary to do so. In that case the filter transfer function can be rearranged to correspond to the frequency assignments of the elements of the FFT output.

It is also possible to produce normal-looking FFT outputs (with dc at the center between negative and positive frequencies) by "modulating" the data prior to taking the FFT. Suppose we multiply the data with $(-1)^n$ to produce a new sequence x'_n

$$x'_n = x_n(-1)^n. \qquad (63)$$

Let X'_u designate the FFT of this new sequence. Substituting (63) in (43), we obtain

$$X'_u = X_{u-N/2} \qquad (64)$$

for $u = 0, 1, 2, \cdots, N - 1$. This implies the following equivalences

$$X'_0 = X_{-N/2} \qquad (65)$$
$$X'_1 = X_{-N/2+1} \qquad (66)$$
$$X'_2 = X_{-N/2+2} \qquad (67)$$
$$\vdots \qquad (68)$$
$$X'_{N/2} = X_0 \qquad (69)$$
$$\vdots \qquad (70)$$
$$X'_{N-1} = X_{N/2-1}. \qquad (71)$$

2.1.8 How to Increase the Display Resolution in the Frequency Domain

The right column of Fig. 2.12 shows the magnitude of the FFT output (the dc is centered) of the sequence that represents a rectangular function as shown in the left column. As was mentioned before, the Fourier transform of a discrete sequence contains all frequencies, although it is periodic, and the FFT output represents the samples of one period. For many situations, the

22 COMPUTERIZED TOMOGRAPHIC IMAGING

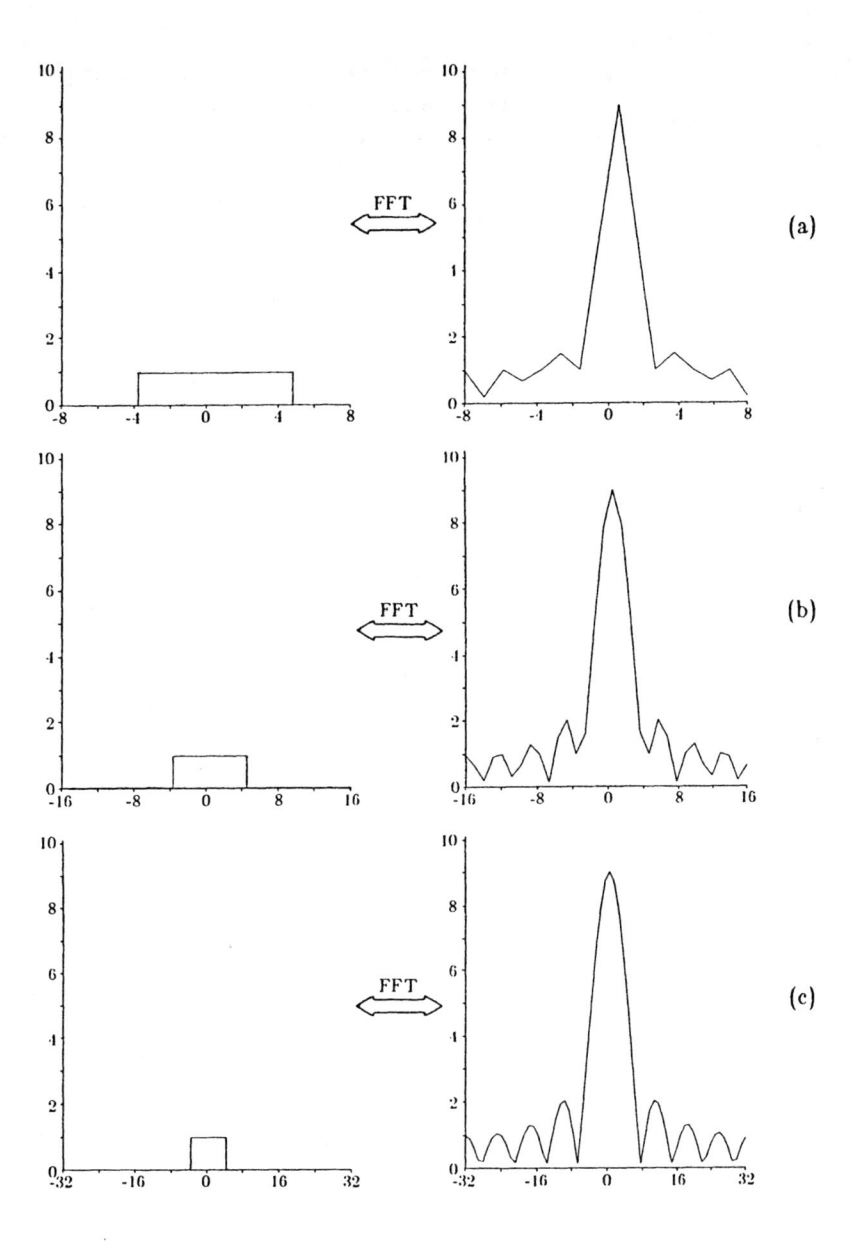

Fig. 2.12: *As shown here, padding a sequence of data with zeros increases the resolution in the frequency domain. The sequence in (a) has only 16 points, (b) has 32 points, while (c) has 64 points.*

frequency domain samples supplied by the FFT, although containing practically all the information for the reconstruction of the continuous Fourier transform, are hard to interpret visually. This is evidenced by Fig. 2.12(a), where for part of the display we have only one sample associated with an oscillation in the frequency domain. It is possible to produce smoother-looking outputs by what is called zero-padding the data before taking the FFT. For example, if the sequence of Fig. 2.12(a) is extended with zeros to twice its length, the FFT of the resulting 32 element sequence will be as shown in Fig. 2.12(b), which is visually smoother looking than the pattern in Fig. 2.12(a). If we zero-pad the data to four times its original length, the output is as shown in Fig. 2.12(c).

That zero-padding a data sequence yields frequency domain points that are more closely spaced can be shown by the following derivation. Again let x_1, $x_2, \cdots, x_{N-1}$ represent the original data. By zero-padding the data we will define a new x' sequence:

$$x'_n = x_n \quad \text{for } n = 0, 1, 2, \cdots, N-1 \tag{72}$$

$$= 0 \quad \text{for } n = N, N+1, \cdots, 2N-1. \tag{73}$$

Let X'_u be the FFT of the new sequence x'_n. Therefore,

$$X'_u = \sum_{0}^{2N-1} x'_n e^{-j(2\pi/2N)un} \tag{74}$$

which in terms of the original data is equal to

$$X'_u = \sum_{0}^{N-1} x_n e^{-j(2\pi/2N)un}. \tag{75}$$

If we evaluate this expression at even values of u, that is when

$$u = 2m \quad \text{where } m = 0, 1, 2, \cdots, N-1 \tag{76}$$

we get

$$X'_{2m} = \sum_{0}^{N-1} x_n e^{-j(2\pi/N)mn} \tag{77}$$

$$= X_m. \tag{78}$$

In Fig. 2.13 is illustrated the equality between the even-numbered elements of the new transform and the original transform. That $X'_1, X'_3, \cdots$, etc. are the interpolated values between X_0 and X_1; between X_1 and X_2; etc. can be seen from the summations in (43) and (74) written in the following form

$$X'_u = X'\left(m \frac{2\pi}{2N\tau}\right) = \sum_{n=0}^{N-1} x(n\tau) e^{-j((2\pi/2N\tau)m)n\tau} \tag{79}$$

$$X_m = X\left(m \frac{2\pi}{N\tau}\right) = \sum_{n=0}^{N-1} x(n\tau) e^{-j(2\pi m/N\tau)n\tau}. \tag{80}$$

Comparing the two summations, we see that the upper one simply represents the sampled DFT with half the sampling interval.

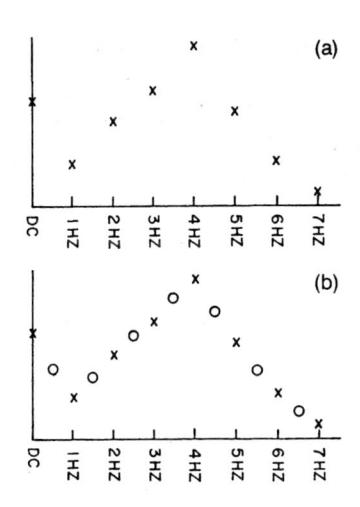

Fig. 2.13: *When a data sequence is padded with zeros the effect is to increase the resolution in the frequency domain. The points in (a) are also in the longer sequence shown in (b), but there are additional points, as indicated by circles, that provide interpolated values of the FFT.*

So we have the following conclusion: to increase the display resolution in the frequency domain, we must zero-extend the time domain signal. This also means that if we are comparing the transforms of sequences of *different* lengths, they must all be zero-extended to the *same* number, so that they are all plotted with the same display resolution. This is because the upper summation, (79), has a sampling interval in the frequency domain of $2\pi/2N\tau$ while the lower summation, (80), has a sampling interval that is twice as long or $2\pi/N\tau$.

2.1.9 How to Deal with Data Defined for Negative Time

Since the forward and the inverse FFT relationships, (43) and (46), are symmetrical, the periodicity property described in (62) also applies in time domain. What is being said here is that if a time domain sequence and its transform obey (43) and (46), then an N element data sequence in the time domain must satisfy the following property

$$x_{-n} = x_{N-n}. \tag{81}$$

To explain the implications of this property, consider the case of $N = 8$, for which the data sequence may be written down as

$$x_0, \ x_1, \ x_2, \ x_3, \ x_4, \ x_5, \ x_6, \ x_7. \tag{82}$$

By the property under discussion, this sequence should be interpreted as

$$x_0, \ x_1, \ x_2, \ x_3, \ x_4 \ (\text{or } x_{-4}), \ x_{-3}, \ x_{-2}, \ x_{-1}. \tag{83}$$

Then if our data are defined for negative indices (times), and, say, are of the following form

$$x_{-3}, \ x_{-2}, \ x_{-1}, \ x_0, \ x_1, \ x_2, \ x_3, \ x_4 \tag{84}$$

they should be fed into an FFT program as

$$x_0, x_1, x_2, x_3, x_4, x_{-3}, x_{-2}, x_{-1}. \tag{85}$$

To further drive home the implications of the periodicity property in (62), consider the following example, which consists of taking an 8 element FFT of the data

$$0.9 \quad 0.89 \quad 0.88 \quad 0.87 \quad 0.86 \quad 0.85 \quad 0.84 \quad 0.83. \tag{86}$$

We insist for the sake of explaining a point, that only an 8 element FFT be taken. If the given data have no association with time, then the data should be fed into the program as they are presented. However, if it is definitely known that the data are ZERO before the first element, then the sequence presented to the FFT program should look like

$$\underbrace{0.9 \quad 0.89 \quad 0.88 \quad 0.87}_{} \quad \underbrace{\frac{0.86+0}{2} \quad 0 \quad 0 \quad 0.}_{} \tag{87}$$

$$\text{positive time} \tag{88}$$

$$\text{negative time} \tag{89}$$

This sequence represents the given fact that at $t = -1, -2$ and -3 the data are supposed to be zero. Also, since the fifth element represents both x_4 and x_{-4} (these two elements are supposed to be equal for ideal data), and since in the given data the element x_{-4} is zero, we simply replace the fifth element by the average of the two. Note that in the data fed into the FFT program, the sharp discontinuity at the origin, as represented by the transition from 0 to 0.9, has been retained. This discontinuity will contribute primarily to the high frequency content of the transform of the signal.

2.1.10 How to Increase Frequency Domain Display Resolution of Signals Defined for Negative Time

Let's say that we have an eight element sequence of data defined for both positive and negative times as follows:

$$x_{-3} \ x_{-2} \ x_{-1} \ x_0 \ x_1 \ x_2 \ x_3 \ x_4. \tag{90}$$

It can be fed into an FFT algorithm after it is rearranged to look like

$$x_0 \ x_1 \ x_2 \ x_3 \ x_4 \ x_{-3} \ x_{-2} \ x_{-1}. \tag{91}$$

If x_{-4} was also defined in the original sequence, we have three options: we can either ignore x_{-4}, or ignore x_4 and retain x_{-4} for the fifth from left position in the above sequence, or, better yet, use $(x_{-4} + x_4)/2$ for the fifth position. Note we are making use of the property that due to the data periodicity properties assumed by the FFT algorithm, the fifth element corresponds to both x_4 and x_{-4} and in the ideal case they are supposed to be equal to each other.

Now suppose we wish to double the display resolution in the frequency domain; we must then zero-extend the data as follows

$$x_0 \; x_1 \; x_2 \; x_3 \; x_4 \; 0 \; 0 \; 0 \; 0 \; 0 \; 0 \; x_{-4} \; x_{-3} \; x_{-2} \; x_{-1}. \tag{92}$$

Note that we have now given separate identities to x_4 and x_{-4}, since they don't have to be equal to each other anymore. So if they are separately available, they can be used as such.

2.1.11 Data Truncation Effects

To see the data truncation effects, consider a signal defined for all indices n. If $X(\omega)$ is the true DFT of this signal, we have

$$X(\omega) = \sum_{-\infty}^{\infty} x_n e^{-j\omega n T_s}. \tag{93}$$

Suppose we decide to take only a 16 element transform, meaning that of all the x_n's, we will retain only 16.

Assuming that the most significant transitions of the signal occur in the base interval defined by n going from -7 to 8, we may write approximately

$$X(\omega) \simeq \sum_{-7}^{8} x_n e^{-j\omega n T_s}. \tag{94}$$

More precisely, if $X'(\omega)$ denotes the DFT of the truncated data, we may write

$$X'(\omega) = \sum_{-7}^{8} x_n e^{-j\omega n T_s} \tag{95}$$

$$= \sum_{-\infty}^{\infty} x_n I_{16}(n) e^{-j\omega n T_s} \tag{96}$$

where $I_{16}(n)$ is a function that is equal to 1 for n between -7 and 8, and zero outside. By the convolution theorem

$$X'(\omega) = \frac{T_s}{2\pi} X(\omega) * A(\omega) \tag{97}$$

where

$$A(\omega) = \sum_{-7}^{8} e^{-j\omega n T_s} \tag{98}$$

$$= e^{-j\omega(T_s/2)} \frac{\sin \frac{\omega N T_s}{2}}{\sin \frac{\omega T_s}{2}} \tag{99}$$

with $N = 16$. This function is displayed in Fig. 2.14, and illustrates the nature of distortion introduced by data truncation.

2.2 Image Processing

The signal processing concepts described in the first half of this chapter are easily extended to two dimensions. As was done before, we will describe how to represent an image with delta functions, linear operations on images and the use of the Fourier transform.

2.2.1 Point Sources and Delta Functions

Let O be an operation that takes pictures into pictures; given the input picture f, the result of applying O to f is denoted by $O[f]$. Like the 1-dimensional case discussed earlier in this chapter, we call O *linear* if

$$O[af + bg] = aO[f] + bO[g] \tag{100}$$

for all pictures, f, g and all constants a, b.

In the analysis of linear operations on pictures, the concept of a *point*

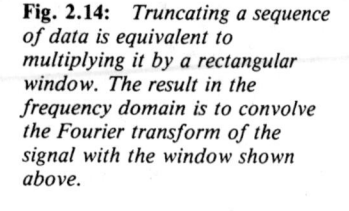

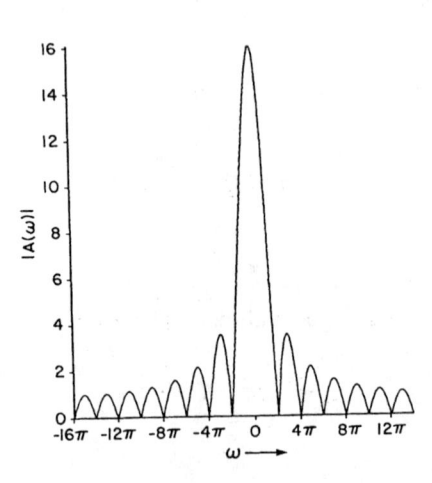

Fig. 2.14: *Truncating a sequence of data is equivalent to multiplying it by a rectangular window. The result in the frequency domain is to convolve the Fourier transform of the signal with the window shown above.*

source is very convenient. If any arbitrary picture *f* could be considered to be a sum of point sources, then a knowledge of the operation's output for a point source input could be used to determine the output for *f*. Whereas for one-dimensional signal processing the response due to a point source input is called the impulse response, in image processing it is usually referred to as the *point spread function* of *O*. If in addition the point spread function is not dependent on the location of the point source input then the operation is said to be space invariant.

A point source can be regarded as the limit of a sequence of pictures whose nonzero values become more and more concentrated spatially. Note that in order for the total brightness to be the same for each of these pictures, their nonzero values must get larger and larger. As an example of such a sequence of pictures, let

$$\text{rect } (x, y) = \begin{cases} 1 & \text{for } |x| \leq \frac{1}{2} \text{ and } |y| \leq \frac{1}{2} \\ 0 & \text{elsewhere} \end{cases} \quad (101)$$

(see Fig. 2.15) and let

$$\delta_n(x, y) = n^2 \text{ rect } (nx, ny), \quad n = 1, 2, \cdots . \quad (102)$$

Thus δ_n is zero outside the $1/n \times 1/n$ square described by $|x| \leq 1/2n$, $|y| \leq 1/2n$ and has constant value n^2 inside that square. It follows that

$$\int\int_{-\infty}^{\infty} \delta_n(x, y) \, dx \, dy = 1 \quad (103)$$

for any *n*.

As $n \to \infty$, the sequence δ_n does not have a limit in the usual sense, but it is convenient to treat it as though its limit existed. This limit, denoted by δ, is

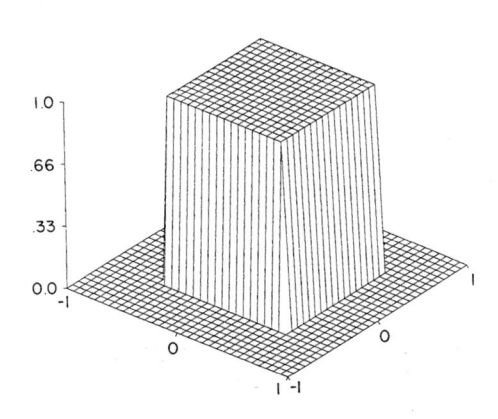

Fig. 2.15: *As in the one-dimensional case, the delta function (δ) is defined as the limit of the rectangle function shown here.*

SIGNAL PROCESSING FUNDAMENTALS 29

called a *Dirac delta function*. Evidently, we have $\delta(x, y) = 0$ for all (x, y) other than $(0, 0)$ where it is infinite. It follows that $\delta(-x, -y) = \delta(x, y)$.

A number of the properties of the one-dimensional delta function described earlier extend easily to the two-dimensional case. For example, in light of (103), we can write

$$\int\int_{-\infty}^{\infty} \delta(x, y)\, dx\, dy = 1. \tag{104}$$

More generally, consider the integral $\int_{-\infty}^{\infty} \int_{-\infty}^{\infty} g(x, y)\delta_n(x, y)\, dx\, dy$. This is just the average of $g(x, y)$ over a $1/n \times 1/n$ square centered at the origin. Thus in the limit we retain just the value at the origin itself, so that we can conclude that the area under the delta function is one and write

$$\int\int_{-\infty}^{\infty} g(x, y)\delta(x, y)\, dx\, dy = g(0, 0). \tag{105}$$

If we shift δ by the amount (α, β), i.e., we use $\delta(x - \alpha, y - \beta)$ instead of $\delta(x, y)$, we similarly obtain the value of g at the point (α, β), i.e.,

$$\int\int_{-\infty}^{\infty} g(x, y)\delta(x - \alpha, y - \beta)\, dx\, dy = g(\alpha, \beta). \tag{106}$$

The same is true for any region of integration containing (α, β). Equation (106) is called the "sifting" property of the δ function.

As a final useful property of δ, we have

$$\int\int_{-\infty}^{\infty} \exp\left[-j2\pi(ux + vy)\right]\, du\, dv = \delta(x, y). \tag{107}$$

For a discussion of this property, see Papoulis [Pap62].

2.2.2 Linear Shift Invariant Operations

Again let us consider a linear operation on images. The point spread function, which is the output image for an input point source at the origin of the xy-plane, is denoted by $h(x, y)$.

A linear operation is said to be *shift invariant* (or space invariant, or position invariant) if the response to $\delta(x - \alpha, y - \beta)$, which is a point source located at (α, β) in the xy-plane, is given by $h(x - \alpha, y - \beta)$. In other words, the output is merely shifted by α and β in the x and y directions, respectively.

Now let us consider an arbitrary input picture $f(x, y)$. By (106) this picture can be considered to be a linear sum of point sources. We can write $f(x, y)$ as

$$f(x, y) = \int_{-\infty}^{\infty} \int_{-\infty}^{\infty} f(\alpha, \beta)\delta(\alpha-x, \beta-y) \, d\alpha \, d\beta. \quad (108)$$

In other words, the image $f(x, y)$ is a linear sum of point sources located at (α, β) in the xy-plane with α and β ranging from $-\infty$ to $+\infty$. In this sum the point source at a particular value of (α, β) has "strength" $f(\alpha, \beta)$. Let the response of the operation to the input $f(x, y)$ be denoted by $O[f]$. If we assume the operation to be shift invariant, then by the interpretation just given to the right-hand side of (108), we obtain

$$O[f(x, y)] = O\left[\int_{-\infty}^{\infty} \int_{-\infty}^{\infty} f(\alpha, \beta)\delta(\alpha-x, \beta-y) \, d\alpha \, d\beta\right] \quad (109)$$

$$= \iint f(\alpha, \beta) O[\delta(\alpha-x, \beta-y)] \, d\alpha \, d\beta \quad (110)$$

by the linearity of the operation, which means that the response to a sum of excitations is equal to the sum of responses to each excitation. As stated earlier, the response to $\delta(\alpha - x, \beta - y) \,[= \delta(x - \alpha, y - \beta)]$, which is a point source located at (α, β), is given by $h(x - \alpha, y - \beta)$ and if $O[f]$ is denoted by g, we obtain

$$g(x, y) = \int_{-\infty}^{\infty} \int_{-\infty}^{\infty} f(\alpha, \beta) h(x-\alpha, y-\beta) \, d\alpha \, d\beta. \quad (111)$$

The right-hand side is called the *convolution* of f and h, and is often denoted by $f * h$. The integrand is a product of two functions $f(\alpha, \beta)$ and $h(\alpha, \beta)$ with the latter rotated about the origin by 180° and shifted by x and y along the x and y directions, respectively. A simple change of variables shows that (111) can also be written as

$$g(x, y) = \int_{-\infty}^{\infty} \int_{-\infty}^{\infty} f(x-\alpha, y-\beta) h(\alpha, \beta) \, d\alpha \, d\beta \quad (112)$$

so that $f * h = h * f$.

Fig. 2.16 shows the effect of a simple blurring operation on two different images. In this case the point response, h, is given by

$$h(x, y) = \begin{cases} 1 & x^2+y^2 < 0.25^2 \\ 0 & \text{elsewhere.} \end{cases} \quad (113)$$

As can be seen in Fig. 2.16 one effect of this convolution is to smooth out the edges of each image.

(a)

(b)

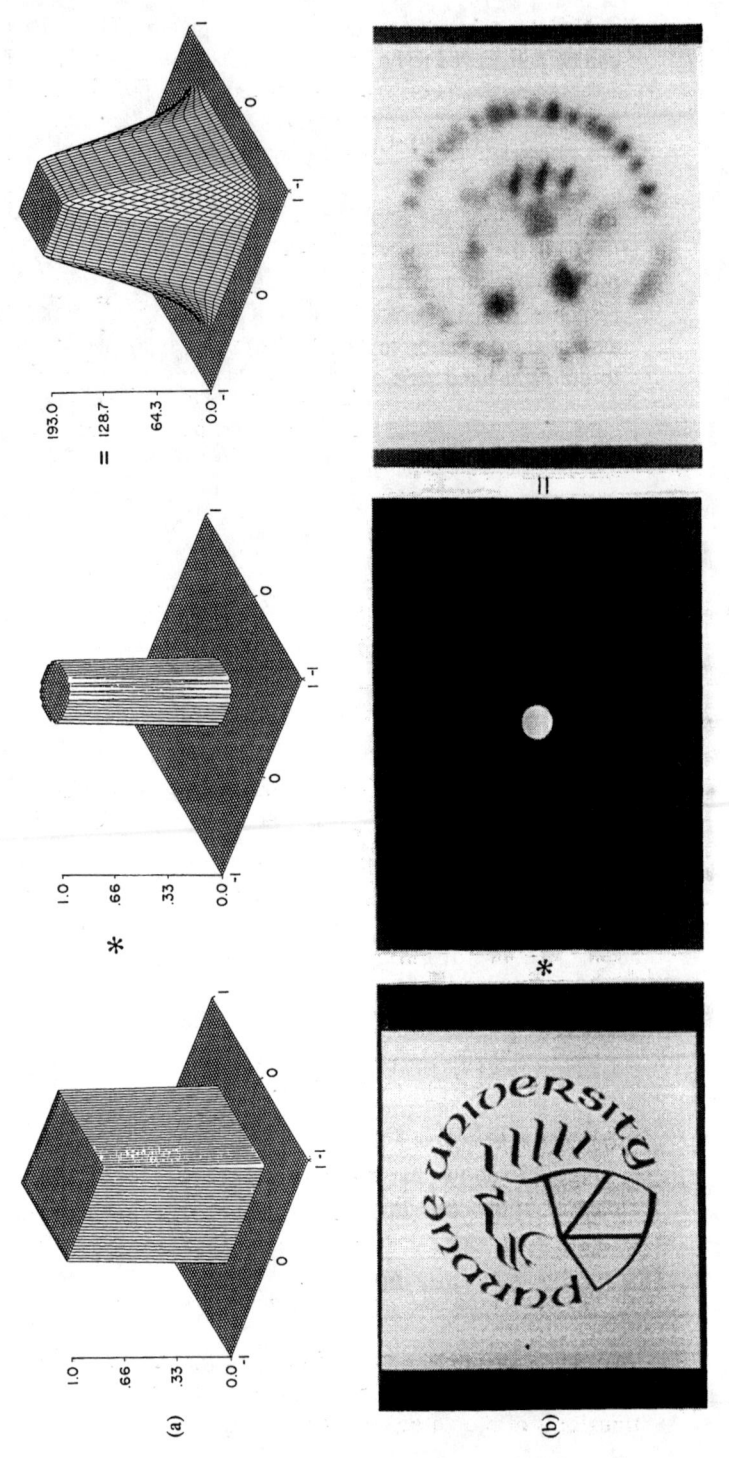

Fig. 2.16: *The two-dimensional convolutions of a circular point spread function and a square (a) and a binary image (b) are shown.*

2.2.3 Fourier Analysis

Representing two-dimensional images in the Fourier domain is as useful as it is in the one-dimensional case. Let $f(x, y)$ be a function of two independent variables x and y; then its *Fourier transform* $F(u, v)$ is defined by

$$F(u, v) = \int_{-\infty}^{\infty} \int_{-\infty}^{\infty} f(x, y) e^{-j2\pi(ux+vy)} \, dx \, dy. \tag{114}$$

In the definition of the one- and two-dimensional Fourier transforms we have used slightly different notations. Equation (26) represents the frequency in terms of radians per unit length while the above equation represents frequency in terms of cycles per unit length. The two forms are identical except for a scaling and either form can be converted to the other using the relation

$$f = u = v = 2\pi\omega. \tag{115}$$

By splitting the exponential into two halves it is easy to see that the two-dimensional Fourier transform can be considered as two one-dimensional transforms; first with respect to x and then y

$$F(u, v) = \int_{-\infty}^{\infty} e^{-j2\pi vy} \, dy \int_{-\infty}^{\infty} f(x, y) e^{-j2\pi ux} \, dx. \tag{116}$$

In general, F is a complex-valued function of u and v. As an example, let $f(x, y) = \text{rect}(x, y)$. Carrying out the integration indicated in (114) we find

$$F(u, v) = \int_{-1/2}^{1/2} \int_{-1/2}^{1/2} e^{-j2\pi(ux+vy)} \, dx \, dy \tag{117}$$

$$= \frac{\sin \pi u}{\pi u} \int_{-1/2}^{1/2} e^{-j2\pi vy} \, dy \tag{118}$$

$$= \frac{\sin \pi u}{\pi u} \frac{\sin \pi v}{\pi v}. \tag{119}$$

This last function is usually denoted by sinc (u, v) and is illustrated in Fig. 2.17. More generally, using the change of variables $x' = nx$ and $y' = ny$, it is easy to show that the Fourier transform of rect (nx, ny) is

$$(1/n^2) \text{ sinc } (u/n, v/n). \tag{120}$$

Given the definition of the Dirac delta function as a limit of a sequence of the functions n^2 rect (nx, ny); by the arguments in Section 2.1.3, the Fourier transform of the Dirac delta function is the limit of the sequence of Fourier

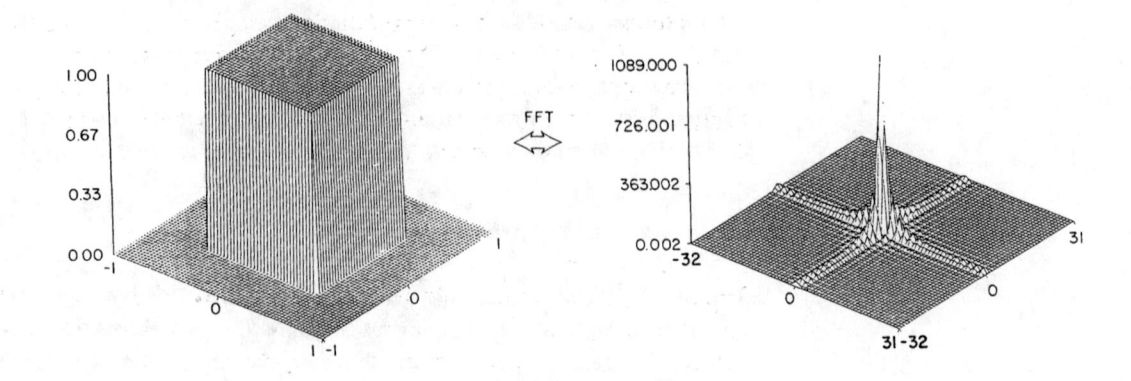

Fig. 2.17: *The two-dimensional Fourier transform of the rectangle function is shown here.*

transforms sinc $(u/n, v/n)$. In other words, when

$$f(x, y) = \delta(x, y) \tag{121}$$

then

$$F(u, v) = \lim_{n \to \infty} \text{sinc } (u/n, v/n) = 1. \tag{122}$$

The inverse Fourier transform of $F(u, v)$ is found by multiplying both sides of (114) by $e^{j2\pi(ux+v\beta)}$ and integrating with respect to u and v to find

$$\int_{-\infty}^{\infty} \int_{-\infty}^{\infty} F(u, v) \exp\left[-j2\pi(ux+v\beta)\right] du\, dv$$

$$= \int_{-\infty}^{\infty} \int_{-\infty}^{\infty} \int_{-\infty}^{\infty} \int_{-\infty}^{\infty} f(x, y) e^{j2\pi(u\alpha+v\beta)} e^{j2\pi(ux+v\beta)} du\, dv\, dx\, dy \tag{123}$$

or

$$= \int_{-\infty}^{\infty} \int_{-\infty}^{\infty} \int_{-\infty}^{\infty} \int_{-\infty}^{\infty} f(x, y) e^{-j2\pi[u(x-\alpha)+v(y-\beta)]} du\, dv\, dx\, dy. \tag{124}$$

Making use of (107) it is easily shown that

$$\int_{-\infty}^{\infty} \int_{-\infty}^{\infty} F(u, v) \exp\left[j2\pi(ux+v\beta)\right] du\, dv$$

$$= \int_{-\infty}^{\infty} \int_{-\infty}^{\infty} f(x, y)\delta(x-\alpha, y-\beta)\, dx\, dy \tag{125}$$

$$= f(\alpha, \beta) \tag{126}$$

or equivalently

$$f(x, y) = \int_{-\infty}^{\infty} \int_{-\infty}^{\infty} F(u, v) \exp\left[j2\pi(ux+vy)\right] du\, dv. \tag{127}$$

This integral is called the *inverse Fourier transform* of $F(u, v)$. By (114) and (127), $f(x, y)$ and $F(u, v)$ form a *Fourier transform pair*.

If x and y represent spatial coordinates, (127) can be used to give a physical interpretation to the Fourier transform $F(u, v)$ and to the coordinates u and v. Let us first examine the function

$$e^{j2\pi(ux+vy)}. \tag{128}$$

The real and imaginary parts of this function are $\cos 2\pi(ux + vy)$ and $\sin 2\pi(ux + vy)$, respectively. In Fig. 2.18(a), we have shown $\cos 2\pi(ux + vy)$. It is clear that if one took a section of this two-dimensional pattern parallel to the x-axis, it goes through u cycles per unit distance, while a section parallel to the y-axis goes through v cycles per unit distance. This is the reason why u and v are called the *spatial frequencies* along the x- and y-axes, respectively. Also, from the figure it can be seen that the spatial period of the pattern is $(u^2 + v^2)^{-1/2}$. The plot for $\sin 2\pi(ux + vy)$ looks similar to the one in Fig. 2.18(a) except that it is displaced by a quarter period in the direction of maximum rate of change.

From the preceding discussion it is clear that $e^{j2\pi(ux+vy)}$ is a two-dimensional pattern, the sections of which, parallel to the x- and y-axes, are spatially periodic with frequencies u and v, respectively. The pattern itself has a spatial period of $(u^2 + v^2)^{-1/2}$ along a direction that subtends an angle $\tan^{-1}(v/u)$ with the x-axis. By changing u and v, one can generate patterns with spatial periods ranging from 0 to ∞ in any direction in the xy-plane.

Equation (127) can, therefore, be interpreted to mean that $f(x, y)$ is a linear combination of elementary periodic patterns of the form $e^{j2\pi(ux+vy)}$. Evidently, the function, $F(u, v)$, is simply a weighting factor that is a measure of the relative contribution of the elementary pattern to the total sum. Since u and v are the spatial frequency of the pattern in the x and y directions, $F(u, v)$ is called the *frequency spectrum* of $f(x, y)$.

2.2.4 Properties of Fourier Transforms

Several properties of the two-dimensional Fourier transform follow easily from the defining integrals equation. Let $F\{f\}$ denote the Fourier transform of a function $f(x, y)$. Then $F\{f(x, y)\} = F(u, v)$. We will now present without proof some of the more common properties of Fourier transforms. The proofs are, for the most part, left for the reader (see the books by Goodman [Goo68] and Papoulis [Pap62]).

1) Linearity:

$$F\{af_1(x, y) + bf_2(x, y)\} = aF\{f_1(x, y)\} + bF\{f_2(x, y)\} \tag{129}$$

$$= aF_1(u, v) + bF_2(u, v). \tag{130}$$

This follows from the linearity of the integration operation.

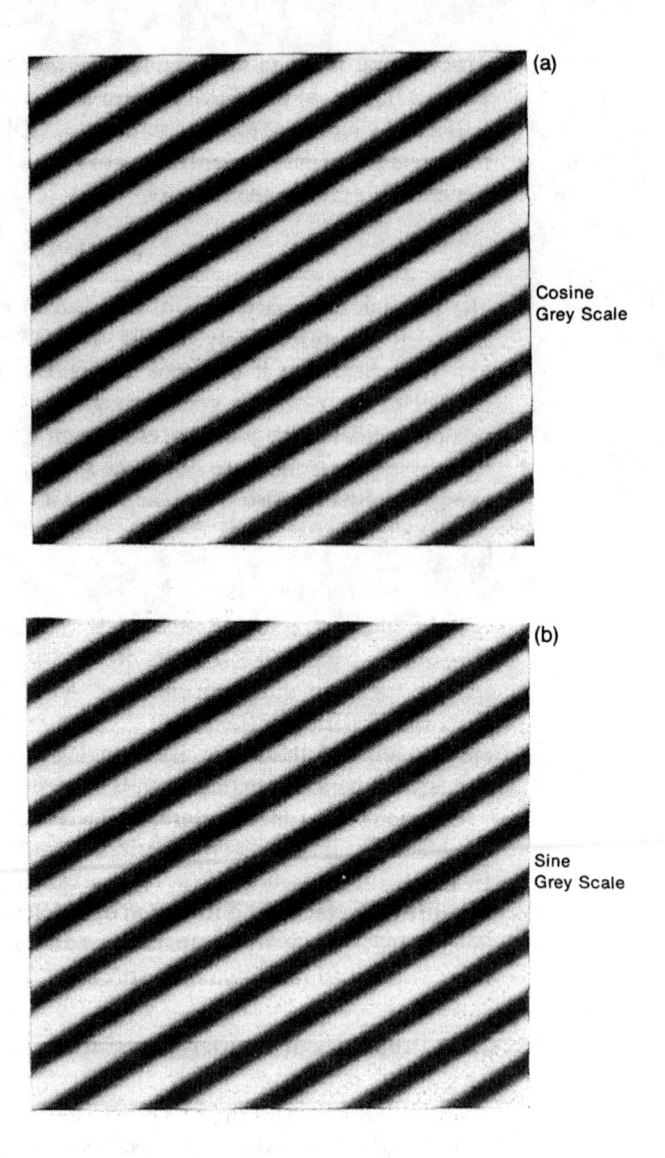

Fig. 2.18: *The Fourier transform represents an image in terms of exponentials of the form $e^{j2\pi(ux+vy)}$. Here we have shown the real (cosine) and the imaginary (sine) parts of one such exponential.*

2) *Scaling:*

$$F\{f(\alpha x, \beta y)\} = \frac{1}{|\alpha\beta|} F\left(\frac{u}{\alpha}, \frac{v}{\beta}\right). \tag{131}$$

To see this, introduce the change of variables $x' = \alpha x$, $y' = \beta y$. This property is illustrated in Fig. 2.19.

3) *Shift Property:*

$$F\{f(x-\alpha, y-\beta)\} = F(u, v)e^{-j2\pi(u\alpha+v\beta)}. \tag{132}$$

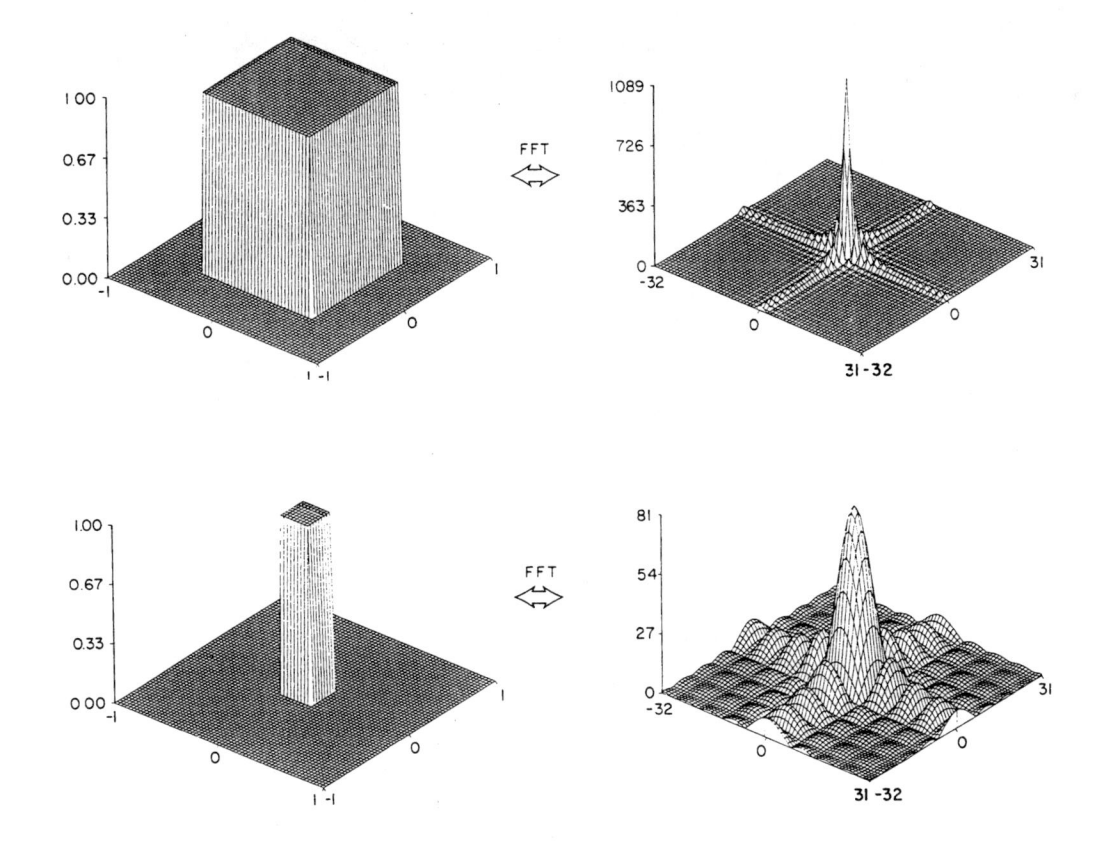

Fig. 2.19: *Scaling the size of an image leads to compression and amplification in the Fourier domain.*

This too follows immediately if we make the change of variables $x' = x - \alpha$, $y' = y - \beta$. The corresponding property for a shift in the frequency domain is

$$F\{\exp[j2\pi(u_0 x + v_0 y)]f(x, y)\} = F(u - u_0, v - v_0). \quad (133)$$

4) Rotation by Any Angle: In polar coordinates we can write

$$F\{f(r, \theta)\} = F(\omega, \phi). \quad (134)$$

If the function, f, is rotated by an angle α then the following result follows

$$F\{f(r, \theta + \alpha)\} = F(\omega, \phi + \alpha). \quad (135)$$

This property is illustrated in Fig. 2.20.

5) Rotational Symmetry: If $f(x, y)$ is a circularly symmetric function, i.e., $f(r, \theta)$ is only a function of r, then its frequency spectrum is also

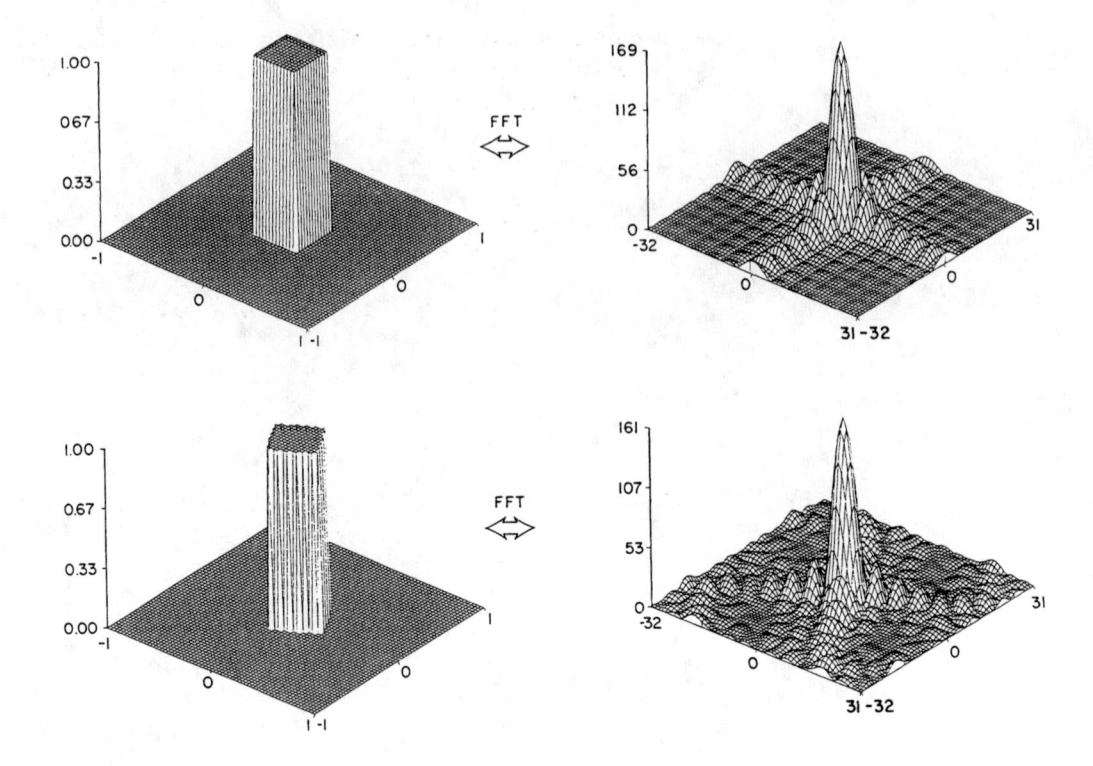

Fig. 2.20: *Rotation of an object by 30° leads to a similar rotation in the Fourier transform of the image.*

circularly symmetric and is given by

$$F(u, v) = F(p) = 2\pi \int_0^\infty r f(r) J_0(2\pi r p) \, dr. \tag{136}$$

The inverse relationship is given by

$$f(r) = 2\pi \int_0^\infty p F(p) J_0(2\pi r p) \, dp \tag{137}$$

where

$$r = \sqrt{x^2 + y^2}, \; \theta = \tan^{-1}(y/x), \; p = \sqrt{u^2 + v^2}, \; \phi = \tan^{-1}(v/u) \tag{138}$$

and

$$J_0(x) = (1/2\pi) \int_0^{2\pi} \exp\left[-jx \cos(\theta - \phi)\right] d\theta \tag{139}$$

is the zero-order Bessel function of the first kind. The transformation in (136) is also called the *Hankel transform of zero order*.

6) 180° Rotation:

$$F\{F\{f(x, y)\}\} = f(-x, -y). \tag{140}$$

7) Convolution:

$$F\left\{\int_{-\infty}^{\infty}\int_{-\infty}^{\infty} f_1(\alpha, \beta) f_2(x-\alpha, y-\beta)\, d\alpha\, d\beta\right\}$$

$$= F\{f_1(x, y)\} F\{f_2(x, y)\} \tag{141}$$

$$= F_1(u, v) F_2(u, v). \tag{142}$$

Note that the convolution of two functions in the space domain is equivalent to the very simple operation of multiplication in the spatial frequency domain. The corresponding property for convolution in the spatial frequency domain is given by

$$F\{f_1(x, y) f_2(x, y)\} = \int\int_{-\infty}^{\infty} F_1(u-s, v-t) F_2(s, t)\, ds\, dt. \tag{143}$$

A useful example of this property is shown in Figs. 2.21 and 2.22. By the Fourier convolution theorem we have chosen a frequency domain function, H, such that all frequencies above Ω cycles per picture are zero. In the space domain the convolution of x and h is a simple linear filter while in the frequency domain it is easy to see that all frequency components above Ω cycles/picture have been eliminated.

8) Parseval's Theorem:

$$\int_{-\infty}^{\infty}\int_{-\infty}^{\infty} f_1(x, y) f_2^*(x, y)\, dx\, dy = \int_{-\infty}^{\infty}\int_{-\infty}^{\infty} F_1(u, v) F_2^*(u, v)\, du\, dy$$

$$\tag{144}$$

where the asterisk denotes the complex conjugate. When $f_1(x, y) = f_2(x, y) = f(x, y)$, we have

$$\int_{-\infty}^{\infty}\int_{-\infty}^{\infty} |f(x, y)|^2\, dx\, dy = \int_{-\infty}^{\infty}\int_{-\infty}^{\infty} |F(u, v)|^2\, du\, dv. \tag{145}$$

In this form, this property is interpretable as a statement of conservation of energy.

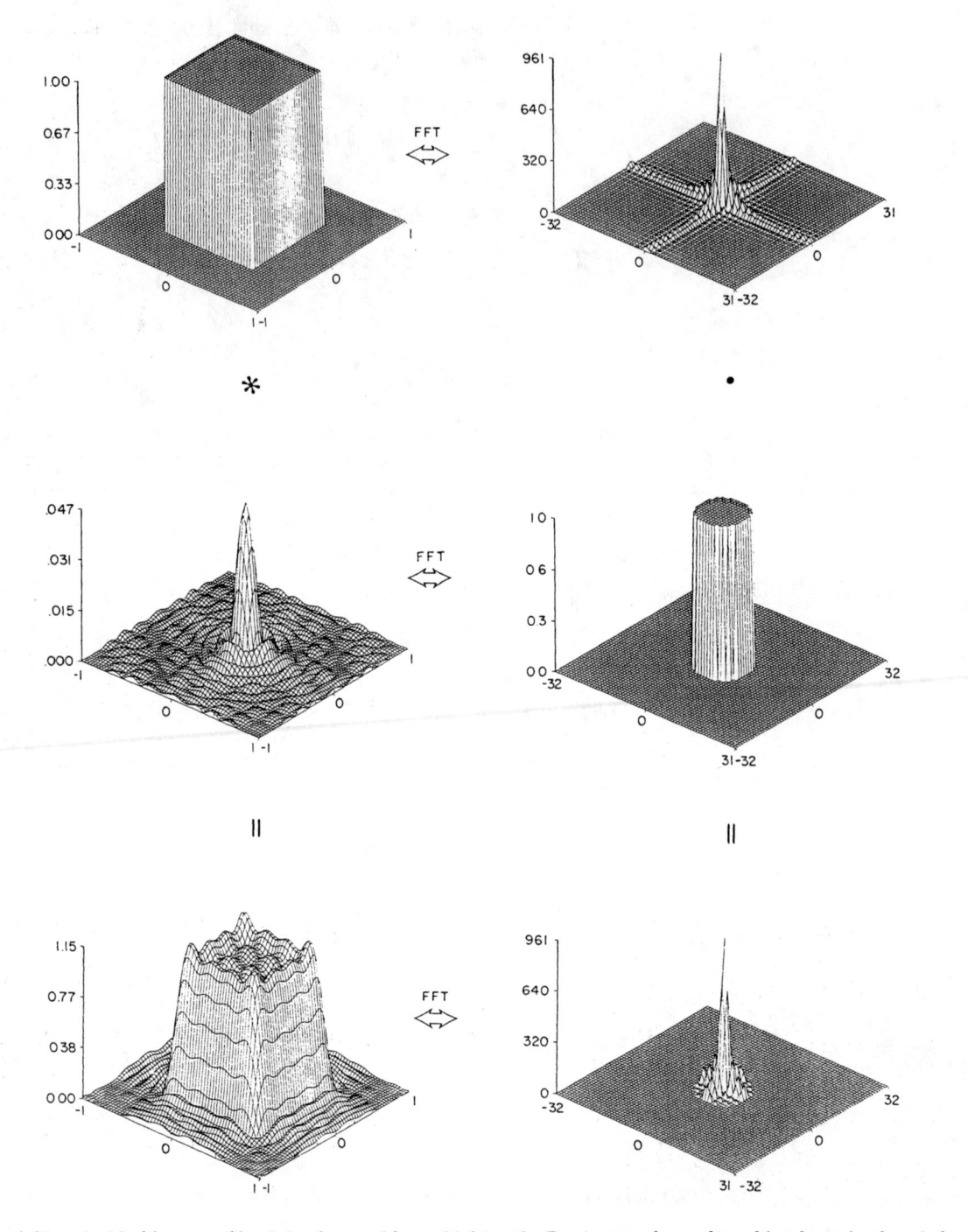

Fig. 2.21: *An ideal low pass filter is implemented by multiplying the Fourier transform of an object by a circular window.*

40   COMPUTERIZED TOMOGRAPHIC IMAGING

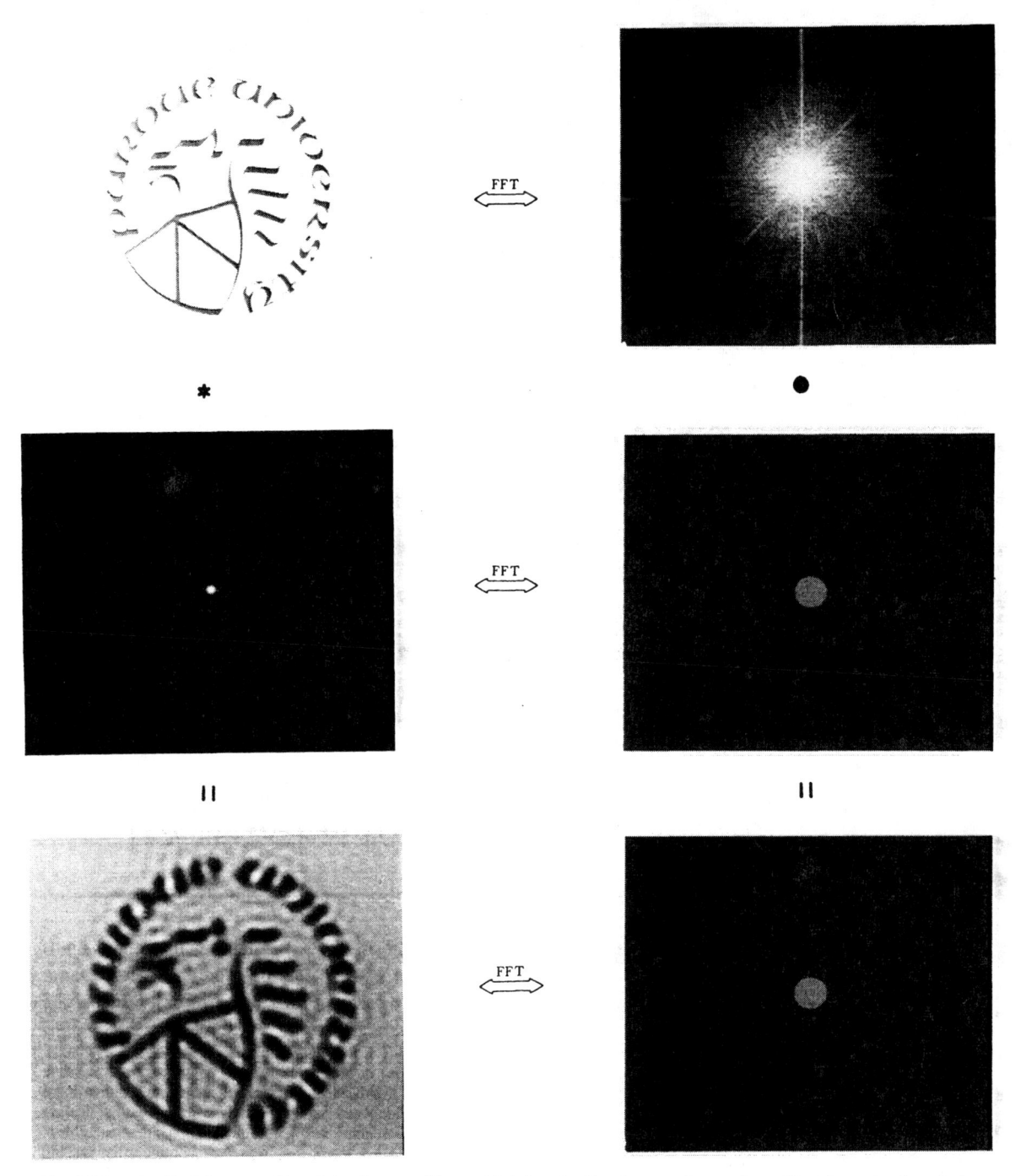

Fig. 2.22: *An ideal low pass filter is implemented by multiplying the Fourier transform of an object by a circular window.*

SIGNAL PROCESSING FUNDAMENTALS 41

2.2.5 The Two-Dimensional Finite Fourier Transform

Let $f(m, n)$ be a sampled version of a continuous two-dimensional function f. The finite Fourier transform (FFT) is defined as the summation[2]

$$F(u, v) = \frac{1}{MN} \sum_{m=0}^{M-1} \sum_{n=0}^{N-1} f(m, n) \exp\left[-j2\pi\left(\frac{mu}{M} + \frac{nv}{N}\right)\right] \quad (146)$$

for $u = 0, 1, 2, \cdots, M - 1$; $v = 0, 1, 2, \cdots, N - 1$.

The inverse FFT (IFFT) is given by the summation

$$f(m, n) = \sum_{u=0}^{M-1} \sum_{r=0}^{N-1} F(u, v) \exp\left[j2\pi\left(\frac{mu}{M} + \frac{nv}{N}\right)\right] \quad (147)$$

for $m = 0, 1, \cdots, M - 1$; $n = 0, 1, \cdots, N - 1$. It is easy to verify that the summations represented by the FFT and IFFT are inverses by noting that

$$\sum_{m=0}^{J-1} \exp\left[\frac{-j2\pi}{J} km\right] \exp\left[\frac{j2\pi}{J} mn\right] = \begin{cases} J, & k = n \\ 0, & k \neq n. \end{cases} \quad (148)$$

This is the discrete version of (107). That the inverse FFT undoes the effect of the FFT is seen by substituting (43) into (147) for the inverse DFT to find

$$f(m, n) = \frac{1}{MN} \sum_{u=0}^{M-1} \sum_{r=0}^{N-1} \sum_{m=0}^{M-1} \sum_{n=0}^{N-1} f(m, n)$$

$$\cdot \exp\left[-j2\pi\left(\frac{mu}{M} + \frac{nv}{N}\right)\right] \exp\left[j2\pi\left(\frac{mu}{M} + \frac{nv}{N}\right)\right]. \quad (149)$$

The desired result is made apparent by rearranging the order of summation and using (148).

In (146) the discrete Fourier transform $F(u, v)$ is defined for u between 0 and $M - 1$ and for v between 0 and $N - 1$. If, however, we use the same equation to evaluate $F(\pm u, \pm v)$, we discover that the periodicity properties

---

[2] To be consistent with the notation in the one-dimensional case, we should express the space and frequency domain arrays as $f_{m,n}$ and $F_{u,v}$. However, we feel that for the two-dimensional case, the math looks a bit neater with the style chosen here, especially when one starts dealing with negative indices and other extensions. Also, note that the variables u and v are indices here, which is contrary to their usage in Section 2.2.3 where they represent continuously varying spatial frequencies.

of the exponential factor imply that

$$F(u, -v) = F(u, N-v) \tag{150}$$

$$F(-u, v) = F(M-u, v) \tag{151}$$

$$F(-u, -v) = F(M-u, N-v). \tag{152}$$

Similarly, using (147) we can show that

$$f(-m, n) = f(M-m, n) \tag{153}$$

$$f(m, -n) = f(m, N-n) \tag{154}$$

$$f(-m, -n) = f(M-m, N-n). \tag{155}$$

Another related consequence of the periodicity properties of the exponential factors in (28) and (147) is that

$$F(aM+u, bN+v) = F(u, v) \text{ and } f(aM+m, bN+n) = f(m, n) \tag{156}$$

for $a = 0, \pm 1, \pm 2, \cdots, b = 0, \pm 1, \pm 2, \cdots$. Therefore, we have the following conclusion: if a finite array of numbers $f_{m,n}$ and its Fourier transform $F_{u,v}$ are related by (28) and (147), then if it is desired to extend the definition of $f(m, n)$ and $F(u, v)$ beyond the original domain as given by [0 ≤ (m and u) ≤ $M - 1$] and [0 ≤ (n and v) ≤ $N - 1$], this extension must be governed by (151), (154) and (156). In other words, the extensions are periodic repetitions of the arrays.

It will now be shown that this periodicity has important consequences when we compute the convolution of two $M \times N$ arrays, $f(m, n)$ and $d(m, n)$, by multiplying their finite Fourier transforms, $F(u, v)$ and $D(u, v)$. The convolution of two arrays $f(m, n)$ and $d(m, n)$ is given by

$$g(\alpha, \beta) = \frac{1}{MN} \sum_{m=0}^{M-1} \sum_{n=0}^{N-1} f(m, n) d(\alpha - m, \beta - n) \tag{157}$$

$$= \frac{1}{MN} \sum_{m=0}^{M-1} \sum_{n=0}^{N-1} f(\alpha - m, \beta - n) d(m, n) \tag{158}$$

for $\alpha = 0, 1, \cdots, M - 1, \beta = 0, 1, \cdots, N - 1$, where we insist that when the values of $f(m, n)$ and $d(m, n)$ are required for indices outside the ranges 0 ≤ m ≤ $M - 1$ and 0 ≤ n ≤ $N - 1$, for which $f(m, n)$ and $d(m, n)$ are defined, then they should be obtained by the rules given in (151), (154) and (156). With this condition, the convolution previously defined becomes a circular or cyclic convolution.

As in the 1-dimensional case, the FFT of (157) can be written as the product of the two Fourier transforms. By making use of (147), we obtain

$$g(\alpha, \beta) = \frac{1}{MN} \sum_{m=0}^{M-1} \sum_{n=0}^{N-1} f(m, n) d(\alpha - m, \beta - n) \quad (159)$$

expanding f and d in terms of their DFTs

$$= \frac{1}{MN} \sum_{m=0}^{M-1} \sum_{n=0}^{N-1} \left\{ \sum_{u=0}^{M-1} \sum_{v=0}^{N-1} F(u, v) \exp\left[j2\pi\left(\frac{mu}{M} + \frac{nv}{N}\right)\right] \right\}$$

$$\cdot \left\{ \sum_{w=0}^{M-1} \sum_{z=0}^{N-1} D(w, z) \exp\left[j2\pi\left((\alpha - m)\frac{w}{M} + \frac{(\beta - n)z}{N}\right)\right] \right\} \quad (160)$$

and then rearranging the summations

$$= \frac{1}{MN} \sum_{u=0}^{M-1} \sum_{v=0}^{N-1} \sum_{w=0}^{M-1} \sum_{z=0}^{N-1} \left\{ F(u, v) D(w, z) \exp\left[j2\pi\left(\frac{\alpha w}{M} + \frac{\beta z}{N}\right)\right] \right.$$

$$\left. \cdot \sum_{m=0}^{M-1} \sum_{n=0}^{N-1} \exp\left[j2\pi \frac{m(u-w)}{M}\right] \exp\left[j2\pi \frac{n(v-z)}{N}\right] \right\}. \quad (161)$$

Using the orthogonality relationship (148) we find

$$= \sum_{u=0}^{M-1} \sum_{v=0}^{N-1} F(u, v) D(u, v) \exp\left[j2\pi\left(\frac{\alpha u}{M} + \frac{\beta v}{N}\right)\right]. \quad (162)$$

Thus we see that the convolution of the two-dimensional arrays f and d can be expressed as a simple multiplication in the frequency domain.

The discrete version of Parseval's theorem is an often used property of the finite Fourier transform. In the continuous case this theorem is given by (144) while for the discrete case

$$\sum_{m=0}^{M-1} \sum_{n=0}^{N-1} f(m, n) g^*(m, n) = MN \sum_{u=0}^{M-1} \sum_{v=0}^{N-1} F(u, v) G^*(u, v). \quad (163)$$

The following relationship directly follows from (163):

$$\sum_{m=0}^{M-1} \sum_{n=0}^{N-1} |f(m, n)|^2 = MN \sum_{u=0}^{M-1} \sum_{v=0}^{N-1} |F(u, v)|^2. \quad (164)$$

As in the one-dimensional and the continuous two-dimensional cases Parseval's theorem states that the energy in the space domain and that in the frequency domain are equal.

As in a one-dimensional case, a two-dimensional image must be sampled at a rate greater than the Nyquist frequency to prevent errors due to aliasing. For a moment, going back to the interpretation of u and v as continuous frequencies (see Section 2.2.3), if the Fourier transform of the image is zero for all frequencies greater than B, meaning that $F(u, v) = 0$ for all u and v such that $|u| \geq B$ and $|v| \geq B$, then there will be no aliasing if samples of the image are taken on a rectangular grid with intervals of less than $\frac{1}{2B}$. A pictorial representation of the effect of aliasing on two-dimensional images is shown in Fig. 2.23. Further discussion on aliasing in two-dimensional sampling can be found in [Ros82].

2.2.6 Numerical Implementation of the Two-Dimensional FFT

Before we end this chapter, we would like to say a few words about the numerical implementation of the two-dimensional finite Fourier transform. Equation (28) may be written as

$$F(u, v) = \frac{1}{M} \sum_{m=0}^{M-1} \left[\frac{1}{N} \sum_{n=0}^{N-1} f(m, n) \exp\left(-j\frac{2\pi}{N} nv\right) \right]$$

$$\cdot \exp\left(-j\frac{2\pi}{M} mu\right),$$

$$u = 0, \cdots, M-1, \ v = 0, \cdots, N-1. \tag{165}$$

The expression within the square brackets is the one-dimensional FFT of the mth row of the image, which may be implemented by using a standard FFT (fast Fourier transform) computer program (in most instances N is a power of 2). Therefore, to compute $F(u, v)$, we *replace each row in the image by its one-dimensional FFT, and then perform the one-dimensional FFT of each column.*

Ordinarily, when a 2-D FFT is computed in the manner described above, the frequency domain origin will not be at the center of the array, which if displayed as such can lead to difficulty in interpretation. Note, for example, that in a 16 × 16 image the indices $u = 15$ and $v = 0$ correspond to a negative frequency of one cycle per image width. This can be seen by substituting $u = 1$ and $v = 0$ in the second equation in (151). To display the frequency domain origin at approximately the center of the array (a precise center does not exist when either M or N is an even number), the image data $f(m, n)$ are first multiplied by $(-1)^{m+n}$ and then the finite Fourier transformation is performed. To prove this, let us define a new array $f'(m, n)$ as follows:

$$f'(m, n) = f(m, n)(-1)^{m+n} \tag{166}$$

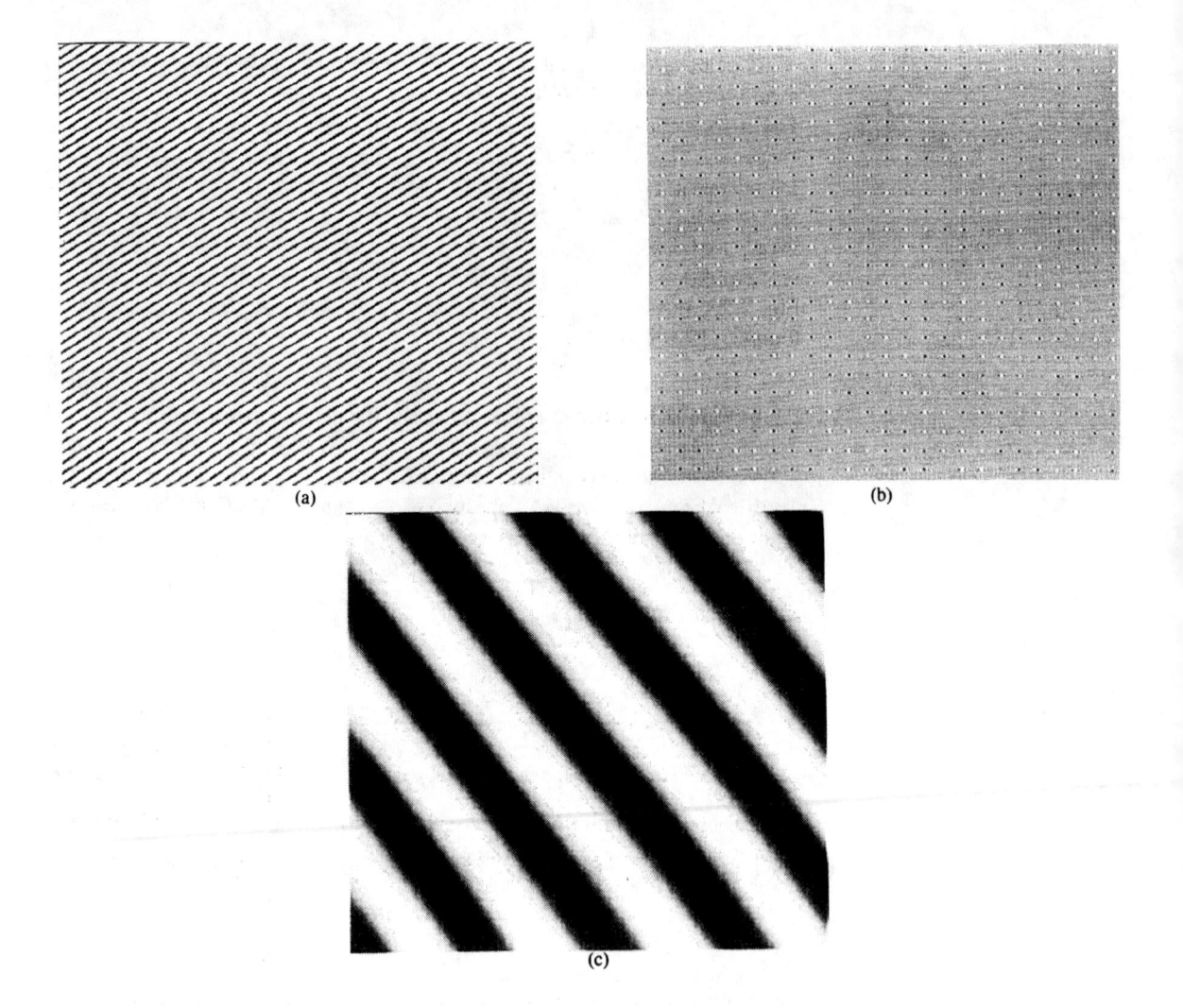

Fig. 2.23: *The effect of aliasing in two-dimensional images is shown here. (This is often known as the Moiré effect.) In (a) a high-frequency sinusoid is shown. In (b) this sinusoid is sampled at a rate much lower than the Nyquist rate and the sampled values are shown as black and white dots (gray is used to represent the area between the samples). Finally, in (c) the sampled data shown in (b) are low pass filtered at the Nyquist rate. Note that both the direction and frequency of the sinusoid have changed due to aliasing.*

and let $F'(u, v)$ be its finite Fourier transform:

$$F'(u, v) = \frac{1}{MN} \sum_{m=0}^{M-1} \sum_{n=0}^{N-1} f(m, n)(-1)^{m+n}$$
$$\cdot \exp\left[-j2\pi\left(\frac{mu}{M} + \frac{nv}{N}\right)\right]. \quad (167)$$

Rewriting this expression as

$$F(u, v) = \frac{1}{MN} \sum_{m=0}^{M-1} \sum_{n=0}^{N-1} f(m, n)$$

$$\cdot \exp\left\{j2\pi\left[\frac{(M/2)m}{M}+\frac{(N/2)n}{N}\right]\right\} \qquad (168)$$

$$\cdot \exp\left[-j2\pi\left(\frac{mu}{M}+\frac{nv}{N}\right)\right] \qquad (169)$$

it is easy to show that

$$F(u, v) = F\left(u-\frac{M}{2},\ v-\frac{N}{2}\right),$$
$$u = 0, 1, \cdots, M-1;\ v = 0, 1, \cdots, N-1. \qquad (170)$$

Therefore, when the array $F'(u, v)$ is displayed, the location at $u = M/2$ and $v = N/2$ will contain $F(0, 0)$.

We have by no means discussed all the important properties of continuous, discrete and finite Fourier transforms; the reader is referred to the cited literature for further details.

2.3 References

[Bri74] E. O. Brigham, *The Fast Fourier Transform*. Englewood Cliffs, NJ: Prentice-Hall, 1974.
[Dud84] D. E. Dudgeon and R. M. Mersereau, *Multidimensional Digital Signal Processing*. Englewood Cliffs, NJ: Prentice-Hall, 1984.
[Gon77] R. C. Gonzalez, *Digital Image Processing*. Reading, MA: Addison-Wesley, 1977.
[Goo68] J. W. Goodman, *Introduction to Fourier Optics*. San Francisco, CA: McGraw-Hill Book Company, 1968.
[Lig60] M. J. Lighthill, *Introduction to Fourier Analysis and Generalized Functions*. London and New York: Cambridge Univ. Press, 1960.
[McG74] C. D. McGillem and G. R. Cooper, *Continuous and Discrete Signal and System Analysis*. New York, NY: Holt, Rinehart and Winston, 1974.
[Opp75] A. V. Oppenheim and R. V. Schafer, *Digital Signal Processing*. Englewood Cliffs, NJ: Prentice-Hall, 1975.
[Pap62] A. Papoulis, *The Fourier Integral and Its Applications*. New York, NY: McGraw-Hill, 1962.
[Pra78] W. K. Pratt, *Digital Image Processing*. New York, NY: J. Wiley, 1978.
[Rab75] L. R. Rabiner and B. Gold, *Theory and Applications of Digital Signal Processing*. Englewood Cliffs, NJ: Prentice-Hall, 1975.
[Ros82] A. Rosenfeld and A. C. Kak, *Digital Picture Processing*, 2nd ed. New York, NY: Academic Press, 1982.
[Sch75] M. Schwartz and L. Shaw, *Signal Processing: Discrete Spectral Analysis, Detection, and Estimation*. New York, NY: McGraw-Hill, 1975.

3 Algorithms for Reconstruction with Nondiffracting Sources

In this chapter we will deal with the mathematical basis of tomography with nondiffracting sources. We will show how one can go about recovering the image of the cross section of an object from the projection data. In ideal situations, projections are a set of measurements of the integrated values of some parameter of the object—integrations being along straight lines through the object and being referred to as line integrals. We will show that the key to tomographic imaging is the Fourier Slice Theorem which relates the measured projection data to the two-dimensional Fourier transform of the object cross section.

This chapter will start with the definition of line integrals and how they are combined to form projections of an object. By finding the Fourier transform of a projection taken along parallel lines, we will then derive the Fourier Slice Theorem. The reconstruction algorithm used depends on the type of projection data measured; we will discuss algorithms based on parallel beam projection data and two types of fan beam data.

3.1 Line Integrals and Projections

A line integral, as the name implies, represents the integral of some parameter of the object along a line. In this chapter we will not concern ourselves with the physical phenomena that generate line integrals, but a typical example is the attenuation of x-rays as they propagate through biological tissue. In this case the object is modeled as a two-dimensional (or three-dimensional) distribution of the x-ray attenuation constant and a line integral represents the total attenuation suffered by a beam of x-rays as it travels in a straight line through the object. More details of this process and other examples will be presented in Chapter 4.

We will use the coordinate system defined in Fig. 3.1 to describe line integrals and projections. In this example the object is represented by a two-dimensional function $f(x, y)$ and each line integral by the (θ, t) parameters.

The equation of line AB in Fig. 3.1 is

$$x \cos \theta + y \sin \theta = t \tag{1}$$

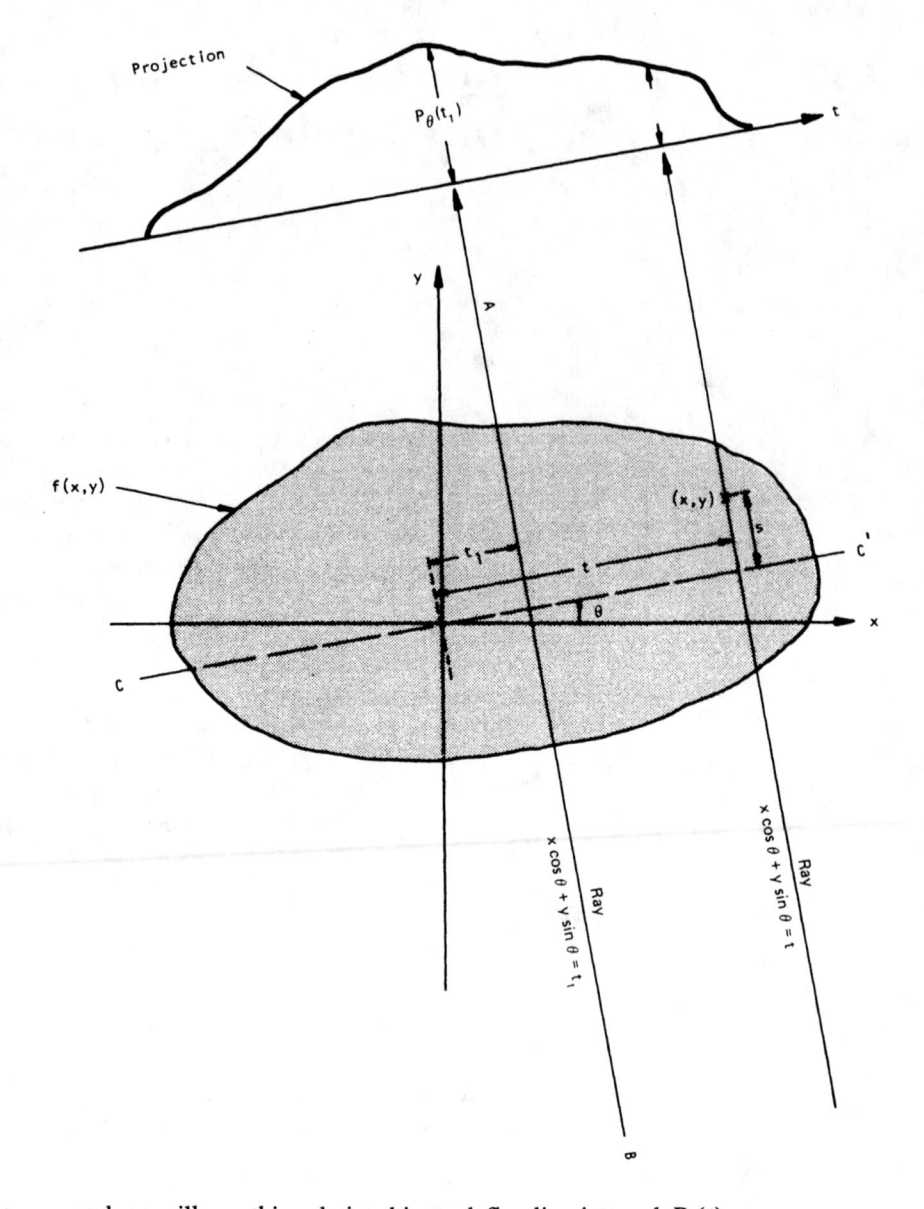

Fig. 3.1: An object, $f(x, y)$, and its projection, $P_\theta(t_1)$, are shown for an angle of θ. (From [Kak79].)

and we will use this relationship to define line integral $P_\theta(t)$ as

$$P_\theta(t) = \int_{(\theta,t)\text{ line}} f(x, y)\, ds. \qquad (2)$$

Using a delta function, this can be rewritten as

$$P_\theta(t) = \int_{-\infty}^{\infty} \int_{-\infty}^{\infty} f(x, y)\delta(x\cos\theta + y\sin\theta - t)\, dx\, dy. \qquad (3)$$

The function $P_\theta(t)$ is known as the Radon transform of the function $f(x, y)$.

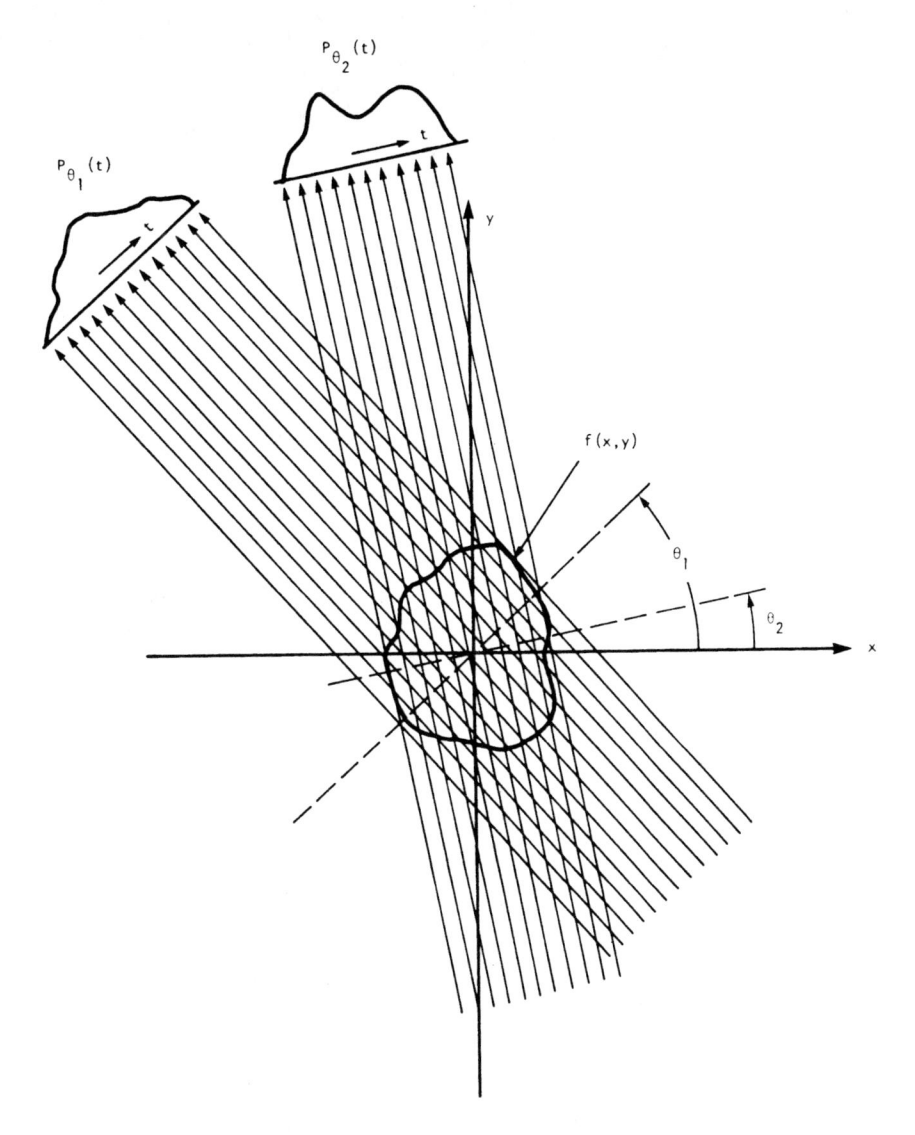

Fig. 3.2: *Parallel projections are taken by measuring a set of parallel rays for a number of different angles. (From [Ros82].)*

A projection is formed by combining a set of line integrals. The simplest projection is a collection of parallel ray integrals as is given by $P_\theta(t)$ for a constant θ. This is known as a parallel projection and is shown in Fig. 3.2. It could be measured, for example, by moving an x-ray source and detector along parallel lines on opposite sides of an object.

Another type of projection is possible if a single source is placed in a fixed position relative to a line of detectors. This is shown in Fig. 3.3 and is known as a fan beam projection because the line integrals are measured along fans.

Most of the computer simulation results in this chapter will be shown for the image in Fig. 3.4. This is the well-known Shepp and Logan [She74]

ALGORITHMS FOR RECONSTRUCTION WITH NONDIFFRACTING SOURCES

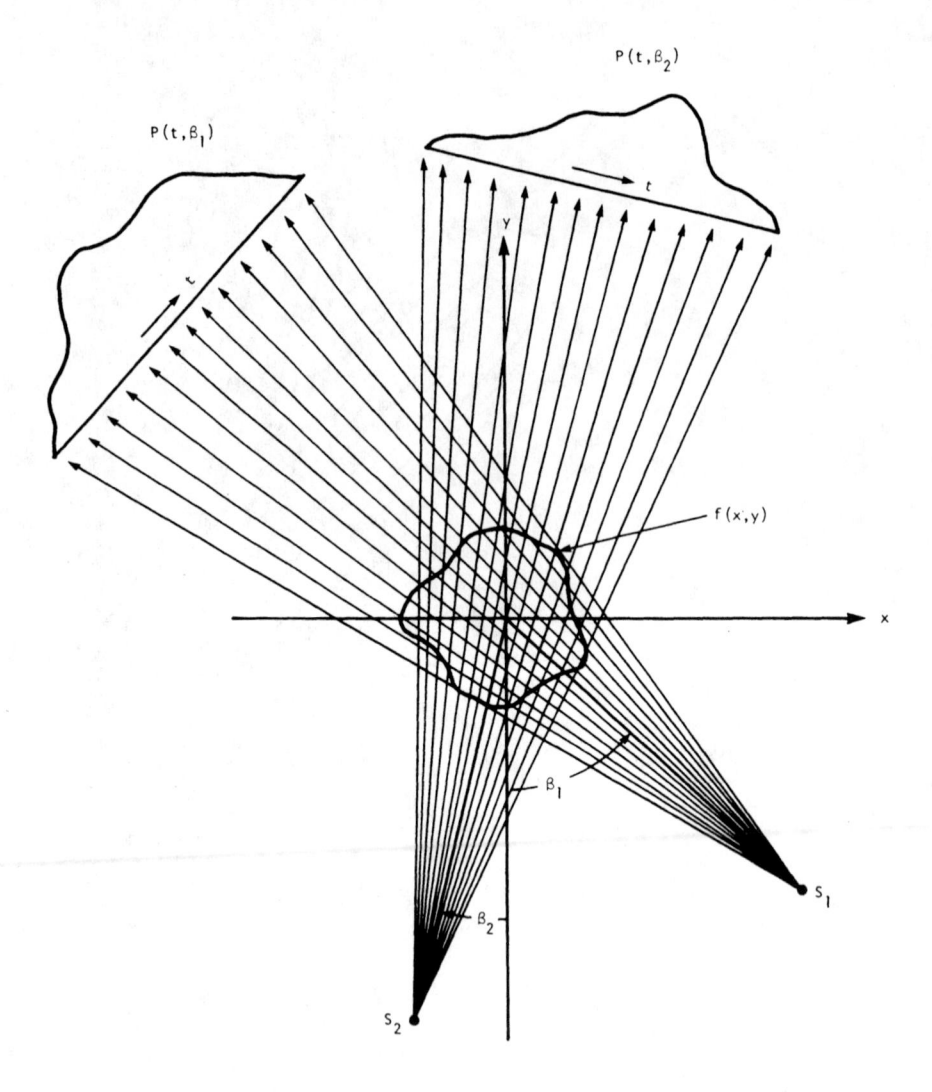

Fig. 3.3: *A fan beam projection is collected if all the rays meet in one location. (From [Ros82].)*

"head phantom," so called because of its use in testing the accuracy of reconstruction algorithms for their ability to reconstruct cross sections of the human head with x-ray tomography. (The human head is believed to place the greatest demands on the numerical accuracy and the freedom from artifacts of a reconstruction method.) The image in Fig. 3.4(a) is composed of 10 ellipses, as illustrated in Fig. 3.4(b). The parameters of these ellipses are given in Table 3.1.

A major advantage of using an image like that in Fig. 3.4(a) for computer simulation is that now one can write analytical expressions for the projections. Note that the projection of an image composed of a number of ellipses is simply the sum of the projections for each of the ellipses; this follows from the linearity of the Radon transform. We will now present

(b)

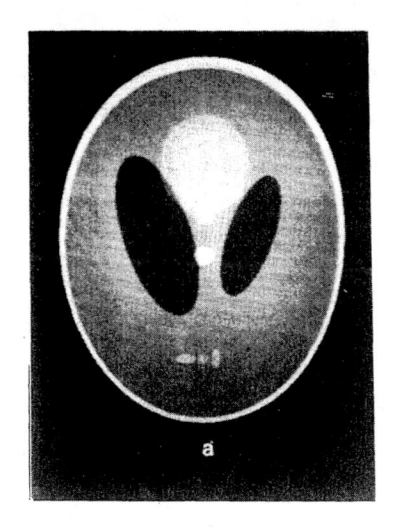

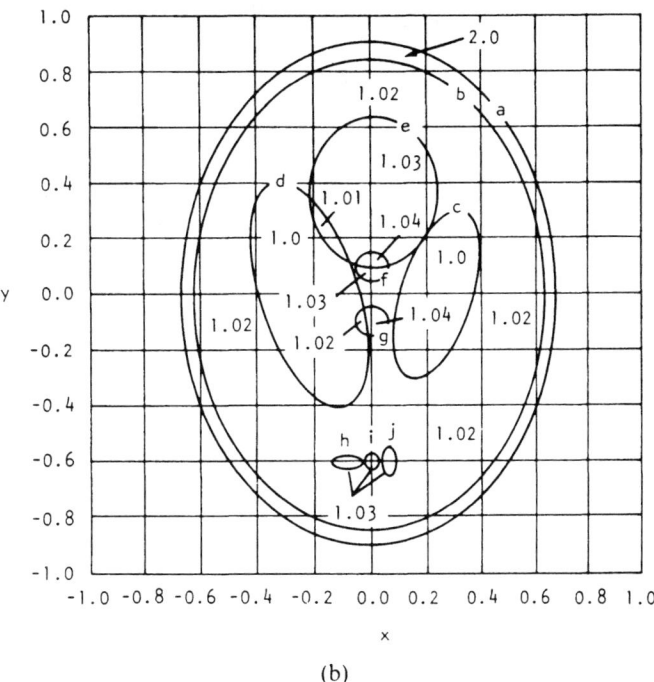

Fig. 3.4: *The Shepp and Logan "head phantom" is shown in (a). Most of the computer simulated results in this chapter were generated using this phantom. The phantom is a superposition of 10 ellipses, each with a size and magnitude as shown in (b). (From [Ros82].)*

expressions for the projections of a single ellipse. Let $f(x, y)$ be as shown in Fig. 3.5(a), i.e.,

$$f(x, y) = \begin{cases} \rho & \text{for } \dfrac{x^2}{A^2} + \dfrac{y^2}{B^2} \leq 1 \quad \text{(inside the ellipse)} \\ 0 & \text{otherwise} \quad \text{(outside the ellipse).} \end{cases} \quad (4)$$

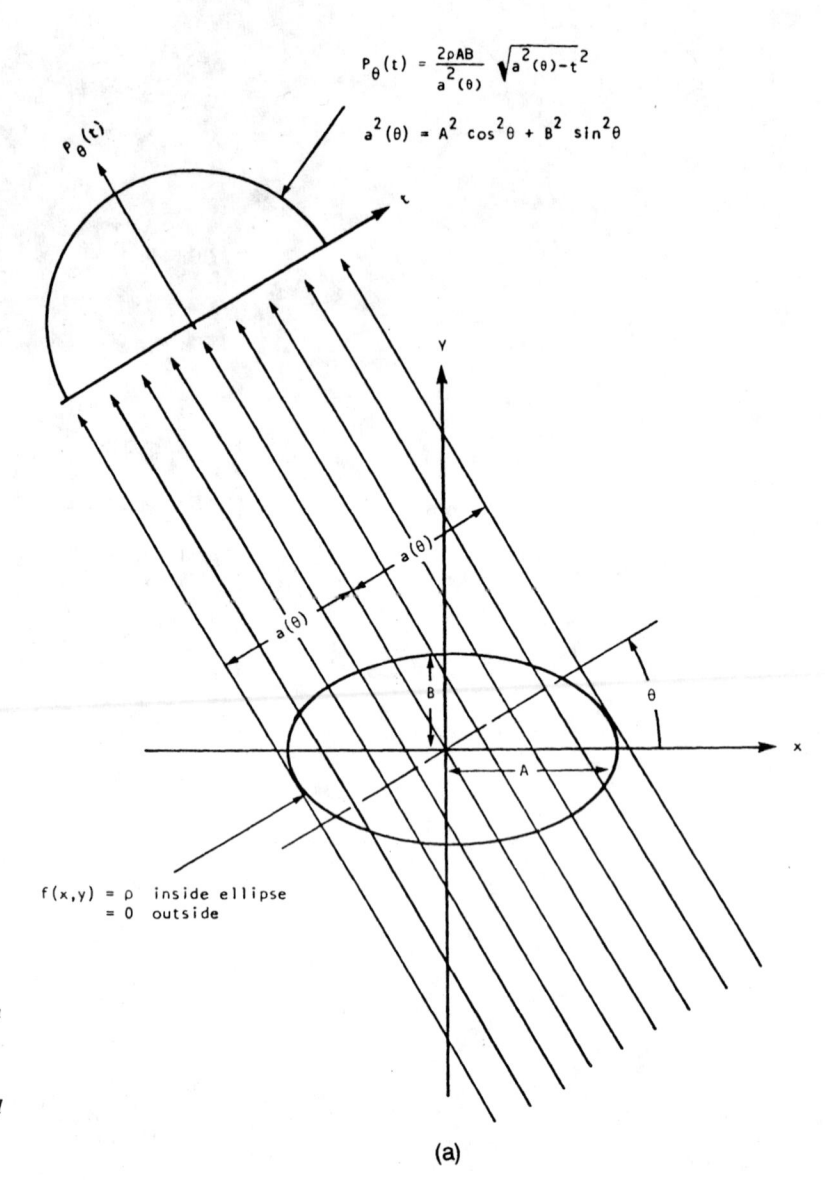

Fig. 3.5: *(a) An analytic expression is shown for the projection of an ellipse. For computer simulations a projection can be generated by simply summing the projection of each individual ellipse. (b) Shown here is an ellipse with its center located at (x_1, y_1) and its major axis rotated by α. (From [Ros82].)*

(a)

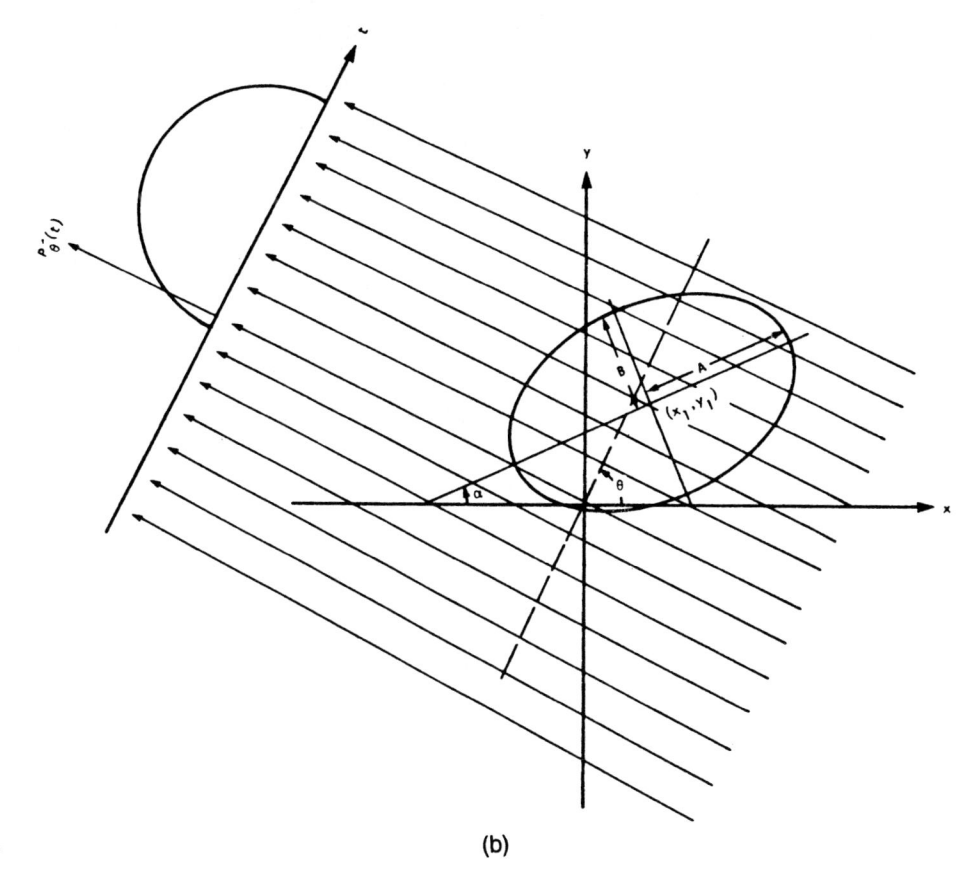

Fig. 3.5: *Continued.* (b)

Table 3.1: Summary of parameters for tomography simulations.

Center Coordinate	Major Axis	Minor Axis	Rotation Angle	Refractive Index
(0, 0)	0.92	0.69	90	2.0
(0, −0.0184)	0.874	0.6624	90	−0.98
(0.22, 0)	0.31	0.11	72	−0.02
(−0.22, 0)	0.41	0.16	108	−0.02
(0, 0.35)	0.25	0.21	90	0.01
(0, 0.1)	0.046	0.046	0	0.01
(0, −0.1)	0.046	0.046	0	0.01
(−0.08, −0.605)	0.046	0.023	0	0.01
(0, −0.605)	0.023	0.023	0	0.01
(0.06, −0.605)	0.046	0.023	90	0.01

It is easy to show that the projections of such a function are given by

$$P_\theta(t) = \begin{cases} \dfrac{2\rho AB}{a^2(\theta)} \sqrt{a^2(\theta) - t^2} & \text{for } |t| \leq a(\theta) \\ 0 & |t| > a(\theta) \end{cases} \qquad (5)$$

where $a^2(\theta) = A^2 \cos^2 \theta + B^2 \sin^2 \theta$. Note that $a(\theta)$ is equal to the projection half-width as shown in Fig. 3.5(a).

Now consider the ellipse described above centered at (x_1, y_1) and rotated by an angle α as shown in Fig. 3.5(b). Let $P'(\theta, t)$ be the resulting projections. They are related to $P_\theta(t)$ in (5) by

$$P_\theta(t) = P_{\theta - \alpha}(t - s \cos(\gamma - \theta)) \qquad (6)$$

where $s = \sqrt{x_1^2 + y_1^2}$ and $\gamma = \tan^{-1}(y_1/x_1)$.

3.2 The Fourier Slice Theorem

We derive the Fourier Slice Theorem by taking the one-dimensional Fourier transform of a parallel projection and noting that it is equal to a slice of the two-dimensional Fourier transform of the original object. It follows that given the projection data, it should then be possible to estimate the object by simply performing a two-dimensional inverse Fourier transform.

We start by defining the two-dimensional Fourier transform of the object function as

$$F(u, v) = \int_{-\infty}^{\infty} \int_{-\infty}^{\infty} f(x, y) e^{-j2\pi(ux + vy)} \, dx \, dy. \qquad (7)$$

Likewise define a projection at an angle θ, $P_\theta(t)$, and its Fourier transform by

$$S_\theta(w) = \int_{-\infty}^{\infty} P_\theta(t) e^{-j2\pi wt} \, dt. \qquad (8)$$

The simplest example of the Fourier Slice Theorem is given for a projection at $\theta = 0$. First, consider the Fourier transform of the object along the line in the frequency domain given by $v = 0$. The Fourier transform integral now simplifies to

$$F(u, 0) = \int_{-\infty}^{\infty} \int_{-\infty}^{\infty} f(x, y) e^{-j2\pi ux} \, dx \, dy \qquad (9)$$

but because the phase factor is no longer dependent on y we can split the integral into two parts,

$$F(u, 0) = \int_{-\infty}^{\infty} \left[\int_{-\infty}^{\infty} f(x, y) \, dy \right] e^{-j2\pi ux} \, dx. \qquad (10)$$

From the definition of a parallel projection, the reader will recognize the term in brackets as the equation for a projection along lines of constant x or

$$P_{\theta=0}(x) = \int_{-\infty}^{\infty} f(x, y) \, dy. \qquad (11)$$

Substituting this in (10) we find

$$F(u, 0) = \int_{-\infty}^{\infty} P_{\theta=0}(x) e^{-j2\pi ux} \, dx. \qquad (12)$$

The right-hand side of this equation represents the one-dimensional Fourier transform of the projection $P_{\theta=0}$; thus we have the following relationship between the vertical projection and the 2-D transform of the object function:

$$F(u, 0) = S_{\theta=0}(u). \qquad (13)$$

This is the simplest form of the Fourier Slice Theorem. Clearly this result is independent of the orientation between the object and the coordinate system. If, for example, as shown in Fig. 3.6 the (t, s) coordinate system is rotated by an angle θ, the Fourier transform of the projection defined in (11) is equal to the two-dimensional Fourier transform of the object along a line rotated by θ. This leads to the Fourier Slice Theorem which is stated as [Kak85]:

The Fourier transform of a parallel projection of an image $f(x, y)$ taken at angle θ gives a slice of the two-dimensional transform, $F(u, v)$, subtending an angle θ with the u-axis. In other words, the Fourier transform of $P_\theta(t)$ gives the values of $F(u, v)$ along line BB in Fig. 3.6.

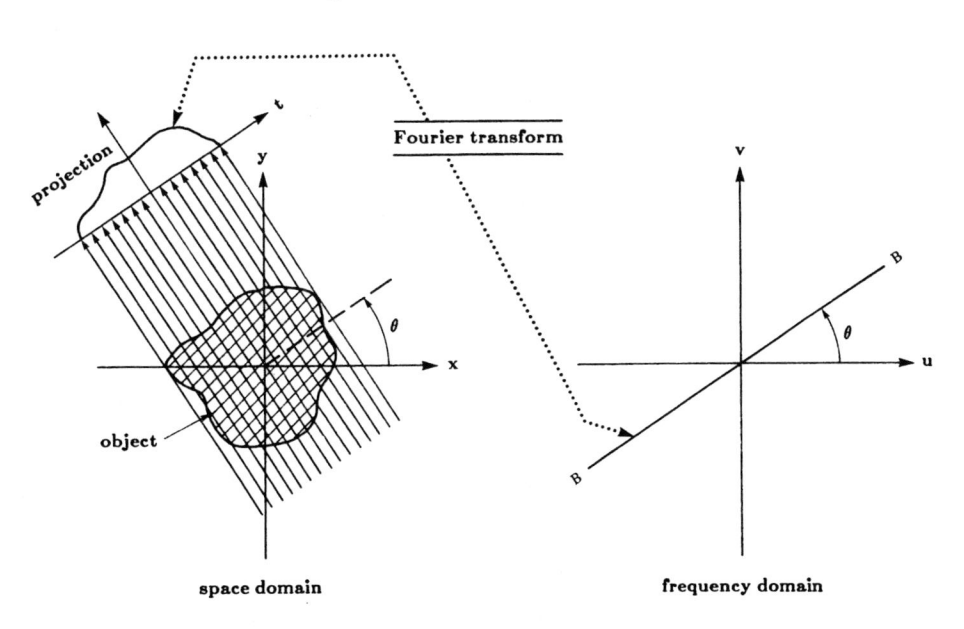

Fig. 3.6: *The Fourier Slice Theorem relates the Fourier transform of a projection to the Fourier transform of the object along a radial line. (From [Pan83].)*

The derivation of the Fourier Slice Theorem can be placed on a more solid foundation by considering the (t, s) coordinate system to be a rotated version of the original (x, y) system as expressed by

$$\begin{bmatrix} t \\ s \end{bmatrix} = \begin{bmatrix} \cos\theta & \sin\theta \\ -\sin\theta & \cos\theta \end{bmatrix} \begin{bmatrix} x \\ y \end{bmatrix}. \tag{14}$$

In the (t, s) coordinate system a projection along lines of constant t is written

$$P_\theta(t) = \int_{-\infty}^{\infty} f(t, s)\, ds \tag{15}$$

and from (8) its Fourier transform is given by

$$S_\theta(w) = \int_{-\infty}^{\infty} P_\theta(t) e^{-j2\pi wt}\, dt. \tag{8}$$

Substituting the definition of a projection into the above equation we find

$$S_\theta(w) = \int_{-\infty}^{\infty} \left[\int f(t, s)\, ds \right] e^{-j2\pi wt}\, dt. \tag{16}$$

This result can be transformed into the (x, y) coordinate system by using the relationships in (14), the result being

$$S_\theta(w) = \int_{-\infty}^{\infty} \int_{-\infty}^{\infty} f(x, y) e^{-j2\pi w(x\cos\theta + y\sin\theta)}\, dx\, dy. \tag{17}$$

The right-hand side of this equation now represents the two-dimensional Fourier transform at a spatial frequency of $(u = w\cos\theta, v = w\sin\theta)$ or

$$S_\theta(w) = F(w, \theta) = F(w\cos\theta, w\sin\theta). \tag{18}$$

This equation is the essence of straight ray tomography and proves the Fourier Slice Theorem.

The above result indicates that by taking the projections of an object function at angles $\theta_1, \theta_2, \cdots, \theta_k$ and Fourier transforming each of these, we can determine the values of $F(u, v)$ on radial lines as shown in Fig. 3.6. If an infinite number of projections are taken, then $F(u, v)$ would be known at all points in the uv-plane. Knowing $F(u, v)$, the object function $f(x, y)$ can be recovered by using the inverse Fourier transform:

$$f(x, y) = \int_{-\infty}^{\infty} \int_{-\infty}^{\infty} F(u, v) e^{j2\pi(ux+vy)}\, du\, dv. \tag{19}$$

If the function $f(x, y)$ is bounded by $-A/2 < x < A/2$ and $-A/2 < y < A/2$, for the purpose of computation (19) can be written as

$$f(x, y) = \frac{1}{A^2} \sum_m \sum_n F\left(\frac{m}{A}, \frac{n}{A}\right) e^{j2\pi((m/A)x + (n/A)y)} \tag{20}$$

for
$$-\frac{A}{2}<x<\frac{A}{2} \text{ and } -\frac{A}{2}<y<\frac{A}{2}. \qquad (21)$$

Since in practice only a finite number of Fourier components will be known, we can write

$$f(x,y) \approx \frac{1}{A^2} \sum_{m=-N/2}^{N/2} \sum_{n=-N/2}^{N/2} F\left(\frac{m}{A},\frac{n}{A}\right) e^{j2\pi((m/A)x+(n/A)y)} \qquad (22)$$

for
$$-\frac{A}{2}<x<\frac{A}{2} \text{ and } -\frac{A}{2}<y<\frac{A}{2} \qquad (23)$$

where we arbitrarily assume N to be an even integer. It is clear that the spatial resolution in the reconstructed picture is determined by N. Equation (22) can be rapidly implemented by using the fast Fourier transform (FFT) algorithm provided the N^2 Fourier coefficients $F(m/A, n/A)$ are known.

In practice only a finite number of projections of an object can be taken. In that case it is clear that the function $F(u, v)$ is only known along a finite number of radial lines such as in Fig. 3.7. In order to be able to use (22) one must then interpolate from these radial points to the points on a square grid. Theoretically, one can exactly determine the N^2 coefficients required in (22) provided as many values of the function $F(u, v)$ are known on some radial lines [Cro70]. This calculation involves solving a large set of simultaneous equations often leading to unstable solutions. It is more common to determine the values on the square grid by some kind of nearest neighbor or linear interpolation from the radial points. Since the density of the radial points becomes sparser as one gets farther away from the center, the interpolation error also becomes larger. This implies that there is greater error in the

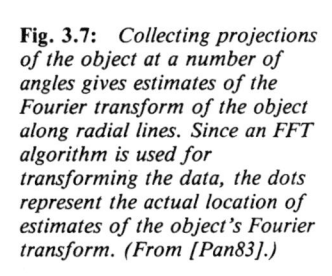

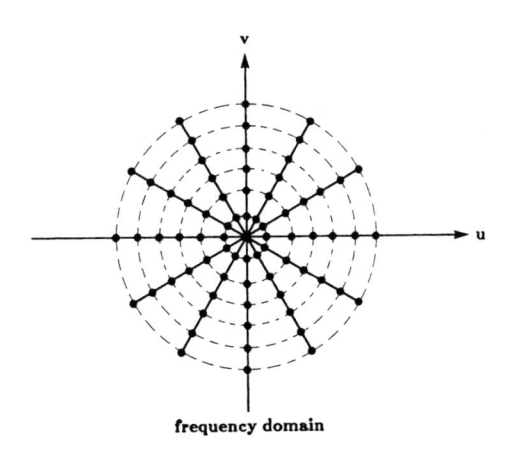

Fig. 3.7: *Collecting projections of the object at a number of angles gives estimates of the Fourier transform of the object along radial lines. Since an FFT algorithm is used for transforming the data, the dots represent the actual location of estimates of the object's Fourier transform. (From [Pan83].)*

calculation of the high frequency components in an image than in the low frequency ones, which results in some image degradation.

3.3 Reconstruction Algorithms for Parallel Projections

The Fourier Slice Theorem relates the Fourier transform of a projection to the Fourier transform of the object along a single radial. Thus given the Fourier transform of a projection at enough angles the projections could be assembled into a complete estimate of the two-dimensional transform and then simply inverted to arrive at an estimate of the object. While this provides a simple conceptual model of tomography, practical implementations require a different approach.

The algorithm that is currently being used in almost all applications of straight ray tomography is the filtered backprojection algorithm. It has been shown to be extremely accurate and amenable to fast implementation and will be derived by using the Fourier Slice Theorem. This theorem is brought into play by rewriting the inverse Fourier transform in polar coordinates and rearranging the limits of the integration therein. *The derivation of this algorithm is perhaps one of the most illustrative examples of how we can obtain a radically different computer implementation by simply rewriting the fundamental expressions for the underlying theory.*

In this chapter, derivations and implementation details will be presented for the backprojection algorithms for three types of scanning geometries, parallel beam, equiangular fan beam, and equispaced fan beam. The computer implementation of these algorithms requires the projection data to be sampled and then filtered. Using FFT algorithms we will show algorithms for fast computer implementation. Before launching into the mathematical derivations of the algorithms, we will first provide a bit of intuitive rationale behind the filtered backprojection type of approach. If the reader finds this presentation excessively wordy, he or she may go directly to Section 3.3.2.

3.3.1 The Idea

The filtered backprojection algorithm can be given a rather straightforward intuitive rationale because each projection represents a nearly independent measurement of the object. This isn't obvious in the space domain but if the Fourier transform is found of the projection at each angle then it follows easily by the Fourier Slice Theorem. We say that the projections are nearly independent (in a loose intuitive sense) because the only common information in the Fourier transforms of the two projections at different angles is the dc term.

To develop the idea behind the filtered backprojection algorithm, we note that because of the Fourier Slice Theorem the act of measuring a projection can be seen as performing a two-dimensional filtering operation. Consider a single projection and its Fourier transform. By the Fourier Slice Theorem, this projection gives the values of the object's two-dimensional Fourier transform along a single line. If the values of the Fourier transform of this projection are inserted into their proper place in the object's two-dimensional Fourier domain then a simple (albeit very distorted) reconstruction can be formed by assuming the other projections to be zero and finding the two-dimensional inverse Fourier transform. The point of this exercise is to show that the reconstruction so formed is equivalent to the original object's Fourier transform multiplied by the simple filter shown in Fig. 3.8(b).

What we really want from a simple reconstruction procedure is the sum of projections of the object filtered by pie-shaped wedges as shown in Fig. 3.8(a). It is important to remember that this summation can be done in either the Fourier domain or in the space domain because of the linearity of the Fourier transform. As will be seen later, when the summation is carried out in the space domain, this constitutes the backprojection process.

As the name implies, there are two steps to the filtered backprojection algorithm: the filtering part, which can be visualized as a simple weighting of each projection in the frequency domain, and the backprojection part, which is equivalent to finding the elemental reconstructions corresponding to each wedge filter mentioned above.

The first step mentioned above accomplishes the following: A simple weighting in the frequency domain is used to take each projection and estimate a pie-shaped wedge of the object's Fourier transform. Perhaps the simplest way to do this is to take the value of the Fourier transform of the projection, $S_\theta(w)$, and multiply it by the width of the wedge at that frequency. Thus if there are K projections over 180° then at a given frequency w, each wedge has a width of $2\pi|w|/K$. Later when we derive the theory more rigorously, we will see that this factor of $|w|$ represents the Jacobian for a change of variable between polar coordinates and the rectangular coordinates needed for the inverse Fourier transform.

The effect of this weighting by $2\pi|w|/K$ is shown in Fig. 3.8(c). Comparing this to that shown in (a) we see that at each spatial frequency, w, the weighted projection, $(2\pi|w|/K)S_\theta(w)$, has the same "mass" as the pie-shaped wedge. Thus the weighted projections represent an approximation to the pie-shaped wedge but the error can be made as small as desired by using enough projections.

The final reconstruction is found by adding together the two-dimensional inverse Fourier transform of each weighted projection. Because each

Fig. 3.8: *This figure shows the frequency domain data available from one projection. (a) is the ideal situation. A reconstruction could be formed by simply summing the reconstruction from each angle until the entire frequency domain is filled. What is actually measured is shown in (b). As predicted by the Fourier Slice Theorem, a projection gives information about the Fourier transform of the object along a single line. The filtered backprojection algorithm takes the data in (b) and applies a weighting in the frequency domain so that the data in (c) are an approximation to those in (a).*

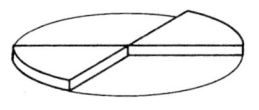

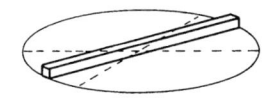

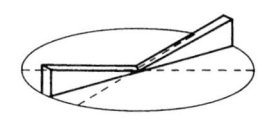

(a)　　　　　　(b)　　　　　　(c)

projection only gives the values of the Fourier transform along a single line, this inversion can be performed very fast. This step is commonly called a backprojection since, as we will show in the next section, it can be perceived as the smearing of each filtered projection over the image plane.

The complete filtered backprojection algorithm can therefore be written as:

> Sum for each of the K angles, θ, between 0 and 180°
> Measure the projection, $P_\theta(t)$
> Fourier transform it to find $S_\theta(w)$
> Multiply it by the weighting function $2\pi|w|/K$
> Sum over the image plane the inverse Fourier transforms of the filtered projections (the backprojection process).

There are two advantages to the filtered backprojection algorithm over a frequency domain interpolation scheme. Most importantly, the reconstruction procedure can be started as soon as the first projection has been measured. This can speed up the reconstruction procedure and reduce the amount of data that must be stored at any one time. To appreciate the second advantage, the reader must note (this will become clearer in the next subsection) that in the filtered backprojection algorithm, when we compute the contribution of each filtered projection to an image point, interpolation is often necessary; it turns out that it is usually more accurate to carry out interpolation in the space domain, as part of the backprojection or smearing process, than in the frequency domain. Simple linear interpolation is often adequate for the backprojection algorithm while more complicated approaches are needed for direct Fourier domain interpolation [Sta81].

In Fig. 3.9(a) we show the projection of an ellipse as calculated by (5). To perform a reconstruction it is necessary to filter the projection and then backproject the result as shown in Fig. 3.9(b). The result due to backproject-

Fig. 3.9: *A projection of an ellipse is shown in (a). (b) shows the projection after it has been filtered in preparation for backprojection.*

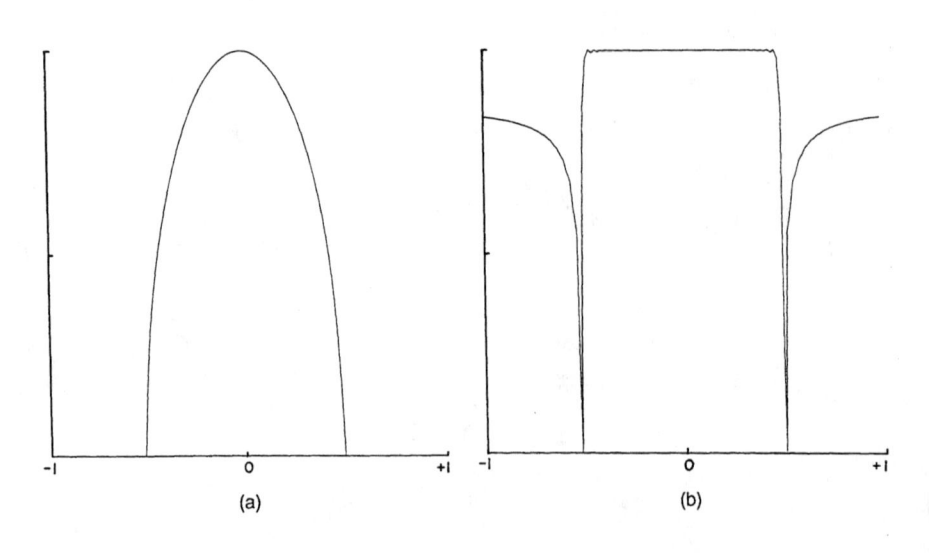

ing one projection is shown in Fig. 3.10. It takes many projections to accurately reconstruct an object; Fig. 3.10 shows the result of reconstructing an object with up to 512 projections.

3.3.2 Theory

We will first present the backprojection algorithm for parallel beam projections. Recalling the formula for the inverse Fourier transform, the object function, $f(x, y)$, can be expressed as

$$f(x, y) = \int_{-\infty}^{\infty} \int_{-\infty}^{\infty} F(u, v) e^{j2\pi(ux+vy)} \, du \, dv. \tag{24}$$

Exchanging the rectangular coordinate system in the frequency domain, (u, v), for a polar coordinate system, (w, θ), by making the substitutions

$$u = w \cos \theta \tag{25}$$

$$v = w \sin \theta \tag{26}$$

and then changing the differentials by using

$$du \, dv = w \, dw \, d\theta \tag{27}$$

Fig. 3.10: *The result of backprojecting the projection in Fig. 3.9 is shown here. (a) shows the result of backprojecting for a single angle, (b) shows the effect of backprojecting over 4 angles, (c) shows 64 angles, and (d) shows 512 angles.*

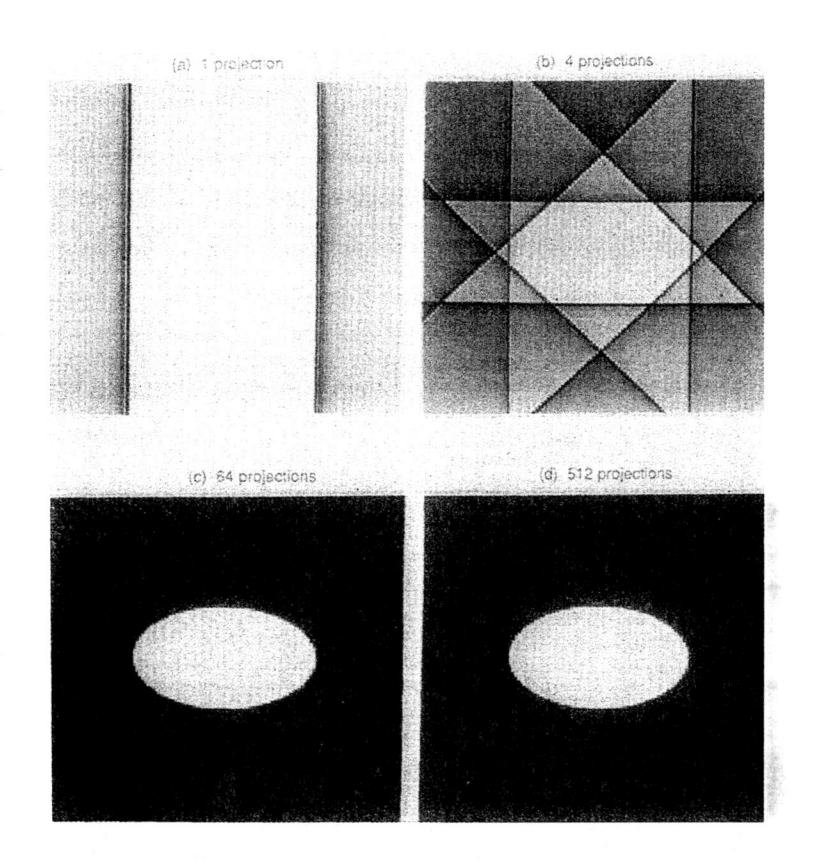

ALGORITHMS FOR RECONSTRUCTION WITH NONDIFFRACTING SOURCES

we can write the inverse Fourier transform of a polar function as

$$f(x, y) = \int_0^{2\pi} \int_0^{\infty} F(w, \theta) e^{j2\pi w(x \cos \theta + y \sin \theta)} w \, dw \, d\theta. \tag{28}$$

This integral can be split into two by considering θ from 0° to 180° and then from 180° to 360°,

$$f(x, y) = \int_0^{\pi} \int_0^{\infty} F(w, \theta) e^{j2\pi w(x \cos \theta + y \sin \theta)} w \, dw \, d\theta$$

$$+ \int_0^{\pi} \int_0^{\infty} F(w, \theta + 180°) e^{j2\pi w[x \cos (\theta + 180°) + y \sin (\theta + 180°)]} w \, dw \, d\theta, \tag{29}$$

and then using the property

$$F(w, \theta + 180°) = F(-w, \theta) \tag{30}$$

the above expression for $f(x, y)$ may be written as

$$f(x, y) = \int_0^{\pi} \left[\int_{-\infty}^{\infty} F(w, \theta) |w| e^{j2\pi wt} \, dw \right] d\theta. \tag{31}$$

Here we have simplified the expression by setting

$$t = x \cos \theta + y \sin \theta. \tag{32}$$

If we substitute the Fourier transform of the projection at angle θ, $S_\theta(w)$, for the two-dimensional Fourier transform $F(w, \theta)$, we get

$$f(x, y) = \int_0^{\pi} \left[\int_{-\infty}^{\infty} S_\theta(w) |w| e^{j2\pi wt} \, dw \right] d\theta. \tag{33}$$

This integral in (33) may be expressed as

$$f(x, y) = \int_0^{\pi} Q_\theta(x \cos \theta + y \sin \theta) \, d\theta \tag{34}$$

where

$$Q_\theta(t) = \int_{-\infty}^{\infty} S_\theta(w) |w| e^{j2\pi wt} \, dw. \tag{35}$$

This estimate of $f(x, y)$, given the projection data transform $S_\theta(w)$, has a simple form. Equation (35) represents a filtering operation, where the frequency response of the filter is given by $|w|$; therefore $Q_\theta(w)$ is called a "filtered projection." The resulting projections for different angles θ are then added to form the estimate of $f(x, y)$.

Equation (34) calls for each filtered projection, Q_θ, to be "backprojected." This can be explained as follows. To every point (x, y) in the image plane there corresponds a value of $t = x \cos \theta + y \sin \theta$ for a given value of θ, and the filtered projection Q_θ contributes to the reconstruction its value at t ($= x \cos \theta + y \sin \theta$). This is further illustrated in Fig. 3.11. It is easily shown that for the indicated angle θ, the value of t is the same for all (x, y) on the line LM. *Therefore, the filtered projection, Q_θ, will make the same contribution to the reconstruction at all of these points.* Therefore, one could say that in the reconstruction process each filtered projection, Q_θ, is smeared back, or backprojected, over the image plane.

The parameter w has the dimension of spatial frequency. The integration in (35) must, in principle, be carried out over all spatial frequencies. In practice the energy contained in the Fourier transform components above a certain frequency is negligible, so for all practical purposes the projections may be considered to be bandlimited. If W is a frequency higher than the highest frequency component in each projection, then by the sampling theorem the projections can be sampled at intervals of

$$T = \frac{1}{2W} \quad (36)$$

without introducing any error. If we also assume that the projection data are equal to zero for large values of $|t|$ then a projection can be represented as

$$P_\theta(mT), \quad m = \frac{-N}{2}, \cdots, 0, \cdots, \frac{N}{2} - 1 \quad (37)$$

for some (large) value of N. An FFT algorithm can then be used to

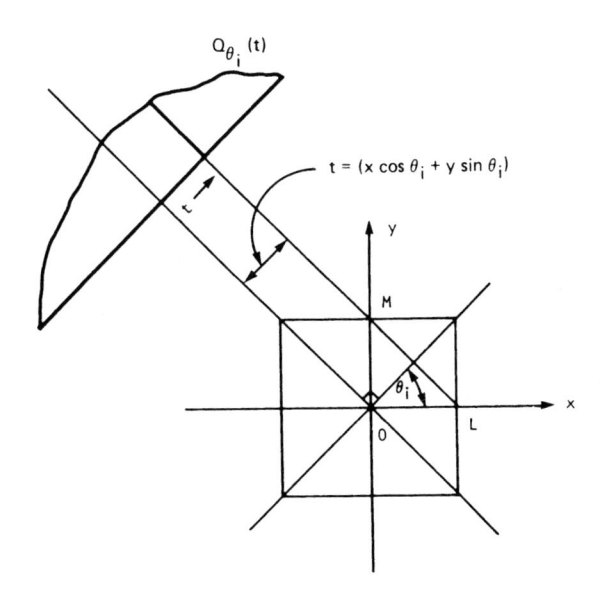

Fig. 3.11: *Reconstructions are often done using a procedure known as backprojection. Here a filtered projection is smeared back over the reconstruction plane along lines of constant t. The filtered projection at a point t makes the same contribution to all pixels along the line LM in the x-y plane. (From [Ros82].)*

approximate the Fourier transform $S_\theta(w)$ of a projection by

$$S_\theta(w) \approx S\left(m\frac{2W}{N}\right) = \frac{1}{2W} \sum_{k=-N/2}^{N/2-1} P_\theta\left(\frac{k}{2W}\right) e^{-j2\pi(mk/N)}. \quad (38)$$

Given the samples of a projection, (38) gives the samples of its Fourier transform. The next step is to evaluate the "modified projection" $Q_\theta(t)$ digitally. Since the Fourier transforms $S_\theta(w)$ have been assumed to be bandlimited, (35) can be approximated by

$$Q_\theta(t) = \int_{-W}^{W} S_\theta(w)|w|e^{j2\pi wt}\,dw \quad (39)$$

$$\approx \frac{2W}{N} \sum_{m=-N/2}^{N/2} S_\theta\left(m\frac{2W}{N}\right)\left|m\frac{2W}{N}\right| e^{j2\pi m(2W/N)t} \quad (40)$$

provided N is large enough. Again, if we want to determine the projections $Q_\theta(t)$ for only those t at which the projections $P_\theta(t)$ are sampled, we get

$$Q_\theta\left(\frac{k}{2W}\right) \approx \left(\frac{2W}{N}\right) \sum_{m=-N/2}^{N/2} S_\theta\left(m\frac{2W}{N}\right)\left|m\frac{2W}{N}\right| e^{j2\pi(mk/N)} \quad (41)$$

$$k = -N/2, \cdots, -1, 0, 1, \cdots, N/2. \quad (42)$$

By the above equation the function $Q_\theta(t)$ at the sampling points of the projection functions is given (approximately) by the inverse DFT of the product of $S_\theta(m(2W/N))$ and $|m(2W/N)|$. From the standpoint of noise in the reconstructed image, superior results are usually obtained if one multiplies the filtered projection, $S_\theta(2W/N)|m(2W/N)|$, by a function such as a Hamming window [Ham77]:

$$Q_\theta\left(\frac{k}{2W}\right) \approx \left(\frac{2W}{N}\right) \sum_{n=-N/2}^{N/2} S_\theta\left(m\frac{2W}{N}\right)$$
$$\cdot \left|m\frac{2W}{N}\right| H\left(m\frac{2W}{N}\right) e^{j2\pi(mk/N)} \quad (43)$$

where $H(m(2W/N))$ represents the window function used. The purpose of the window function is to deemphasize high frequencies which in many cases represent mostly observation noise. By the familiar convolution theorem for the case of discrete transforms, (43) can be written as

$$Q_\theta\left(\frac{k}{2W}\right) \approx \frac{2W}{N} P_\theta\left(\frac{k}{2W}\right) * \phi\left(\frac{k}{2W}\right) \quad (44)$$

where $*$ denotes circular (periodic) convolution and where $\phi(k/2W)$ is the inverse DFT of the discrete function $|m(2W/N)|H(m(2W/N))$, $m = -N/2, \cdots, -1, 0, 1, \cdots, N/2$.

Clearly at the sampling points of a projection, the function $Q_\theta(t)$ may be obtained either in the Fourier domain by using (40), or in the space domain by using (44). The reconstructed picture $f(x, y)$ may then be obtained by the discrete approximation to the integral in (34), i.e.,

$$f(x, y) = \frac{\pi}{K} \sum_{i=1}^{K} Q_{\theta_i}(x \cos \theta_i + y \sin \theta_i) \qquad (45)$$

where the K angles θ_i are those for which the projections $P_\theta(t)$ are known.

Note that the value of $x \cos \theta_i + y \sin \theta_i$ in (45) may not correspond to one of the values of t for which Q_{θ_i} is determined in (43) or in (44). However, Q_{θ_i} for such t may be approximated by suitable interpolation; often linear interpolation is adequate.

Before concluding this subsection we would like to make two comments about the filtering operation in (35). First, note that (35) may be expressed in the t-domain as

$$Q_\theta(t) = \int P_\theta(\alpha) p(t - \alpha) \, d\alpha \qquad (46)$$

where $p(t)$ is nominally the inverse Fourier transform of the $|w|$ function in the frequency domain. Since $|w|$ is not a square integrable function, its inverse transform doesn't exist in an ordinary sense. However, one may examine the inverse Fourier transform of

$$|w| e^{-\epsilon |w|} \qquad (47)$$

as $\epsilon \to 0$. The inverse Fourier transform of this function, denoted by $p_\epsilon(t)$, is given by

$$p_\epsilon(t) = \frac{\epsilon^2 - (2\pi t)^2}{(\epsilon^2 + (2\pi t)^2)^2}. \qquad (48)$$

This function is sketched in Fig. 3.12. Note that for large t we get $p_\epsilon(t) \approx -1/(2\pi t)^2$.

Now our second comment about the filtered projection in (35): This equation may also be written as

$$Q_\theta(t) = \int_{-\infty}^{\infty} j2\pi w S_\theta(w) \left[\frac{-j}{2\pi} \text{sgn}(w) \right] e^{j2\pi wt} \, dw \qquad (49)$$

where

$$\text{sgn}(w) = \begin{cases} 1 & \text{for } w > 0 \\ -1 & \text{for } w < 0. \end{cases} \qquad (50)$$

By the standard convolution theorem, this equation may be expressed as

$$Q_\theta(t) = \{\text{IFT of } j2\pi w S_\theta(w)\} * \left\{\text{IFT of } \frac{-j}{2\pi} \text{sgn}(w)\right\} \qquad (51)$$

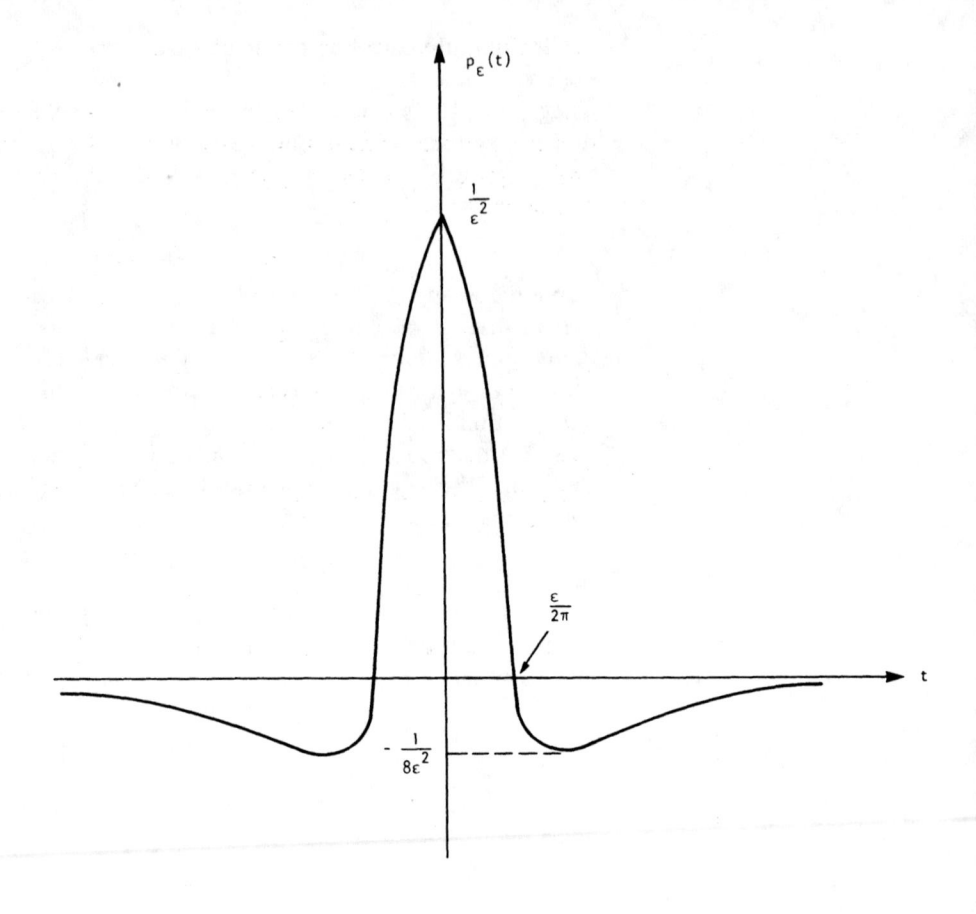

Fig. 3.12: *An approximation to the impulse response of the ideal backprojection filter is shown here. (From [Ros82].)*

where the symbol ∗ denotes convolution and the abbreviation IFT stands for inverse fast Fourier transform. The IFT of $j2\pi w S_\theta(w)$ is $(\partial/\partial t)P_\theta(t)$ while the IFT of $(-j/2\pi)$ sgn (w) is $1/t$. Therefore, the above result may be written as

$$Q_\theta(t) = \frac{1}{2\pi^2 t} * \frac{\partial P_\theta(t)}{\partial t} \tag{52}$$

$$= \text{Hilbert Transform of } \frac{\partial P_\theta(t)}{\partial t} \tag{53}$$

where, expressed as a filtering operation, the Hilbert Transform is usually defined as the following frequency response:

$$H(w) = \begin{cases} -j, & w > 0 \\ j, & w < 0. \end{cases} \tag{54}$$

3.3.3 Computer Implementation of the Algorithm

Let's assume that the projection data are sampled with a sampling interval of τ cm. If there is no aliasing, this implies that in the transform domain the projections don't contain any energy outside the frequency interval $(-W, W)$ where

$$W = \frac{1}{2\tau} \text{ cycles/cm.} \tag{55}$$

Let the sampled projections be represented by $P_\theta(k\tau)$ where k takes integer values. The theory presented in the preceding subsection says that for each sampled projection $P_\theta(k\tau)$ we must generate a filtered $Q_\theta(k\tau)$ by using the periodic (circular) convolution given by (40). Equation (40) is very attractive since it directly conforms to the definition of the DFT and, if N is decomposable, possesses a fast FFT implementation. However, note that (40) is only valid when the projections are of finite bandwidth and finite order. Since these two assumptions (taken together) are never strictly satisfied, computer processing based on (40) usually leads to interperiod interference artifacts created when an aperiodic convolution (required by (35)) is implemented as a periodic convolution. This is illustrated in Fig. 3.13. Fig. 3.13(a) shows a reconstruction of the Shepp and Logan head phantom from 110 projections and 127 rays in each projection using (40) and (45). Equation (40) was implemented with a base 2 FFT algorithm using 128 points. Fig. 3.13(b) shows the reconstructed values on the horizontal line for $y = -0.605$. For comparison we have also shown the values on this line in the original object function.

The comparison illustrated in Fig. 3.13(b) shows that reconstruction based on (42) and (45) introduces a slight "dishing" and a dc shift in the image. These artifacts are partly caused by the periodic convolution implied by (40) and partly by the fact that the implementations in (40) "zero out" all the information in the continuous frequency domain in the cell represented by $m = 0$, whereas the theory (eq. (35)) calls for such "zeroing out" to occur at only *one* frequency, viz. $w = 0$. The contribution to these artifacts by the interperiod interference can be *eliminated* by adequately zero-padding the projection data before using the implementations in (42) or (43).

Zero-padding of the projections also reduces, *but never completely eliminates*, the contribution to the artifacts by the zeroing out of the information in the $m = 0$ cell in (40). This is because zero-padding in the space domain causes the cell size to get smaller in the frequency domain. (If N_{FFT} points are used for performing the discrete Fourier transform, the size of each sampling cell in the frequency domain is equal to $1/N_{FFT}\tau$.) To illustrate the effect of zero-padding, the 127 rays in each projection in the preceding example were padded with 129 zeros to make the data string 256 elements long. These data were transformed by an FFT algorithm and filtered with a $|w|$ function as before. The $y = -0.605$ line through the

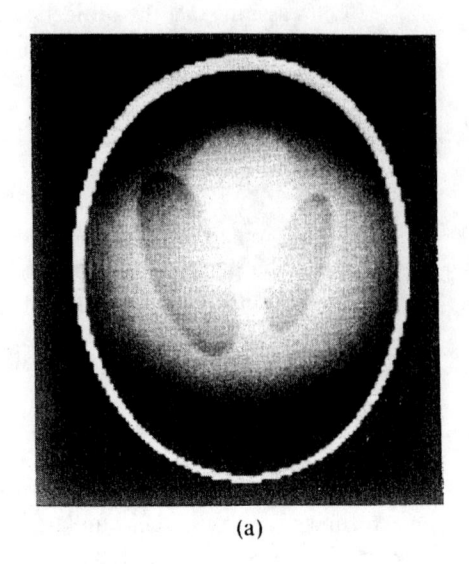

Fig. 3.13: *(a) This reconstruction of the Shepp and Logan phantom shows the artifacts caused when the projection data are not adequately zero-padded and FFTs are used to perform the filtering operation in the filtered backprojection algorithm. The dark regions at the top and the bottom of the reconstruction are the most visible artifacts here. This 128 × 128 reconstruction was made from 110 projections with 127 rays in each projection. (b) A numerical comparison of the true and the reconstructed values on the y = −0.605 line. (For the location of this line see Fig. 3.4.) The "dishing" and the dc shift artifacts are quite evident in this comparison. (c) Shown here are the reconstructed values obtained on the y = −0.605 line if the 127 rays in each projection are zero-padded to 256 points before using the FFTs. The dishing caused by interperiod interference has disappeared; however, the dc shift still remains. (From [Ros82].)*

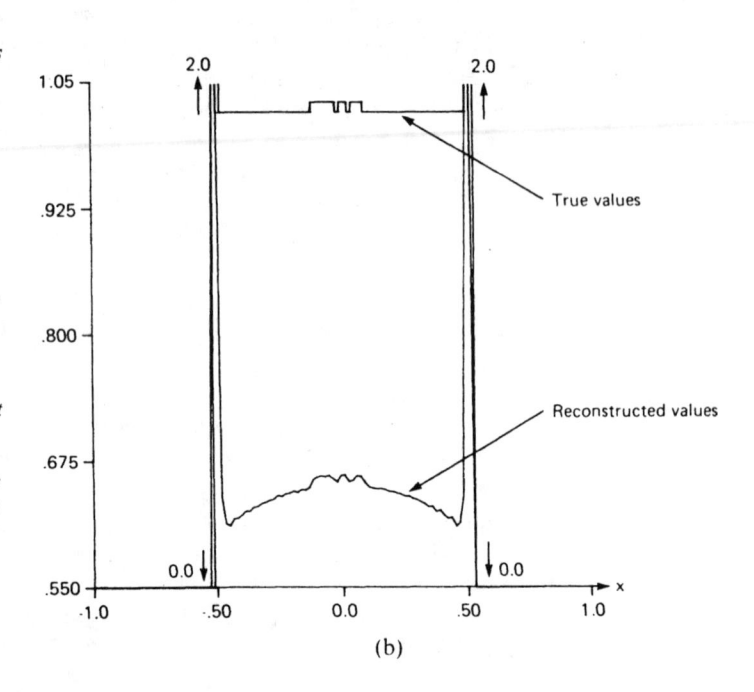

70 COMPUTERIZED TOMOGRAPHIC IMAGING

(c)

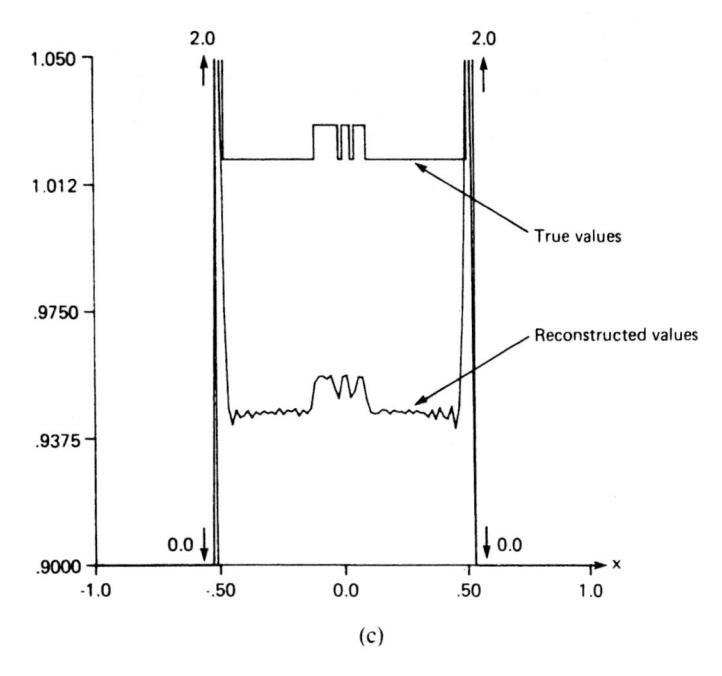

Fig. 3.13: *Continued.*

reconstruction is shown in Fig. 3.13(c), demonstrating that the dishing distortion is now less severe.

We will now show that the artifacts mentioned above can be eliminated by the following alternative implementation of (35) which doesn't require the approximation used in the discrete representation of (40). When the highest frequency in the projections is finite (as given by (55)), (35) may be expressed as

$$Q_\theta(t) = \int_{-\infty}^{\infty} S_\theta(w) H(w) e^{j2\pi wt} \, dw \qquad (56)$$

where

$$H(w) = |w| b_w(w) \qquad (57)$$

where, again,

$$b_W(w) = \begin{cases} 1 & |w| < W \\ 0 & \text{otherwise.} \end{cases} \qquad (58)$$

$H(w)$, shown in Fig. 3.14, represents the transfer function of a filter with which the projections must be processed. The impulse response, $h(t)$, of this filter is given by the inverse Fourier transform of $H(w)$ and is

$$h(t) = \int_{-\infty}^{\infty} H(w) e^{+j2\pi wt} \, dw \qquad (59)$$

$$= \frac{1}{2\tau^2} \frac{\sin 2\pi t/2\tau}{2\pi t/2\tau} - \frac{1}{4\tau^2} \left(\frac{\sin \pi t/2\tau}{\pi t/2\tau} \right)^2 \qquad (60)$$

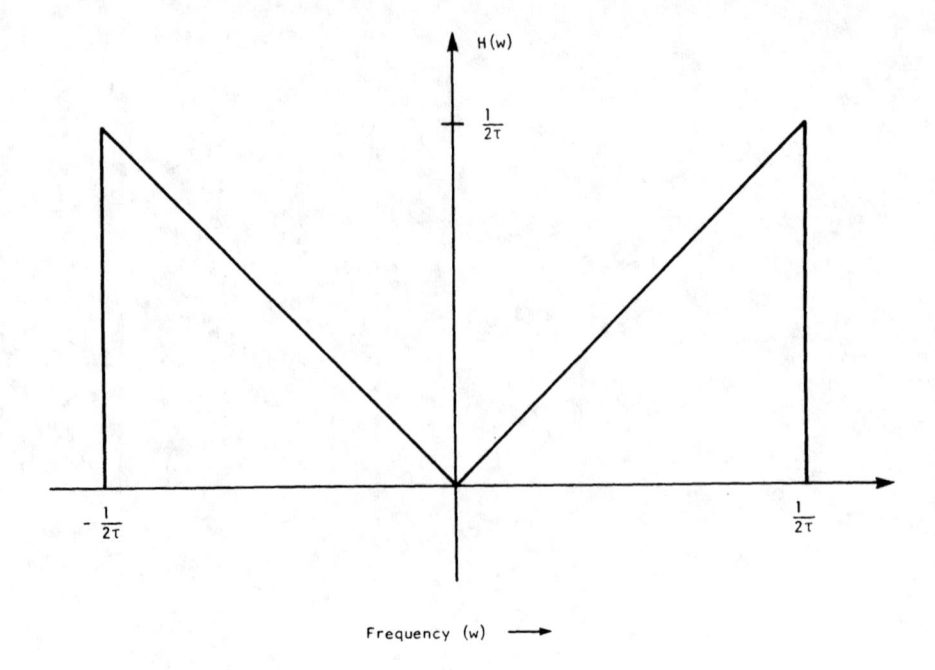

[Graph of H(w) showing triangular filter bandlimited to ±1/2τ with peak 1/2τ]

Fig. 3.14: *The ideal filter response for the filtered backprojection algorithm is shown here. It has been bandlimited to 1/2τ. (From [Ros82].)*

where we have used (55). Since the projection data are measured with a sampling interval of τ, for digital processing the impulse response need only be known with the same sampling interval. The samples, $h(n\tau)$, of $h(t)$ are given by

$$h(n\tau) = \begin{cases} 1/4\tau^2, & n=0 \\ 0, & n \text{ even} \\ -\dfrac{1}{n^2\pi^2\tau^2}, & n \text{ odd.} \end{cases} \quad (61)$$

This function is shown in Fig. 3.15.

Since both $P_\theta(t)$ and $h(t)$ are now bandlimited functions, they may be expressed as

$$P_\theta(t) = \sum_{k=-\infty}^{\infty} P_\theta(k\tau) \frac{\sin 2\pi W(t-k\tau)}{2\pi W(t-k\tau)} \quad (62)$$

$$h(t) = \sum_{k=-\infty}^{\infty} h(k\tau) \frac{\sin 2\pi W(t-k\tau)}{2\pi W(t-k\tau)}. \quad (63)$$

By the convolution theorem the filtered projection (56) can be written as

$$Q_\theta(t) = \int_{-\infty}^{\infty} P_\theta(t')h(t-t')\,dt'. \quad (64)$$

72 COMPUTERIZED TOMOGRAPHIC IMAGING

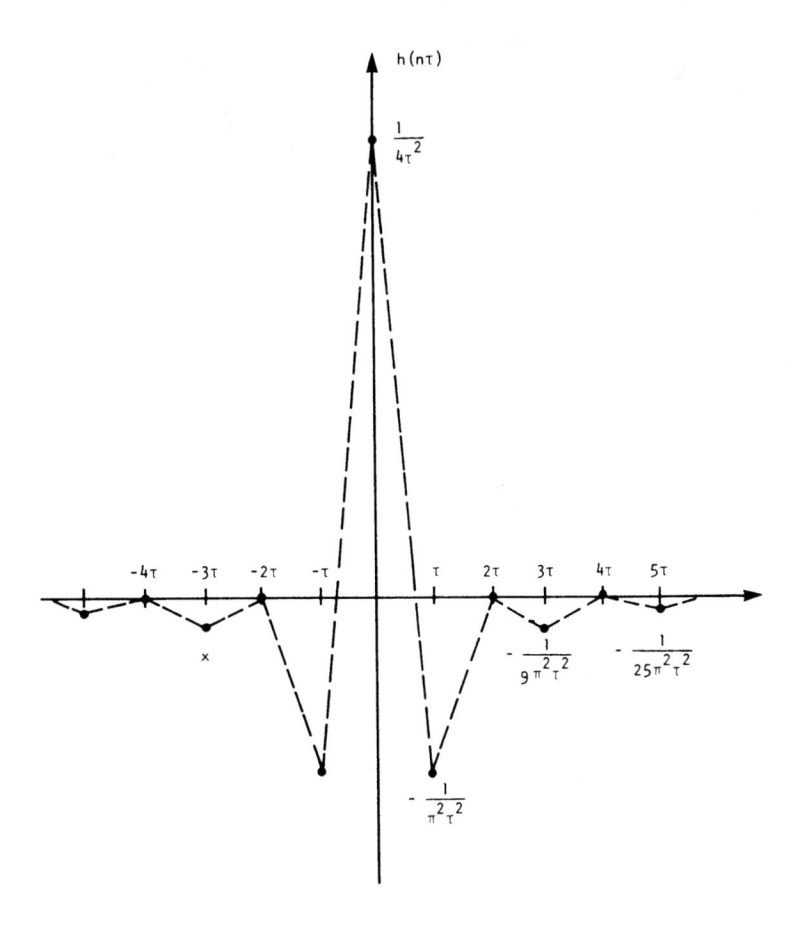

Fig. 3.15: *The impulse response of the filter shown in Fig. 3.14 is shown here. (From [Ros82].)*

Substituting (62) and (63) in (64) we get the following result for the values of the filtered projection at the sampling points:

$$Q_\theta(n\tau) = \tau \sum_{k=-\infty}^{\infty} h(n\tau - k\tau)P_\theta(k\tau). \tag{65}$$

In practice each projection is of only finite extent. Suppose that each $P_\theta(k\tau)$ is zero outside the index range $k = 0, \cdots, N - 1$. We may now write the following two equivalent forms of (65):

$$Q_\theta(n\tau) = \tau \sum_{k=0}^{N-1} h(n\tau - k\tau)P_\theta(k\tau), \qquad n = 0, 1, 2, \cdots, N-1 \tag{66}$$

or

$$Q_\theta(n\tau) = \tau \sum_{k=-(N-1)}^{N-1} h(k\tau)P_\theta(n\tau - k\tau), \qquad n = 0, 1, 2, \cdots, N-1. \tag{67}$$

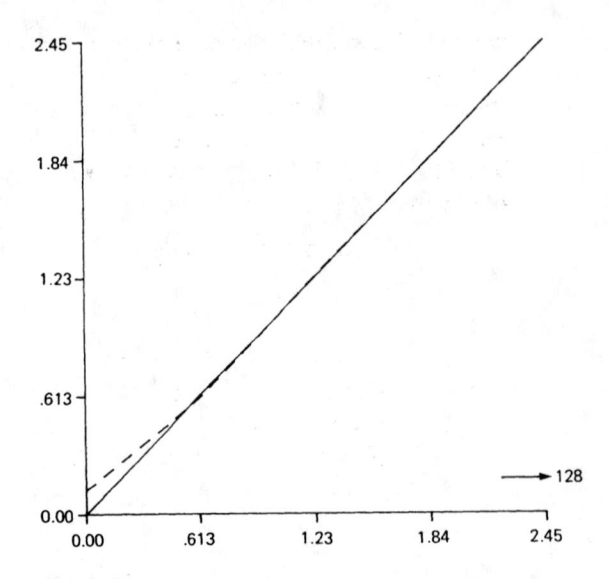

Fig. 3.16: *The DFT of the bandlimited filter (broken line) and that of the ideal filter (solid line) are shown here. Notice the primary difference is in the dc component. (From [Ros82].)*

These equations imply that in order to determine $Q_\theta(n\tau)$ the length of the sequence $h(n\tau)$ used should be from $l = -(N - 1)$ to $l = (N - 1)$. It is important to realize that the results obtained by using (66) or (67) aren't identical to those obtained by using (42). This is because the discrete Fourier transform of the sequence $h(n\tau)$ with n taking values in a finite range [such as when n ranges from $-(N - 1)$ to $(N - 1)$] is not the sequence $|k[(2W)/N]|$. While the latter sequence is zero at $k = 0$, the DFT of $h(n\tau)$ with n ranging from $-(N - 1)$ to $(N - 1)$ is nonzero at this point. This is illustrated in Fig. 3.16.

The discrete convolution in (66) or (67) may be implemented directly on a general purpose computer. However, it is much faster to implement it in the frequency domain using FFT algorithms. [By using specially designed hardware, direct implementation of (66) can be made as fast or faster than the frequency domain implementation.] For the frequency domain implementation one has to keep in mind the fact that one can now only perform periodic (or circular) convolutions, while the convolution required in (66) is aperiodic. To eliminate the interperiod interference artifacts inherent to periodic convolution, we pad the projection data with a sufficient number of zeros. It can easily be shown [Jak76] that if we pad $P_\theta(k\tau)$ with zeros so that it is $(2N - 1)$ elements long, we avoid interperiod interference over the N samples of $Q_\theta(k\tau)$. Of course, if one wants to use the base 2 FFT algorithm, which is most often the case, the sequences $P_\theta(k\tau)$ and $h(k\tau)$ have to be zero-padded so that each is $(2N - 1)_2$ elements long, where $(2N - 1)_2$ is the smallest integer that is a power of 2 and that is greater than $2N - 1$. Therefore, the frequency domain implementation may be expressed as

$$Q_\theta(n\tau) = \tau \times \text{IFFT} \{[\text{FFT } P_\theta(n\tau) \text{ with ZP}] \times [\text{FFT } h(n\tau) \text{ with ZP}]\}, \quad (68)$$

where FFT and IFFT denote, respectively, fast Fourier transform and inverse fast Fourier transform; ZP stands for zero-padding. One usually obtains superior reconstructions when some smoothing is also incorporated in (68). Smoothing may be implemented by multiplying the product of the two FFTs by a Hamming window. When such a window is incorporated, (68) may be rewritten as

$$Q_\theta(n\tau) = \tau \times \text{IFFT} \{[\text{FFT } P_\theta(n\tau) \text{ with ZP}]$$
$$\times [\text{FFT } h(n\tau) \text{ with ZP}] \times \text{smoothing} - \text{window}\}. \quad (69)$$

After the filtered projections $Q_\theta(n\tau)$ are calculated with the alternative method presented here, the rest of the implementation for reconstructing the image is the same as in the preceding subsection. That is, we use (45) for backprojections and their summation. Again for a given (x, y) and θ_i the argument $x \cos \theta_i + y \sin \theta_i$ may not correspond to one of the $k\tau$ at which Q_{θ_i} is known. This will call for interpolation and often linear interpolation is adequate. Sometimes, in order to eliminate the computations required for interpolation, preinterpolation of the functions $Q_\theta(t)$ is also used. In this technique, which can be combined with the computation in (69), prior to backprojection, the function $Q_\theta(t)$ is preinterpolated onto 10 to 1000 times the number of points in the projection data. From this dense set of points one simply retains the nearest neighbor to obtain the value of Q_{θ_i} at $x \cos \theta_i + y \sin \theta_i$. A variety of techniques are available for preinterpolation [Sch73].

One method of preinterpolation, which combines it with the operations in (69), consists of the following: In (69), prior to performing the IFFT, the *frequency domain function* is padded with a large number of zeros. The inverse transform of this sequency yields the preinterpolated Q_θ. It was recently shown [Kea78] that if the data sequence contains "fractional" frequencies this approach may lead to large errors especially near the beginning and the end of the data sequence. Note that with preinterpolation and with appropriate programming, the backprojection for parallel projection data can be accomplished with virtually no multiplications.

Using the implementation in (68), Fig. 3.17(b) shows the reconstructed values on the line $y = -0.605$ for the Shepp and Logan head phantom. Comparing with Fig. 3.13(b), we see that the dc shift and the dishing have been eliminated. Fig. 3.17(a) shows the complete reconstruction. The number of rays used in each projection was 127 and the number of projections 100. To make convolutions aperiodic, the projection data were padded with zeros to make each projection 256 elements long.

3.4 Reconstruction from Fan Projections

The theory in the preceding subsections dealt with reconstructing images from their parallel projections such as those shown in Fig. 3.1. In generating these parallel data a source–detector combination has to linearly scan over the

Fig. 3.17: *(a) Reconstruction obtained by using the filter shown in Fig. 3.16. The 127 rays in the projection were zero-padded so that each projection was 256 elements long. The unit sample response h(nτ) was used with n ranging from −128 to 127, yielding 256 points for this function. The number of projections was 100 and the display matrix size is 128 × 128. (b) A numerical comparison of the y = −0.605 line of the reconstruction in (a) with the true values. Note that the dishing and dc shift artifacts visible in Fig. 3.13 have disappeared. (From [Ros82].)*

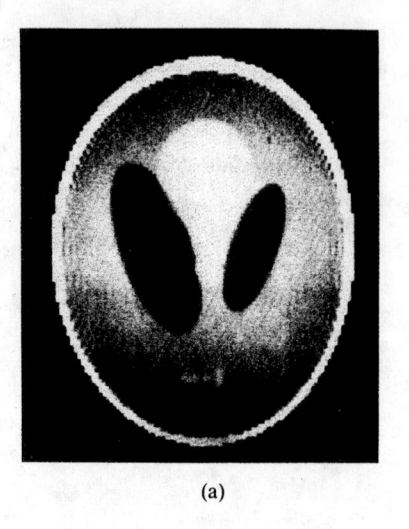

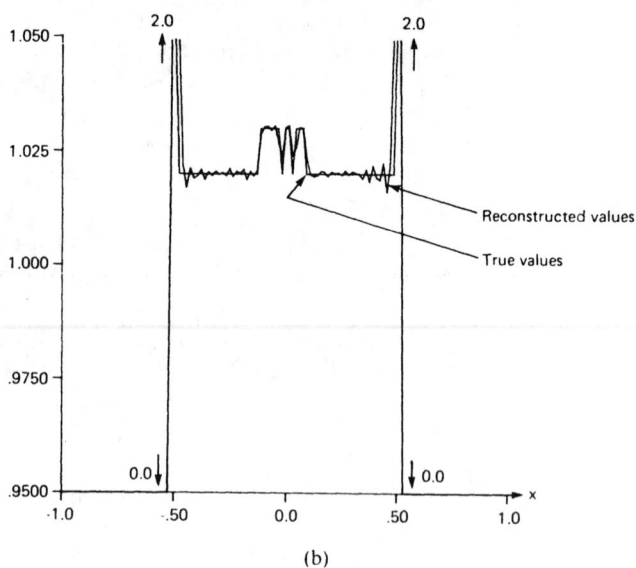

length of a projection, then rotate through a certain angular interval, then scan linearly over the length of the next projection, and so on. This usually results in times that are as long as a few minutes for collecting all the data. A much faster way to generate the line integrals is by using fan beams such as those shown in Fig. 3.3. One now uses a point source of radiation that emanates a fan-shaped beam. On the other side of the object a bank of detectors is used to make all the measurements in one fan simultaneously. The source and the entire bank of detectors are rotated to generate the desired number of fan projections. As might be expected, one has to pay a price for this simpler and faster method of data collection; as we will see later the simple backprojection of parallel beam tomography now becomes a weighted backprojection.

There are two types of fan projections depending upon whether a projection is sampled at equiangular or equispaced intervals. This difference is illustrated in Fig. 3.18. In (a) we have shown an equiangular set of rays. If the detectors for the measurement of line integrals are arranged on the straight line $D_1 D_2$, this implies unequal spacing between them. If, however, the detectors are arranged on the arc of a circle whose center is at S, they may now be positioned with equal spacing along this arc (Fig. 3.18(b)). The second type of fan projection is generated when the rays are arranged such that the detector spacing on a straight line is now equal (Fig. 3.18(c)). The algorithms that reconstruct images from these two different types of fan projections are different and will be separately derived in the following subsection.

3.4.1 Equiangular Rays

Let $R_\beta(\gamma)$ denote a fan projection as shown in Fig. 3.19. Here β is the angle that the source S makes with a reference axis, and the angle γ gives the location of a ray within a fan. Consider the ray SA. If the projection data were generated along a set of parallel rays, then the ray SA would belong to a parallel projection $P_\theta(t)$ for θ and t given by

$$\theta = \beta + \gamma \quad \text{and} \quad t = D \sin \gamma \tag{70}$$

where D is the distance of the source S from the origin O. The relationships in (70) are derived by noting that all the rays in the parallel projection at angle θ are perpendicular to the line PQ and that along such a line the distance OB is equal to the value of t. Now we know that from parallel projections $P_\theta(t)$ we may reconstruct $f(x, y)$ by

$$f(x, y) = \int_0^\pi \int_{-t_m}^{t_m} P_\theta(t) h(x \cos \theta + y \sin \theta - t) \, dt \, d\theta \tag{71}$$

where t_m is the value of t for which $P_\theta(t) = 0$ with $|t| > t_m$ in all projections. This equation only requires the parallel projections to be collected over 180°. However, if one would like to use the projections generated over 360°, this equation may be rewritten as

$$f(x, y) = \frac{1}{2} \int_0^{2\pi} \int_{-t_m}^{t_m} P_\theta(t) h(x \cos \theta + y \sin \theta - t) \, dt \, d\theta. \tag{72}$$

Derivation of the algorithm becomes easier when the point (x, y) (marked C in Fig. 3.20) is expressed in polar coordinates (r, ϕ), that is,

$$x = r \cos \phi \quad y = r \sin \phi. \tag{73}$$

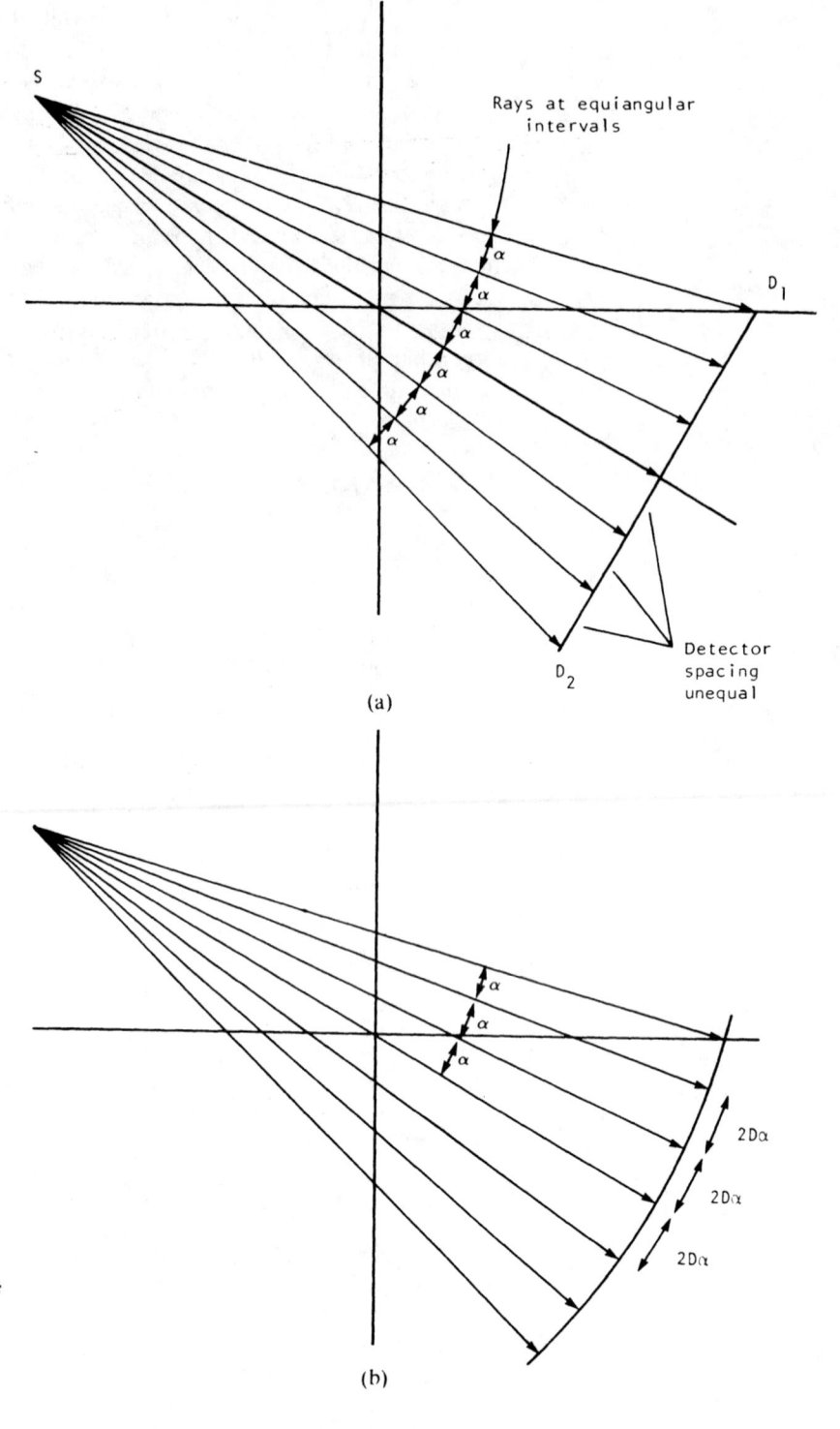

Fig. 3.18: *Two different types of fan beams are shown here. In (a) the angle between rays is constant but the detector spacing is uneven. If the detectors are placed along a circle the spacing will then be equal as shown in (b). As shown in (c) the detectors can be arranged with constant spacing along a line but then the angle between rays is not constant. (From [Ros82].)*

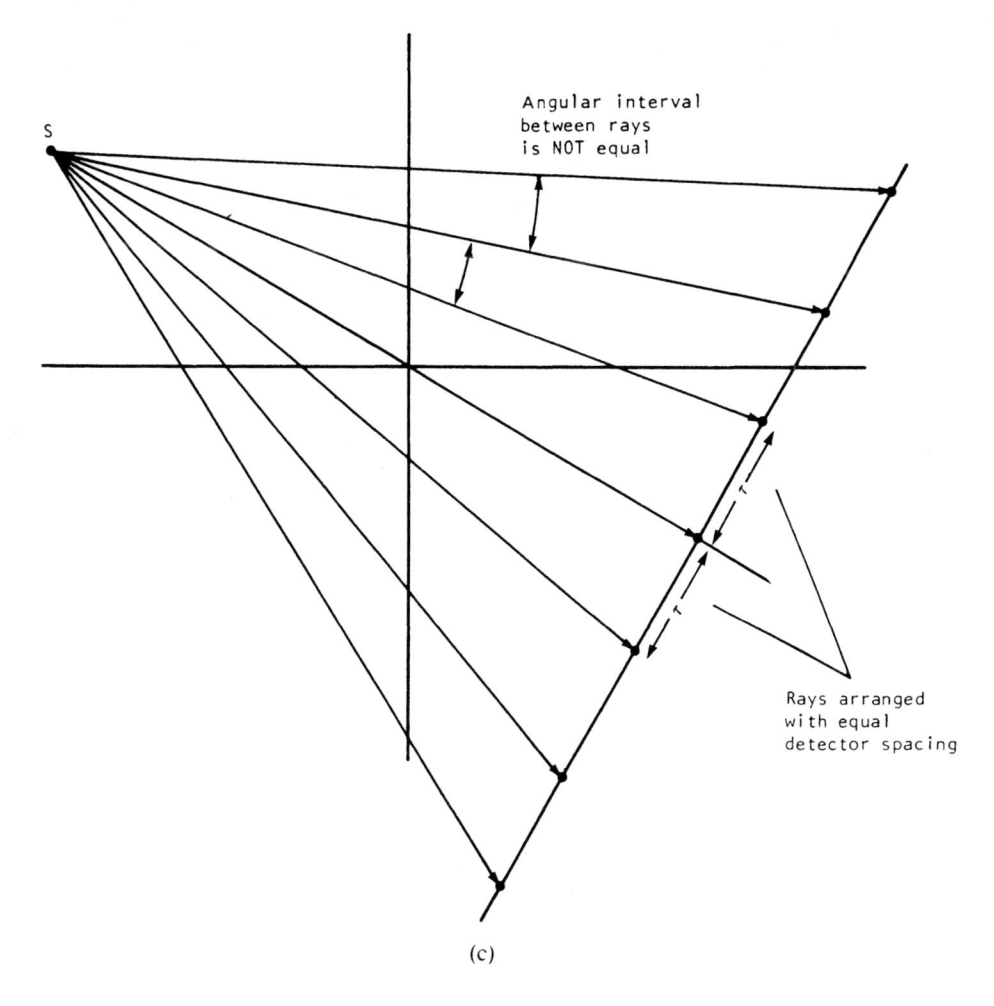

Fig. 3.18: *Continued.*

The expression in (72) can now be written as

$$f(r, \phi) = \frac{1}{2} \int_0^{2\pi} \int_{-t_m}^{t_m} P_\theta(t) h(r \cos(\theta - \phi) - t) \, dt \, d\theta. \quad (74)$$

Using the relationships in (70), the double integration may be expressed in terms of γ and β,

$$f(r, \phi) = \frac{1}{2} \int_{-\gamma}^{2\pi - \gamma} \int_{-\sin^{-1}(t_m/D)}^{\sin^{-1}(t_m/D)} P_{\beta + \gamma}(D \sin \gamma) h(\tau \cos(\beta + \gamma - \phi)$$

$$- d \sin \gamma) D \cos \gamma \, d\gamma \, d\beta \quad (75)$$

where we have used $dt \, d\theta = D \cos \gamma \, d\gamma \, d\beta$. A few observations about this expression are in order. The limits $-\gamma$ to $2\pi - \gamma$ for β cover the entire range of 360°. Since all the functions of β are periodic (with period 2π) these limits

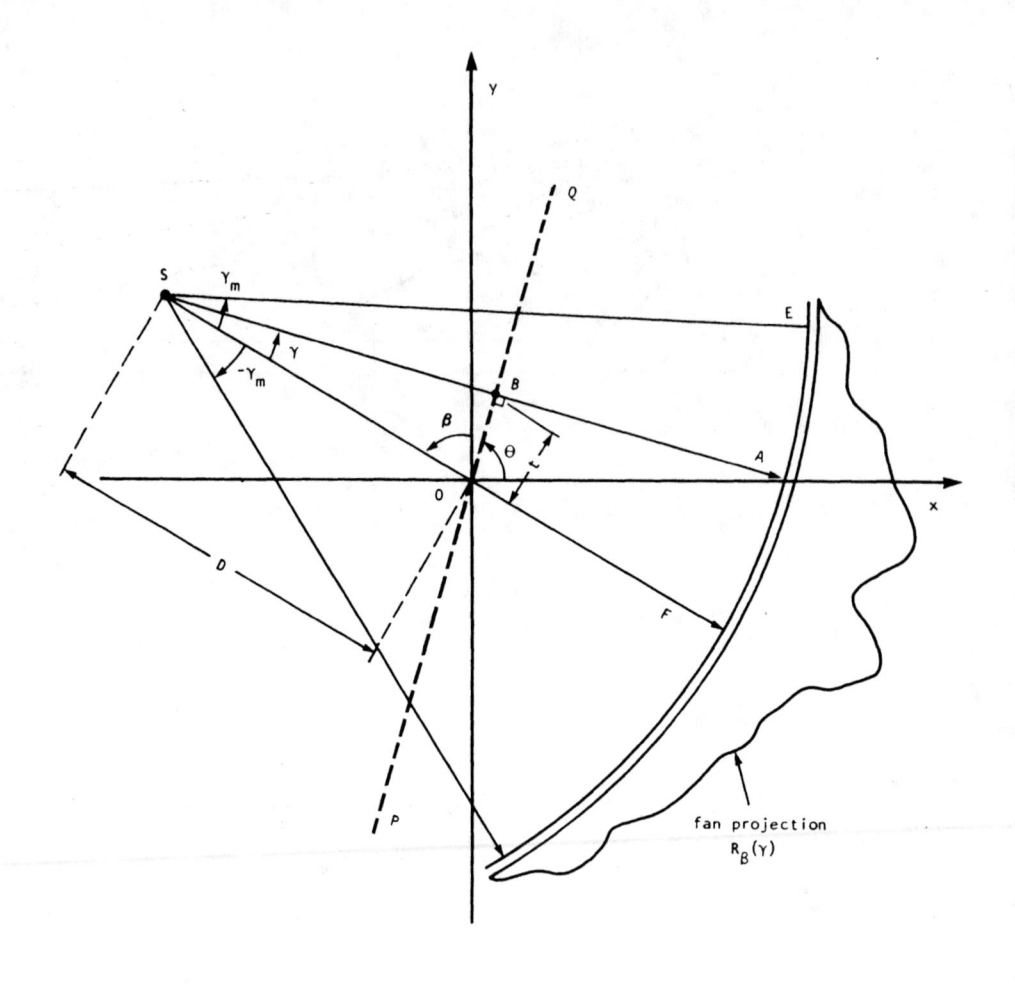

Fig. 3.19: *An equiangular fan is shown here. Each ray is identified by its angle γ from the central ray. (From [Ros82].)*

may be replaced by 0 and 2π, respectively. $\sin^{-1}(t_m/D)$ is equal to the value of γ for the extreme ray SE in Fig. 3.19. Therefore, the upper and lower limits for γ may be written as γ_m and $-\gamma_m$, respectively. The expression $P_{\beta+\gamma}(D \sin \gamma)$ corresponds to the ray integral along SA in the parallel projection data $P_\theta(t)$. The identity of this ray integral in the fan projection data is simply $R_\beta(\gamma)$. Introducing these changes in (75) we get

$$f(r, \phi) = \frac{1}{2} \int_0^{2\pi} \int_{-\gamma_m}^{\gamma_m} R_\beta(\gamma) h(r \cos(\beta + \gamma - \phi) - D \sin \gamma) D \cos \gamma \, d\gamma \, d\beta.$$

(76)

In order to express the reconstruction formula given by (76) in a form that can be easily implemented on a computer we will first examine the argument

80 COMPUTERIZED TOMOGRAPHIC IMAGING

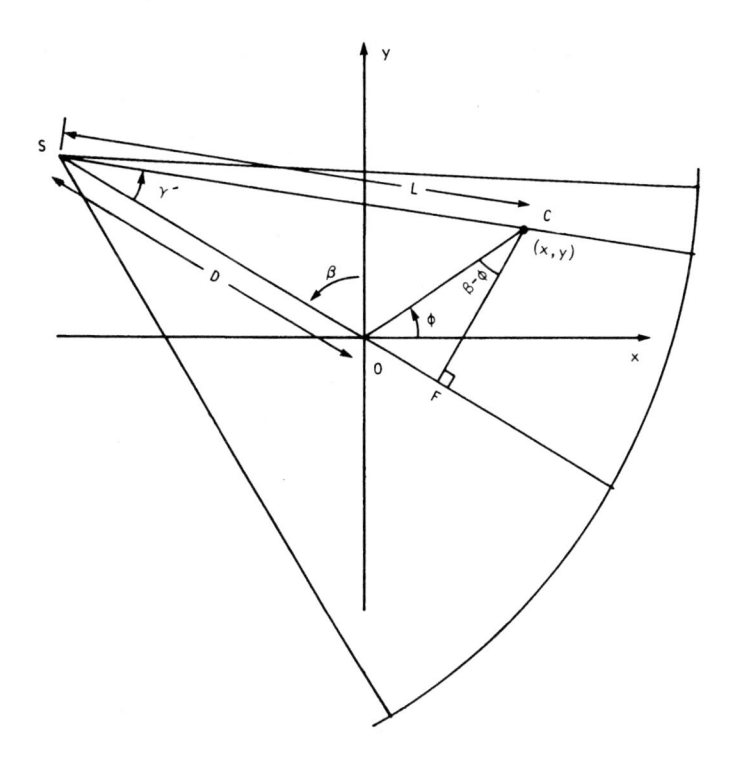

Fig. 3.20: *This figure illustrates that L is the distance of the pixel at location (x, y) from the source S; and γ is the angle that the source-to-pixel line subtends with the central ray. (From [Ros82].)*

of the function h. The argument may be rewritten as

$$r \cos(\beta + \gamma - \phi) - D \sin \gamma$$
$$= r \cos(\beta - \phi) \cos \gamma - [r \sin(\beta - \phi) + D] \sin \gamma. \quad (77)$$

Let L be the distance from the source S to a point (x, y) [or (r, ϕ) in polar coordinates] such as C in Fig. 3.20. Clearly, L is a function of three variables, r, ϕ, and β. Also, let γ' be the angle of the ray that passes through this point (r, ϕ). One can now easily show that

$$L \cos \gamma' = D + r \sin(\beta - \phi)$$
$$L \sin \gamma' = r \cos(\beta - \phi). \quad (78)$$

Note that the pixel location (r, ϕ) and the projection angle β completely determine both L and γ':

$$L(r, \phi, \beta) = \sqrt{[D + r \sin(\beta - \phi)]^2 + [r \cos(\beta - \phi)]^2} \quad (79)$$

and

$$\gamma' = \tan^{-1} \frac{r \cos(\beta - \phi)}{D + r \sin(\beta - \phi)}. \quad (80)$$

ALGORITHMS FOR RECONSTRUCTION WITH NONDIFFRACTING SOURCES

Using (78) in (77) we get for the argument of h

$$r \cos(\beta + \gamma - \phi) - D \sin \gamma = L \sin(\gamma' - \gamma) \qquad (81)$$

and substituting this in (76) we get

$$f(r, \phi) = \frac{1}{2} \int_0^{2\pi} \int_{-\gamma_m}^{\gamma_m} R_\beta(\gamma) h(L \sin(\gamma' - \gamma)) D \cos \gamma \, d\gamma \, d\beta. \qquad (82)$$

We will now express the function $h(L \sin(\gamma' - \gamma))$ in terms of $h(t)$. Note that $h(t)$ is the inverse Fourier transform of $|w|$ in the frequency domain:

$$h(t) = \int_{-\infty}^{\infty} |w| e^{j2\pi wt} \, dw. \qquad (83)$$

Therefore,

$$h(L \sin \gamma) = \int_{-\infty}^{\infty} |w| e^{j2\pi wL \sin \gamma} \, dw. \qquad (84)$$

Using the transformation

$$w' = \frac{wL \sin \gamma}{\gamma} \qquad (85)$$

we can write

$$h(L \sin \gamma) = \left(\frac{\gamma}{L \sin \gamma}\right)^2 \int_{-\infty}^{\infty} |w'| e^{j2\pi w' \gamma} \, dw' \qquad (86)$$

$$= \left(\frac{\gamma}{L \sin \gamma}\right)^2 h(\gamma). \qquad (87)$$

Therefore, (82) may be written as

$$f(r, \phi) = \int_0^{2\pi} \frac{1}{L^2} \int_{-\gamma_m}^{\gamma_m} R_\beta(\gamma) g(\gamma' - \gamma) D \cos \gamma \, d\gamma \, d\beta \qquad (88)$$

where

$$g(\gamma) = \frac{1}{2} \left(\frac{\gamma}{\sin \gamma}\right)^2 h(\gamma). \qquad (89)$$

For the purpose of computer implementation, (88) may be interpreted as a weighted filtered backprojection algorithm. To show this we rewrite (88) as follows:

$$f(r, \phi) = \int_0^{2\pi} \frac{1}{L^2} Q_\beta(\gamma') \, d\beta \qquad (90)$$

where
$$Q_\beta(\gamma) = R'_\beta(\gamma) * g(\gamma) \tag{91}$$
and where
$$R'_\beta(\gamma) = R_\beta(\gamma) \cdot D \cdot \cos \gamma. \tag{92}$$
This calls for reconstructing an image using the following three steps:

Step 1:

Assume that each projection $R_\beta(\gamma)$ is sampled with sampling interval α. The known data then are $R_{\beta_i}(n\alpha)$ where n takes integer values. β_i are the angles at which projections are taken. The first step is to generate for each fan projection $R_{\beta_i}(n\alpha)$ the corresponding $R'_{\beta_i}(n\alpha)$ by
$$R'_{\beta_i}(n\alpha) = R_{\beta_i}(n\alpha) \cdot D \cdot \cos n\alpha. \tag{93}$$
Note that $n = 0$ corresponds to the ray passing through the center of the projection.

Step 2:

Convolve each modified projection $R'_{\beta_i}(n\alpha)$ with $g(n\alpha)$ to generate the corresponding filtered projection:
$$Q_{\beta_i}(n\alpha) = R'_{\beta i}(n\alpha) * g(n\alpha). \tag{94}$$
To perform this discrete convolution using an FFT program the function $R'_{\beta_i}(n\alpha)$ must be padded with a sufficient number of zeros to avoid interperiod interference artifacts. The sequence $g(n\alpha)$ is given by the samples of (89):
$$g(n\alpha) = \frac{1}{2}\left(\frac{n\alpha}{\sin n\alpha}\right)^2 h(n\alpha). \tag{95}$$
If we substitute in this the values of $h(n\alpha)$ from (61), we get for the discrete impulse response

$$g(n\alpha) = \begin{cases} \dfrac{1}{8\alpha^2}, & n = 0 \\ 0, & n \text{ is even} \\ \left(\dfrac{\alpha}{\pi\alpha \sin n\alpha}\right)^2, & n \text{ is odd.} \end{cases} \tag{96}$$

Although, theoretically, no further filtering of the projection data than that called for by (94) is required, in practice superior reconstructions are obtained if a certain amount of smoothing is combined with the required filtering:
$$Q_{\beta_i}(n\alpha) = R'_{\beta i}(n\alpha) * g(n\alpha) * k(n\alpha) \tag{97}$$

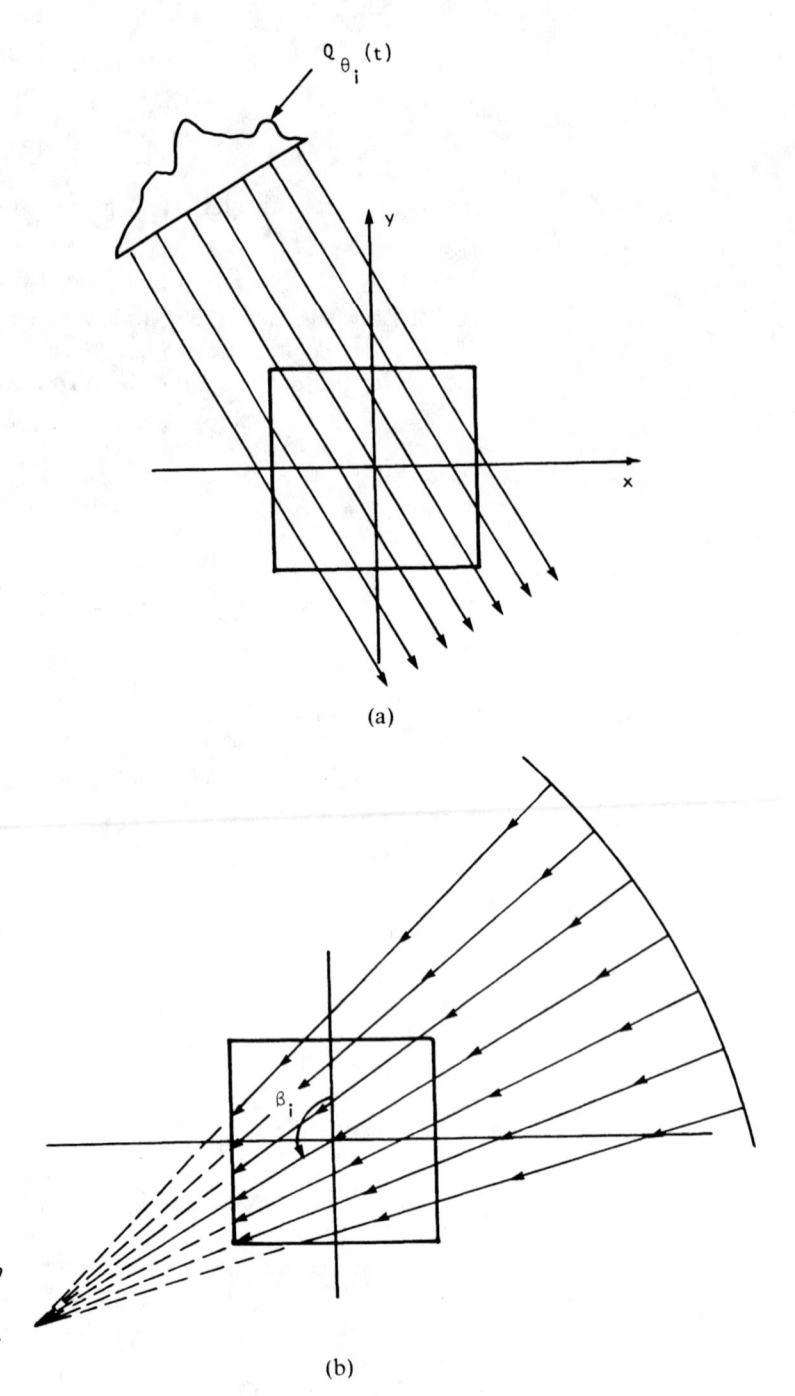

Fig. 3.21: *While the filtered projections are backprojected along parallel lines for the parallel beam case (a), for the fan beam case the backprojection is performed along converging lines (b). (c) This figure illustrates the implementation step that in order to determine the backprojected value at pixel (x, y), one must first compute γ' for that pixel. (From [Ros82].)*

84   COMPUTERIZED TOMOGRAPHIC IMAGING

(c)

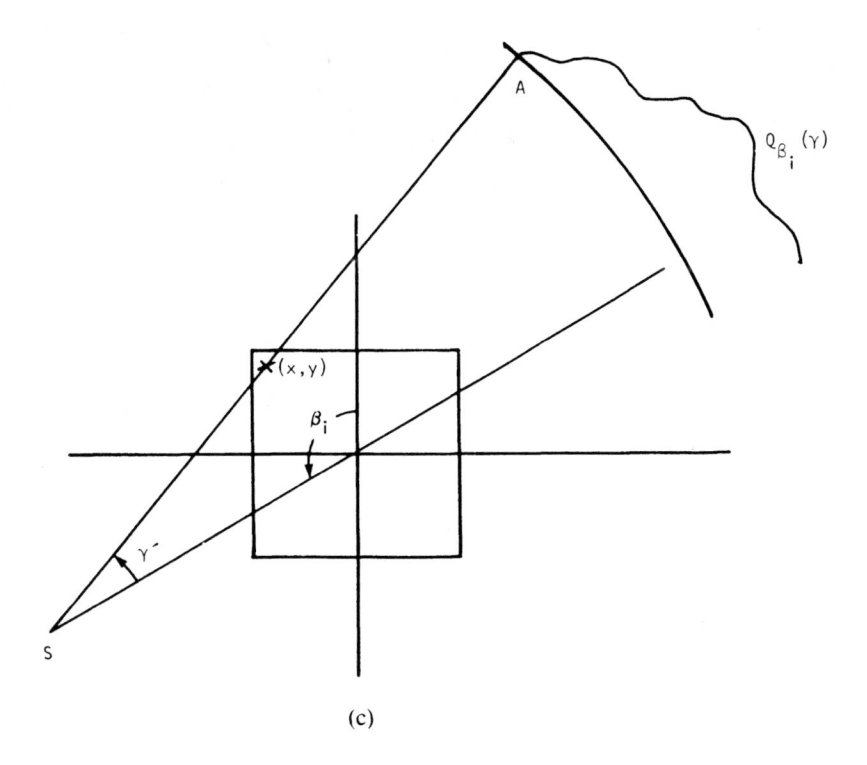

Fig. 3.21: *Continued.*

where $k(n\alpha)$ is the impulse response of the smoothing filter. In the frequency domain implementation this smoothing filter may be a simple cosine function or a Hamming window.

Step 3:

Perform a *weighted* backprojection of each filtered projection *along the fan*. Since the backprojection here is very different from that for the parallel case, we will explain it in some detail. For the parallel case the filtered projection is backprojected along a set of parallel lines as shown in Fig. 3.21(a). For the fan beam case the backprojection is done along the fan (Fig. 3.21(b)). This is dictated by the structure of (90):

$$f(x, y) \approx \Delta\beta \sum_{i=1}^{M} \frac{1}{L^2(x, y, \beta_i)} Q_{\beta_i}(\gamma') \qquad (98)$$

where γ' is the angle of the fan beam ray that passes through the point (x, y) and $\Delta\beta = 2\pi/M$. For β_i chosen in Fig. 3.21(c) in order to find the contribution of $Q_{\beta_i}(\gamma)$ to the point (x, y) shown there one must first find the angle, γ', of the ray SA that passes through that point (x, y). $Q_{\beta_i}(\gamma')$ will then be contributed from the filtered projection at β_i to the point (x, y) under consideration. Of course, the computed value of γ' may not correspond to one of $n\alpha$ for which $Q_{\beta_i}(n\alpha)$ is known. One must then use interpolation. The contribution $Q_{\beta_i}(\gamma')$ at the point (x, y) must then be divided by L^2 where L is the distance from the source S to the point (x, y).

This concludes our presentation of the algorithm for reconstructing projection data measured with detectors spaced at equiangular increments.

3.4.2 Equally Spaced Collinear Detectors

Let $R_\beta(s)$ denote a fan projection as shown in Fig. 3.22, where s is the distance along the straight line corresponding to the detector bank. The principal difference between the algorithm presented in the preceding subsection and the one presented here lies in the way a fan projection is represented, which then introduces differences in subsequent mathematical manipulations. Before, fan projections were sampled at equiangular intervals and we represented them by $R_\beta(\gamma)$ where γ represented the angular location of a ray. Now we represent them by $R_\beta(s)$.

Although the projections are measured on a line such as $D_1 D_2$ in Fig. 3.22,

Fig. 3.22: *For the case of equispaced detectors on a straight line, each projection is denoted by the function $R_\beta(s)$. (From [Ros82].)*

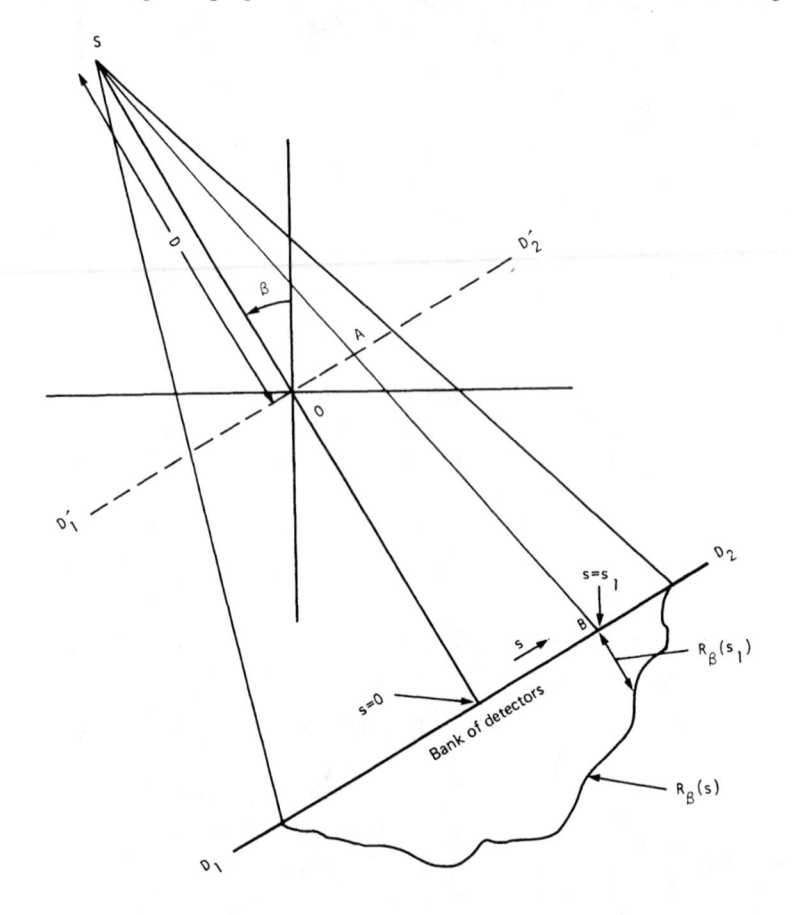

for theoretical purposes it is more efficient to assume the existence of an imaginary detector line $D_1' D_2'$ passing through the origin. We now associate the ray integral along SB with point A on $D_1' D_2'$, as opposed to point B on $D_1 D_2$. Thus in Fig. 3.23 we will associate a fan projection $R_\beta(s)$ with the imaginary detector line $D_1' D_2'$. Now consider a ray SA in the figure; the value of s for this ray is the length of OA. If parallel projection data were generated for the object under consideration, the ray SA would belong to a parallel projection $P_\theta(t)$ with θ and t as shown in the figure. The relationship between β and t for the parallel case is given by

$$t = s \cos \gamma \qquad \theta = \beta + \gamma$$

$$t = \frac{sD}{\sqrt{D^2 + s^2}} \qquad \theta = \beta + \tan^{-1} \frac{s}{D} \qquad (99)$$

where use has been made of the fact that angle AOC is equal to angle OSC, and where D is the distance of the source point S from the origin O.

In terms of the parallel projection data the reconstructed image is given by (74) which is repeated here for convenience:

$$f(r, \phi) = \frac{1}{2} \int_0^{2\pi} \int_{-t_m}^{t_m} P_\theta(t) h(r \cos(\theta - \phi) - t) \, dt \, d\theta \qquad (74)$$

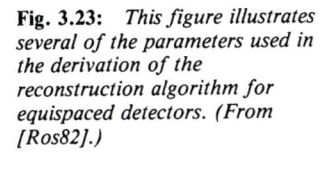

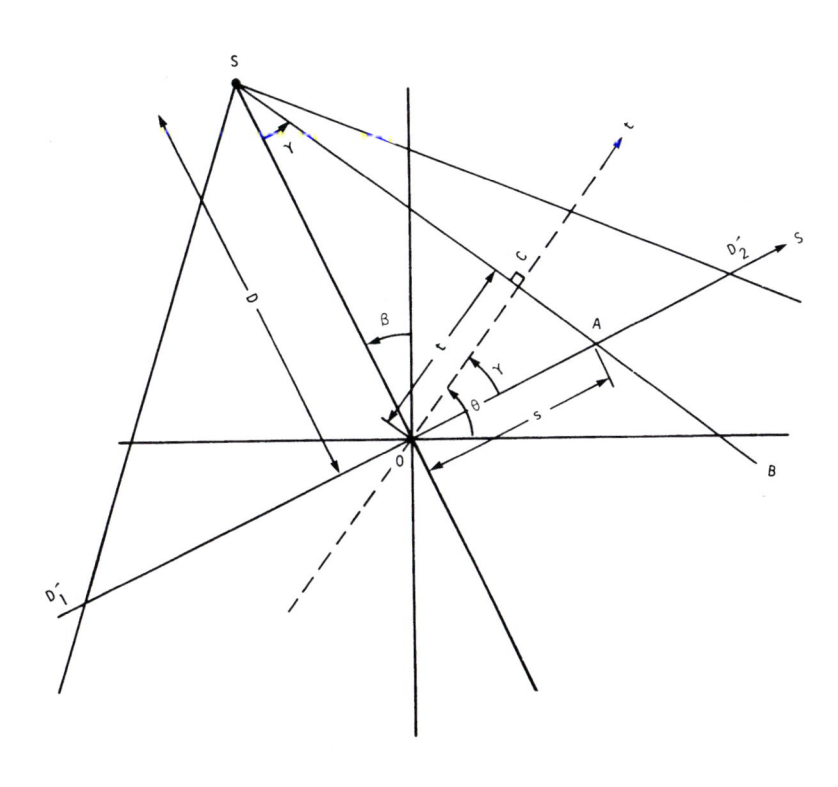

Fig. 3.23: *This figure illustrates several of the parameters used in the derivation of the reconstruction algorithm for equispaced detectors. (From [Ros82].)*

where $f(r, \phi)$ is the reconstructed image in polar coordinates. Using the relationships in (99) the double integration may be expressed as

$$f(r, \phi) = \frac{1}{2} \int_{-\tan^{-1}(S_m/D)}^{2\pi - \tan^{-1}(S_m/D)} \int_{-S_m}^{S_m} P_{\beta+\gamma}\left(\frac{sD}{\sqrt{D^2+s^2}}\right)$$

$$\cdot h\left[r\cos\left(\beta + \tan^{-1}\left(\frac{s}{D}\right) - \phi\right) - \frac{Ds}{\sqrt{D^2+s^2}}\right] \frac{D^3}{(D^2+s^2)^{3/2}} \, ds \, d\beta$$

(100)

where we have used

$$dt \, d\theta = \frac{D^3}{(D^2+s^2)^{3/2}} \, ds \, d\beta. \qquad (101)$$

In (100) s_m is the largest value of s in each projection and corresponds to t_m for parallel projection data. The limits $-\tan^{-1}(S_m/D)$ and $2\pi - \tan^{-1}(S_m/D)$ cover the angular interval of 360°. Since all functions of β in (100) are periodic with period 2π, these limits may be replaced by 0 and 2π, respectively. Also, the expression

$$P_{\beta+\gamma}\left(\frac{sD}{\sqrt{D^2+s^2}}\right) \qquad (102)$$

corresponds to the ray integral along SA in the parallel projection data $P_\theta(t)$. The identity of this ray integral in the fan projection data is simply $R_\beta(s)$. Introducing these changes in (100) we get

$$f(r, \phi) = \frac{1}{2} \int_0^{2\pi} \int_{-S_m}^{S_m} R_\beta(s) h\left(r\cos\left(\beta + \tan^{-1}\frac{s}{D} - \phi\right)\right.$$

$$\left. - \frac{Ds}{\sqrt{D^2+s^2}}\right) \frac{D^3}{(D^2+s^2)^{3/2}} \, ds \, d\beta. \qquad (103)$$

In order to express this formula in a filtered backprojection form we will first examine the argument of h. The argument may be written as

$$r\cos\left(\beta + \tan^{-1}\frac{s}{D} - \phi\right) - \frac{Ds}{\sqrt{D^2+s^2}}$$

$$= r\cos(\beta - \phi)\frac{D}{\sqrt{D^2+s^2}} - (D + r\sin(\beta - \phi))\frac{s}{\sqrt{D^2+s^2}}. \qquad (104)$$

We will now introduce two new variables that are easily calculated in a computer implementation. The first of these, denoted by U, is for each pixel (x, y) the ratio of SP (Fig. 3.24) to the source-to-origin distance. Note that

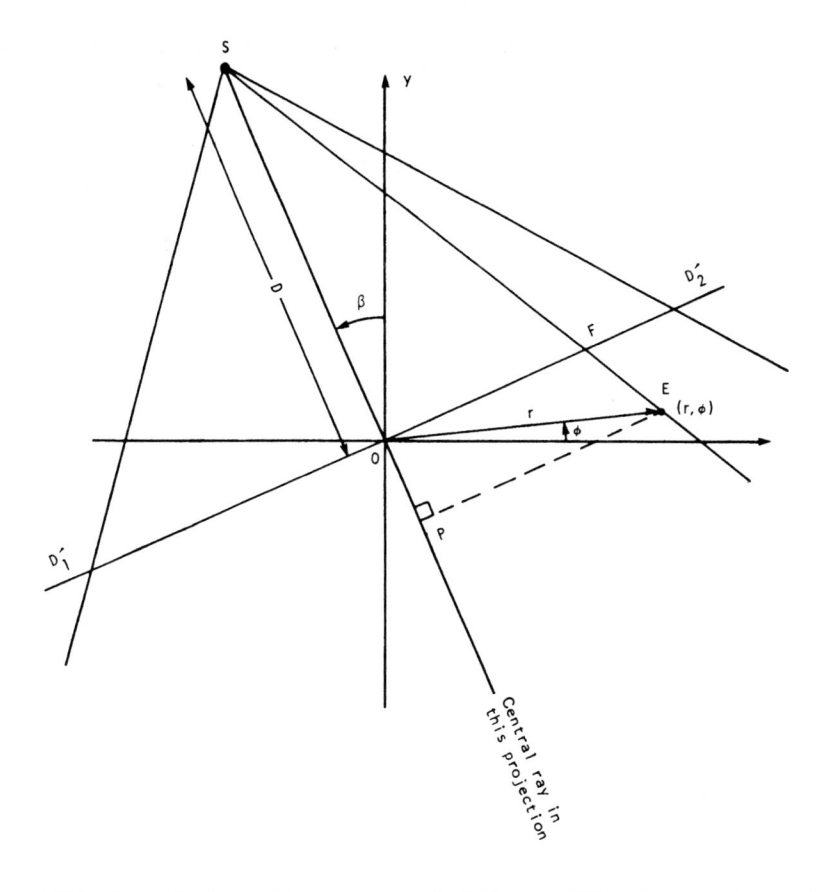

Fig. 3.24: *For a pixel at the polar coordinates (r, ϕ) the variable U is the ratio of the distance SP, which is the projection of the source to pixel line on the central ray, to the source-to-center distance. (Adapted from [Ros82].)*

SP is the projection of the source to pixel distance SE on the central ray. Thus

$$U(r, \phi, \beta) = \frac{\overline{SO} + \overline{OP}}{D} \tag{105}$$

$$= \frac{D + r \sin(\beta - \phi)}{D}. \tag{106}$$

The other parameter we want to define is the value of s for the ray that passes through the pixel (r, ϕ) under consideration. Let s' denote this value of s. Since s is measured along the imaginary detector line $D_1' D_2'$, it is given by the distance OF. Since

$$\frac{s'}{\overline{SO}} = \frac{\overline{EP}}{\overline{SP}} \tag{107}$$

we have

$$s' = D \frac{r \cos(\beta - \phi)}{D + r \sin(\beta - \phi)}. \tag{108}$$

ALGORITHMS FOR RECONSTRUCTION WITH NONDIFFRACTING SOURCES

Equations (106) and (108) can be utilized to express (104) in terms of U and s':

$$r \cos\left(\beta + \tan^{-1}\frac{s}{D} - \phi\right) - \frac{Ds}{\sqrt{D^2+s^2}} = \frac{s'UD}{\sqrt{D^2+s^2}} - \frac{sUD}{\sqrt{D^2+s^2}}. \quad (109)$$

Substituting (109) in (103), we get

$$f(r,\phi) = \frac{1}{2}\int_0^{2\pi}\int_{-S_m}^{S_m} R_\beta(s) h\left[(s'-s)\frac{UD}{\sqrt{D^2+s^2}}\right]\frac{D^3}{(D^2+s^2)^{3/2}}\,ds\,d\beta. \quad (110)$$

We will now express the convolving kernel h in this equation in a form closer to that given by (61). Note that, nominally, $h(t)$ is the inverse Fourier transform of $|w|$ in the frequency domain:

$$h(t) = \int_{-\infty}^{\infty} |w| e^{j2\pi wt}\,dw. \quad (111)$$

Therefore,

$$h\left[(s'-s)\frac{UD}{\sqrt{D^2+s^2}}\right] = \int_{-\infty}^{\infty} |w| e^{j2\pi w(s'-s)(UD/\sqrt{D^2+s^2})}\,dw. \quad (112)$$

Using the transformation

$$w' = w\frac{UD}{\sqrt{D^2+s^2}} \quad (113)$$

we can rewrite (112) as follows:

$$h\left[(s'-s)\frac{UD}{\sqrt{D^2+s^2}}\right] = \frac{D^2+s^2}{U^2D^2}\int_{-\infty}^{\infty}|w'|e^{j2\pi(s'-s)w'}\,dw' \quad (114)$$

$$= \frac{D^2+s^2}{U^2D^2} h(s'-s). \quad (115)$$

Substituting this in (110) we get

$$f(r,\phi) = \int_0^{2\pi}\frac{1}{U^2}\int_{-\infty}^{\infty} R_\beta(s) g(s'-s)\frac{D}{\sqrt{D^2+s^2}}\,ds\,d\beta \quad (116)$$

where

$$g(s) = \frac{1}{2}h(s). \quad (117)$$

For the purpose of computer implementation, (116) may be interpreted as a weighted filtered backprojection algorithm. To show this we rewrite (116) as follows:

$$f(r, \phi) = \int_0^{2\pi} \frac{1}{U^2} Q_\beta(s') \, d\beta \qquad (118)$$

where

$$Q_\beta(s) = R'_\beta(s) * g(s) \qquad (119)$$

and

$$R'_\beta(s) = R_\beta(s) \cdot \frac{D}{\sqrt{D^2 + s^2}}. \qquad (120)$$

Equations (118) through (120) suggest the following steps for computer implementation:

Step 1:

Assume that each projection $R_\beta(s)$ is sampled with a sampling interval of a. The known data then are $R_{\beta_i}(na)$ where n takes integer values with $n = 0$ corresponding to the central ray passing through the origin; β_i are the angles for which fan projections are known. The first step is to generate for each fan projection $R_{\beta_i}(na)$ the corresponding modified projection $R'_{\beta_i}(na)$ given by

$$R'_{\beta_i}(na) = R_{\beta_i}(na) \cdot \frac{D}{\sqrt{D^2 + n^2 a^2}}. \qquad (121)$$

Step 2:

Convolve each modified projection $R'_{\beta_i}(na)$ with $g(na)$ to generate the corresponding filtered projection:

$$Q_{\beta_i}(na) = R'_{\beta_i}(na) * g(na) \qquad (122)$$

where the sequence $g(na)$ is given by the samples of (117):

$$g(na) = \frac{1}{2} h(na). \qquad (123)$$

Substituting in this the values of $h(na)$ given in (61) we get for the impulse response of the convolving filter:

$$g(na) = \begin{cases} \dfrac{1}{8a^2}, & n = 0 \\ 0, & n \text{ even} \\ -\dfrac{1}{2n^2\pi^2 a^2}, & n \text{ odd.} \end{cases} \qquad (124)$$

When the convolution of (122) is implemented in the frequency domain using an FFT algorithm the projection data must be padded with a sufficient number of zeros to avoid distortion due to interperiod interference.

In practice superior reconstructions are obtained if a certain amount of smoothing is included with the convolution in (122). If $k(na)$ is the impulse response of the smoothing filter, we can write

$$Q_{\beta_i}(na) = R_{\beta_i}(na) * g(na) * k(na). \quad (125)$$

In a frequency domain implementation this smoothing may be achieved by a simple multiplicative window such as a Hamming window.

Step 3:

Perform a *weighted* backprojection of each filtered projection along the corresponding fan. The sum of all the backprojections is the reconstructed image

$$f(x, y) = \Delta B \sum_{i=1}^{M} \frac{1}{U^2(x, y, \beta_i)} Q_{\beta_i}(s') \quad (126)$$

where U is computed using (106) and s' identifies the ray that passes through (x, y) in the fan for the source located at angle β_i. Of course, this value of s' may not correspond to one of the values of na at which Q_{β_i} is known. In that case interpolation is necessary.

3.4.3 A Re-sorting Algorithm

We will now describe an algorithm that rapidly re-sorts the fan beam projection data into equivalent parallel beam projection data. After re-sorting one may use the filtered backprojection algorithm for parallel projection data to reconstruct the image. This fast re-sorting algorithm does place constraints on the angles at which the fan beam projections must be taken and also on the angles at which projection data must be sampled within each fan beam projection.

Referring to Fig. 3.19, the relationships between the independent variables of the fan beam projections and parallel projections are given by (70):

$$t = D \sin \gamma \quad \text{and} \quad \theta = \beta + \gamma. \quad (127)$$

If, as before, $R_\beta(\gamma)$ denotes a fan beam projection taken at angle β, and $P_\theta(t)$ a parallel projection taken at angle θ, using (127) we can write

$$R_\beta(\gamma) = P_{\beta+\gamma}(D \sin \gamma). \quad (128)$$

Let $\Delta\beta$ denote the angular increment between successive fan beam projections, and let $\Delta\gamma$ denote the angular interval used for sampling the fan beam projections. We will assume that the following condition is satisfied:

$$\Delta\beta = \Delta\gamma = \alpha. \tag{129}$$

Clearly then β and γ in (128) are equal to $m\alpha$ and $n\alpha$, respectively, for some integer values of the indices m and n. We may therefore write (128) as

$$R_{m\alpha}(n\alpha) = P_{(m+n)\alpha}(D \sin n\alpha). \tag{130}$$

This equation serves as the basis of a fast re-sorting algorithm. It expresses the fact that the nth ray in the mth radial projection is the nth ray in the ($m + n$)th parallel projection. Of course, because of the sin $n\alpha$ factor on the right-hand side of (130), the parallel projections obtained are not uniformly sampled. This can usually be rectified by interpolation.

3.5 Fan Beam Reconstruction from a Limited Number of Views

Simple geometrical arguments should convince the reader that parallel projections that are 180° apart, $P_\theta(t)$ and $P_{\theta+180°}(t)$, are mirror images of each other. That is,

$$P_\theta(t) = P_{\theta+180°}(-t) \tag{131}$$

and thus it is only necessary to measure the projections of an object for angles from 0 to 180°.

We can extend this result by noting that an object is completely specified if the ray integrals of the object are known for

$$\theta_0 \le \theta < \theta_0 + 180° \tag{132}$$

and

$$-t_{max} \le t \le t_{max} \tag{133}$$

where t_{max} is large enough so that each projection is at least as wide as the object at its widest. If each ray integral is represented as a point in a polar coordinate system (t, θ) as shown in Fig. 3.25 then a complete set of ray

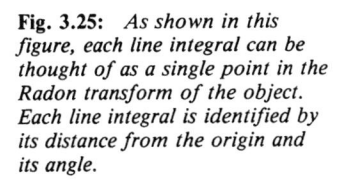

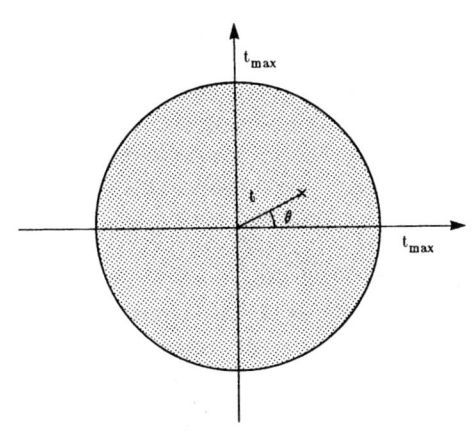

Fig. 3.25: *As shown in this figure, each line integral can be thought of as a single point in the Radon transform of the object. Each line integral is identified by its distance from the origin and its angle.*

(a)   (b)   (c)

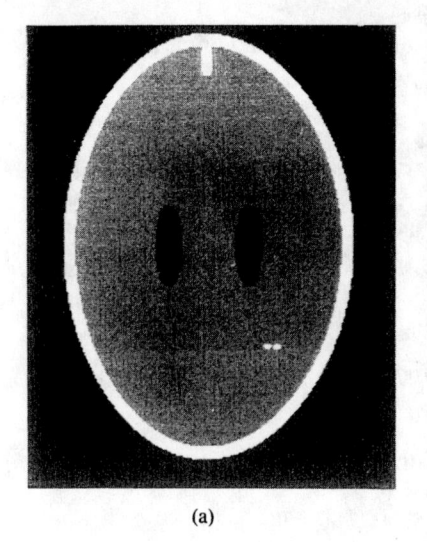

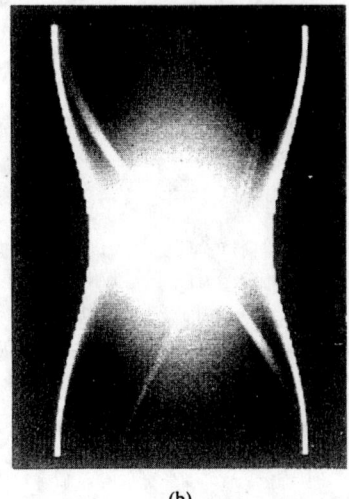

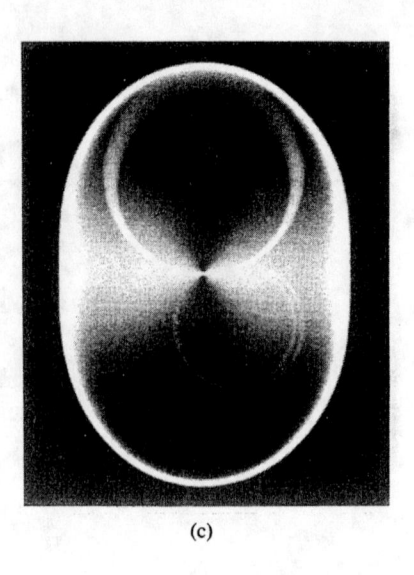

Fig. 3.26: *An object and its Radon transform are shown here. The object in (a) is used to illustrate the short scan algorithm developed by Parker [Par82a]. (b) shows the Radon transform in rectangular coordinates, while (c) represents the Radon transform in polar coordinates. (Reprinted with permission from [Par82a], [Par82b].)*

integrals will completely fill a disk of radius t_{max}. This is commonly known as the Radon transform or a sinogram and is shown for the Shepp and Logan phantom both in polar and rectangular coordinates in Fig. 3.26.

These ideas can also be extended to the fan beam case. From Fig. 3.27 we see that two ray integrals represented by the fan beam angles (β_1, γ_1) and (β_2, γ_2) are identical provided

$$\beta_1 - \gamma_1 = \beta_2 - \gamma_2 + 180° \qquad (134)$$

and

$$\gamma_1 = -\gamma_2. \qquad (135)$$

With fan beam data the coordinate transformation

$$t = D \sin \gamma$$
$$\theta = \beta + \gamma \qquad (136)$$

maps the (β, γ) description of a ray in a fan into its Radon transform equivalent. This transformation can then be used to construct Fig. 3.27, which shows the data available in Radon domain as the projection angle β varies between 0 and 180° with a fan angle of 40° ($\gamma_{max} = 20°$).

Recall that points in Radon space that are periodic with respect to the intervals shown in (132) and (133) represent the same ray integral. Thus the data in Fig. 3.28 for angles $\theta > 180°$ and $t > 0$ are equal to the Radon data for $\theta < 0$ and $t < 0$. These two regions are labeled A in Fig. 3.28. On the other hand, the regions marked B in Fig. 3.28 are areas in the Radon space where there are no measurements of the object. To cover these areas it is necessary to measure projections over an additional $2\gamma_m$ degrees as shown in

94   COMPUTERIZED TOMOGRAPHIC IMAGING

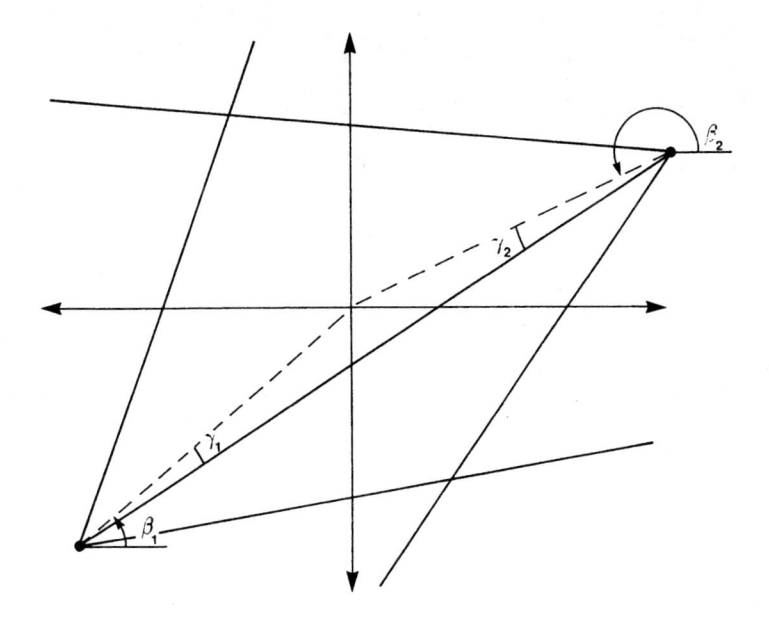

Fig. 3.27: Rays in two fan beams will represent the same line integral if they satisfy the relationship $\beta_1 - \gamma_1 = \beta_2 - \gamma_2 + 180°$.

Fig. 3.28: Collecting projections over 180° gives estimates of the Radon transform between the curved lines as shown on the left. The curved lines represent the most extreme projections for a fan angle of γ_m. On the right is shown the available data in the β-γ coordinate system used in describing fan beams. In both cases the region marked A represents the part of the Radon transform where two estimates are available. On the other hand, for 180° of projections there are no estimates of the Radon transform in the regions marked B.

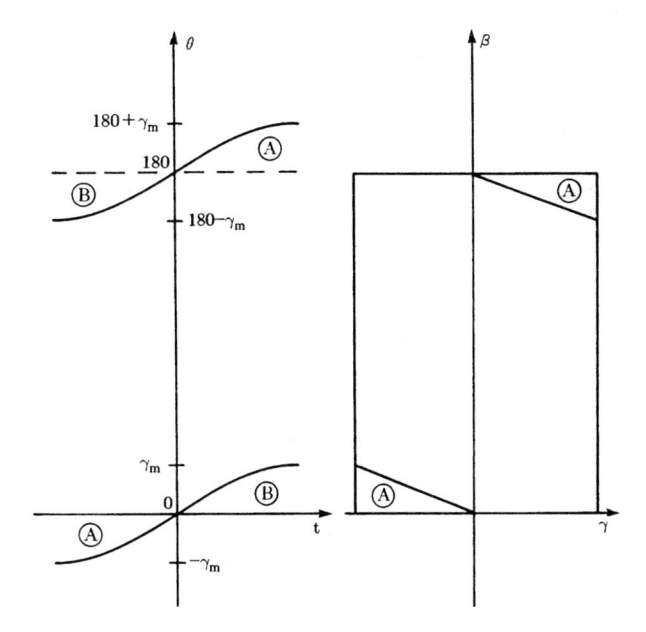

ALGORITHMS FOR RECONSTRUCTION WITH NONDIFFRACTING SOURCES

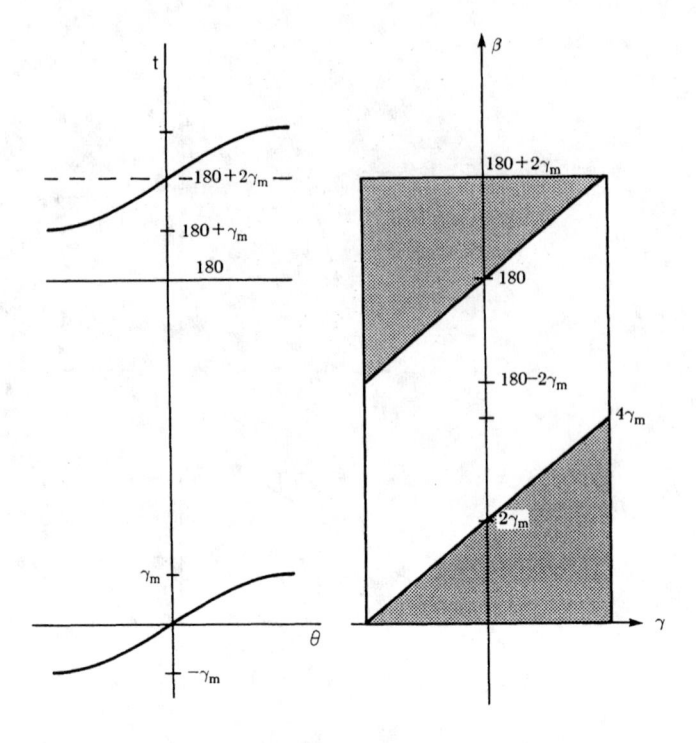

Fig. 3.29: *If projections are gathered over an angle of* $180° + 2\gamma_m$ *then the data illustrated are available. Again on the left is shown the Radon transform while the right shows the available data in the β–γ coordinate system. The line integrals in the shaded regions represent duplicate data and these points must be gradually weighted to obtain good reconstructions.*

Fig. 3.29. Thus it should be possible to reconstruct an object using fan beam projections collected over $180 + 2\gamma_m$ degrees.

Fig. 3.30 shows a "perfect" reconstruction of a phantom used by Parker [Par82a], [Par82b] to illustrate his algorithm for short scan or "180 degree plus" reconstructions. Projection data measured over a full 360° of β were used to generate the reconstruction.

It is more natural to discuss the projection data overlap in the (β, γ) coordinate system. We derive the overlap region in this space by using the relations in (134) and (135) and the limits

$$0 \leq \beta_1 \leq 180° + 2\gamma_m$$
$$0 \leq \beta_2 \leq 180° + 2\gamma_m. \tag{137}$$

Substituting (134) and (135) into the first equation above we find

$$0 \leq \beta_2 - 2\gamma_2 + 180° \leq 180° + 2\gamma_m \tag{138}$$

and then by rearranging

$$-180° + 2\gamma_2 \leq \beta_2 \leq 2\gamma_m - 2\gamma_2. \tag{139}$$

Substituting the same two equations into the second inequality in (137) we find

$$0 \leq \beta_1 - 2\gamma_1 - 180° \leq 180° + 2\gamma_m \tag{140}$$

96 COMPUTERIZED TOMOGRAPHIC IMAGING

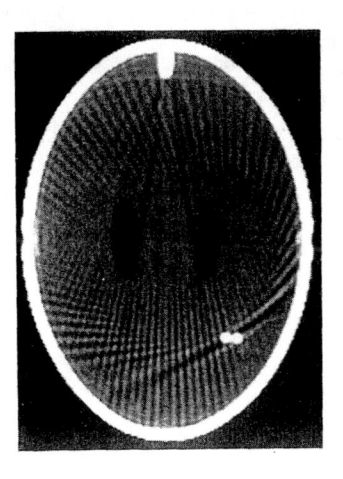

Fig. 3.30: *This figure shows a reconstruction using 360° of fan beam projections and a standard filtered backprojection algorithm. (Reprinted with permission from [Par82a], [Par82b].)*

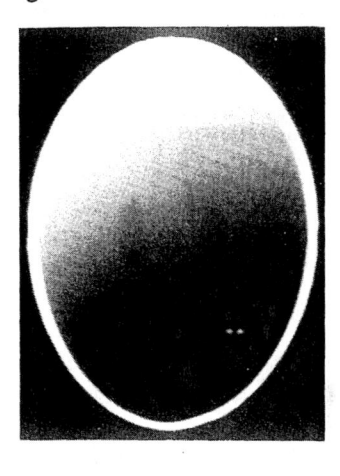

Fig. 3.31: *This reconstruction was generated with a standard filtered backprojection algorithm using 220° of projections. The large artifacts are due to the lack of data in some regions of the Radon transform and duplicate data in others. (Reprinted with permission from [Par82a], [Par82b].)*

and then by rearranging

$$180° + 2\gamma_1 \leq \beta_1 \leq 360° + 2\gamma_m + 2\gamma_1. \tag{141}$$

Since the fan beam angle, γ, is always less then 90°, the overlapping regions are given by

$$0 \leq \beta_2 \leq 2\gamma_m + 2\gamma_2 \tag{142}$$

and

$$180° + 2\gamma_1 \leq \beta_1 \leq 180° + 2\gamma_m \tag{143}$$

as is shown in Fig. 3.29.

If projections are gathered over an angle of $180° + 2\gamma_m$ and a reconstruction is generated using the standard fan beam reconstruction algorithms described in Section 3.4, then the image in Fig. 3.31 is obtained.

In this case a fan angle of 40° ($\gamma_{max} = 20$) was used. As described above, the severe artifacts in this reconstruction are caused by the double coverage of the points in region B of Fig. 3.28.

One might think that the reconstruction can be improved by setting the data to zero in one of the regions of overlap. This can be implemented by multiplying a projection at angle β, $p_\beta(\gamma)$, by a one-zero window, $w_\beta(\gamma)$, given by

$$w_\beta(\gamma) = \begin{cases} 0 & 0 \leq \beta \leq 2\gamma_m + 2\gamma \\ 1 & \text{elsewhere.} \end{cases} \quad (144)$$

As shown by Naparstek [Nap80] using this type of window gives only a small improvement since streaks obscure the resulting image.

While the above filter function properly handles the extra data, better reconstructions can be obtained using a window described in [Par82a]. The sharp cutoff of the one-zero window adds a large high frequency component to each projection which is then enhanced by the $|\omega|$ filter that is used to filter each projection.

More accurate reconstructions are obtained if a "smoother" window is used to filter the data. Mathematically, a "smooth" window is both continuous and has a continuous derivative. Formally, the window, $w_\beta(\gamma)$, must satisfy the following condition:

$$w_{\beta_1}(\gamma_1) + w_{\beta_2}(\gamma_2) = 1 \quad (145)$$

for (β_1, γ_1) and (β_2, γ_2) satisfying the relations in (134) and (135), and

$$w_0(\gamma) = 0 \quad (146)$$

and

$$w_{180° + 2\gamma_m} = 0. \quad (147)$$

To keep the filter function continuous and "smooth" at the boundary between the single and double overlap regions the following constraints are imposed on the derivative of $w_\beta(\gamma)$:

$$\left. \frac{\partial w_\beta(\gamma)}{\partial \beta} \right|_{\beta = 2\gamma_m + 2\gamma} = 0 \quad (148)$$

and

$$\left. \frac{\partial w_\beta(\gamma)}{\partial \beta} \right|_{\beta = 180° + 2\gamma} = 0. \quad (149)$$

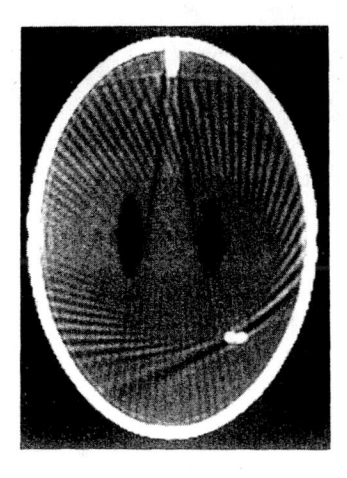

Fig. 3.32: *Using a weighting function that minimizes the discontinuities in the projection this reconstruction is obtained using 220° of projection data. (Reprinted with permission from [Par82a], [Par82b].)*

One such window that satisfies all of these conditions is

$$w_\beta(\gamma) = \begin{cases} \sin^2\left[\dfrac{45°\beta}{\gamma_m - \gamma}\right], & 0 \leq \beta \leq 2\gamma_m - 2\gamma \\ 1, & 2\gamma_m - 2\gamma \leq \beta \leq 180° - 2\gamma \\ \sin^2\left[45°\dfrac{180° + 2\gamma_m - \beta}{\gamma + \gamma_m}\right], & 180° - 2\gamma \leq \beta \leq 180° + 2\gamma_m. \end{cases}$$

(150)

A reconstruction using this weighting function is shown in Fig. 3.32. From this image we see that it is possible to eliminate the overlap without introducing errors by using a smooth window.

3.6 Three-Dimensional Reconstructions[1]

The conventional way to image a three-dimensional object is to illuminate the object with a narrow beam of x-rays and use a two-dimensional reconstruction algorithm. A three-dimensional reconstruction can then be formed by illuminating successive planes within the object and stacking the resulting reconstructions. This is shown in Fig. 3.33.

A more efficient approach, to be considered in this section, is a generalization of the two-dimensional fan beam algorithms presented in Section 3.4.2. Now, instead of illuminating a slice of the object with a fan of x-rays, the entire object is illuminated with a point source and the x-ray flux is measured on a plane. This is called a cone beam reconstruction because the

---

[1] We are grateful for the help of Barry Roberts in the preparation of this material.

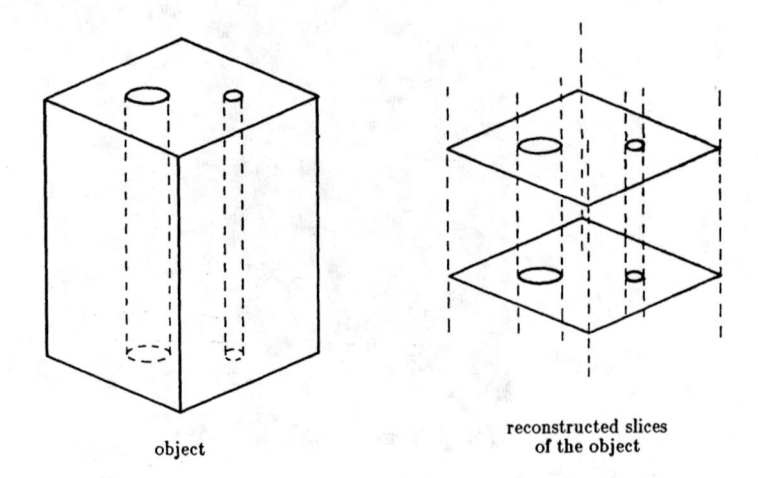

Fig. 3.33: *A three-dimensional reconstruction can be done by repetitively using two-dimensional reconstruction algorithms at different heights along the z-axis. (From [Kak86].)*

rays form a cone as illustrated in Fig. 3.34. Cone beam algorithms have been studied for use with Mayo Clinic's Digital Spatial Reconstructor (DSR) [Rob83] and Imatron's Fifth Generation Scanner [Boy83].

The main advantage of cone beam algorithms is the reduction in data collection time. With a single source, ray integrals are measured through every point in the object in the time it takes to measure a single slice in a conventional two-dimensional scanner. The projection data, $R_\beta(t, r)$, are now a function of the source angle, β, and horizontal and vertical positions on the detector plane, t and r.

3.6.1 Three-Dimensional Projections

A ray in a three-dimensional projection is described by the intersection of two planes

$$t = x \cos \theta + y \sin \theta \tag{151}$$

$$r = -(-x \sin \theta + y \cos \theta) \sin \gamma + z \cos \gamma. \tag{152}$$

A new coordinate system (t, s, r) is obtained by two rotations of the (x, y, z)-axis as shown in Fig. 3.35. The first rotation, as in the two-dimensional case, is by θ degrees around the z-axis to give the (t, s, z)-axes. Then a second rotation is done out of the (t, s)-plane around the t-axis by an angle of γ. In matrix form the required rotations are given by

$$\begin{bmatrix} t \\ s' \\ r \end{bmatrix} = \begin{bmatrix} 1 & 0 & 0 \\ 0 & \cos \gamma & \sin \gamma \\ 0 & -\sin \gamma & \cos \gamma \end{bmatrix} \begin{bmatrix} \cos \theta & \sin \theta & 0 \\ -\sin \theta & \cos \theta & 0 \\ 0 & 0 & 1 \end{bmatrix} \begin{bmatrix} x \\ y \\ z \end{bmatrix}. \tag{153}$$

A three-dimensional parallel projection of the object f is expressed by the

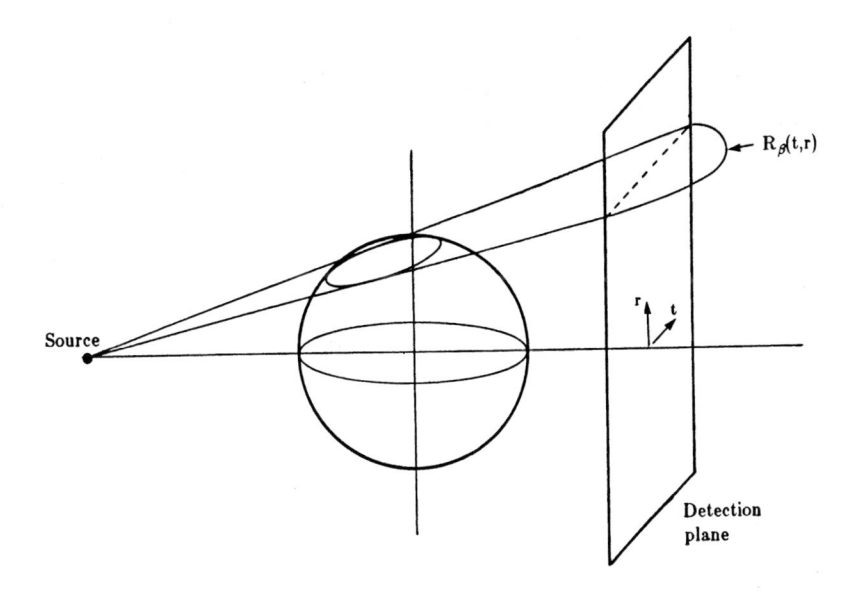

Fig. 3.34: *In cone beam projections the detector measures the x-ray flux over a plane. By rotating the source and detector plane completely around the object all the data necessary for a three-dimensional reconstruction can be gathered in the time a conventional fan beam system collects the data for its two-dimensional reconstruction. (From [Kak86].)*

following integral:

$$P_{\theta,\gamma}(t, r) = \int_{-S_m}^{S_m} f(t, s, r) \, ds. \tag{154}$$

Note that four variables are being used to specify the desired ray; (t, θ) specify the distance and angle in the x–y plane and (r, γ) in the s–z plane.

In a cone beam system the source is rotated by β and ray integrals are measured on the detector plane as described by $R_\beta(p', \zeta')$. To find the equivalent parallel projection ray first define

$$p = \frac{p' D_{SO}}{D_{SO} + D_{DE}} \qquad \zeta = \frac{\zeta' D_{SO}}{D_{SO} + D_{DE}} \tag{155}$$

as was done in Section 3.4.2. Here we have used D_{SO} to indicate the distance from the center of rotation to the source and D_{DE} to indicate the distance from the center of rotation to the detector. For a given cone beam ray, $R_\beta(p, \zeta)$, the parallel projection ray is given by

$$t = p \frac{D_{SO}}{\sqrt{D_{SO}^2 + p^2}} \tag{156}$$

$$\theta = \beta + \tan^{-1}(p/D_{SO}) \tag{157}$$

where t and θ locate a ray in a given tilted fan, and similarly

$$r = \zeta \frac{D_{SO}}{\sqrt{D_{SO}^2 + \zeta^2}} \tag{158}$$

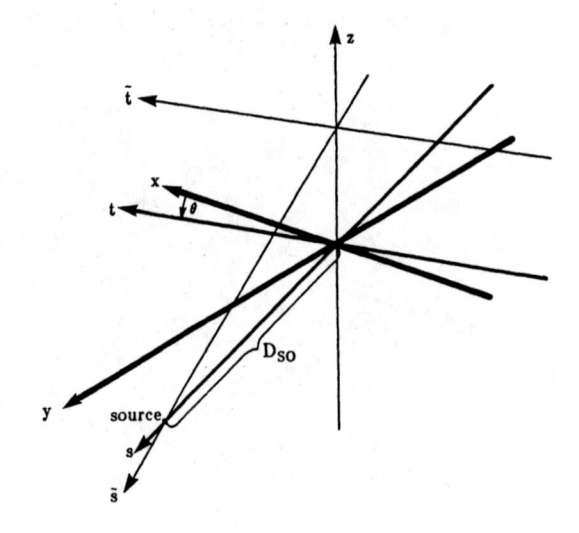

Fig. 3.35: *To simplify the discussion of the cone beam reconstruction the coordinate system is rotated by the angle of the source to give the (s, t)-axis. The r-axis is not shown but is perpendicular to the t- and s-axes. (From [Kak86].)*

$$\gamma = \tan^{-1}(\zeta/D_{SO}). \qquad (159)$$

were r and γ specify the location of the tilted fan itself.

The reconstructions shown in this section will use a three-dimensional version of the Shepp and Logan head phantom. The two-dimensional ellipses of Table 3.1 have been made ellipsoids and repositioned within an imaginary skull. Table 3.2 shows the position and size of each ellipse and Fig. 3.36 illustrates their position.

Because of the linearity of the Radon transform, a projection of an object consisting of ellipsoids is just the sum of the projection of each individual

Table 3.2: Summary of parameters for three-dimensional tomography simulations.

Ellipsoid	Coordinates of the Center (x, y, z)	Axis Lengths (A, B, C)	Rotation Angle β (deg)	Gray Level ρ
a	(0, 0, 0)	(0.69, 0.92, 0.9)	0	2.0
b	(0, 0, 0)	(0.6624, 0.874, 0.88)	0	−0.98
c	(−0.22, 0, −0.25)	(0.41, 0.16, 0.21)	108	−0.02
d	(0.22, 0, −0.25)	(0.31, 0.11, 0.22)	72	−0.02
e	(0, 0.1, −0.25)	(0.046, 0.046, 0.046)	0	0.02
f	(0, 0.1, −0.25)	(0.046, 0.046, 0.046)	0	0.02
g	(−0.8, −0.65, −0.25)	(0.046, 0.023, 0.02)	0	0.01
h	(0.06, −0.065, −0.25)	(0.046, 0.023, 0.02)	90	0.01
i	(0.06, −0.105, 0.625)	(0.56, 0.04, 0.1)	90	0.02
j	(0, 0.1, −0.625)	(0.056, 0.056, 0.1)	0	−0.02

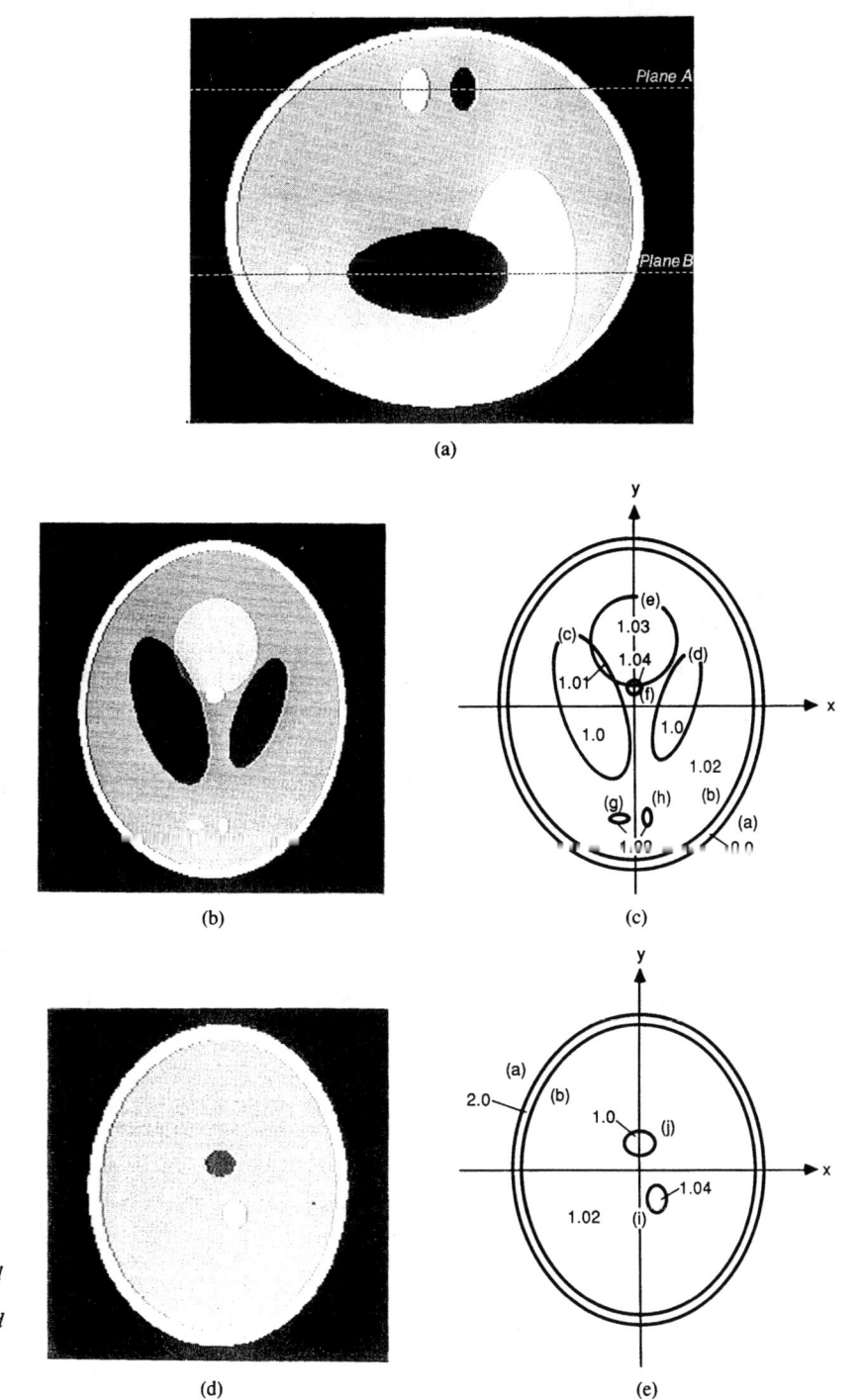

Fig. 3.36: *A three-dimensional version of the Shepp and Logan head phantom is used to test the cone beam reconstruction algorithms in this section. (a) A vertical slice through the object illustrating the position of the two reconstructed planes. (b) An image at plane B ($z = -0.25$) and (c) an illustration of the level of each of the ellipses. (d) An image at plane A ($z = 0.625$) and (e) an illustration of the gray levels with the slice. (From [Kak86].)*

ALGORITHMS FOR RECONSTRUCTION WITH NONDIFFRACTING SOURCES 103 ellipsoid. If the ellipsoid is constant and described by

$$f(x, y, z) = \begin{cases} \rho & \frac{x^2}{A^2} + \frac{y^2}{B^2} + \frac{z^2}{C^2} \leq 1 \\ 0 & \text{otherwise} \end{cases} \qquad (160)$$

then its projection on the detector plane is written

$$P_{\theta,\gamma}(t,r) = \frac{2\rho ABC}{a^2(\theta,\gamma)} \left[a^2(\theta,\gamma) - t^2(C^2 \cos^2 \gamma + (B^2 \cos^2 \theta + A^2 \sin^2 \theta) \sin^2 \gamma) \right.$$

$$- r^2(A^2 \cos^2 \theta + B^2 \sin^2 \theta)\left(\frac{7 + \cos(4\gamma)}{8}\right)$$

$$\left. - 2tr \sin \gamma \cos \theta \sin \theta (B^2 - A^2) \right]^{1/2} \qquad (161)$$

where

$$a^2(\theta, \gamma) = C^2(B^2 \sin^2 \theta + A^2 \cos^2 \theta) \cos^2 \gamma + A^2 B^2 \sin^2 \gamma. \qquad (162)$$

If the tilt angle, γ, is zero then (161) simplifies to (5).

3.6.2 Three-Dimensional Filtered Backprojection

We will present a filtered backprojection algorithm based on analyses presented in [Fel84] and [Kak86]. The reconstruction is based on filtering and backprojecting a single plane within the cone. In other words, each elevation in the cone (described by z or ζ) is considered separately and the final three-dimensional reconstruction is obtained by summing the contribution to the object from all the tilted fan beams.

The cone beam algorithm sketched above is best derived by starting with the filtered backprojection algorithm for equispatial rays. In a three-dimensional reconstruction each fan is angled out of the source–detector plane of rotation. This leads to a change of variables in the backprojection algorithm.

First consider the two-dimensional fan beam reconstruction formula for the point (r, ϕ):

$$g(r, \phi) = \frac{1}{2} \int_0^{2\pi} \frac{1}{U^2} \int_{-\infty}^{\infty} R_\beta(p) h(p' - p) \frac{D_{SO}}{\sqrt{D_{SO}^2 + p^2}} \, dp \, d\beta \qquad (163)$$

$$p' = \frac{D_{SO} r \cos(\beta - \phi)}{D_{SO} + r \sin(\beta - \phi)} \qquad h(p) = \int_{-W}^{W} |\omega| e^{j\omega p} \, d\omega \qquad (164)$$

$$U(r, \phi, \beta) = \frac{D_{SO} + r \sin(\beta - \phi)}{D_{SO}}. \qquad (165)$$

Equation (163) is the same as (116), except that we have now used different names for some of the variables. To further simplify this expression we will replace the (r, ϕ) coordinate system by the rotated coordinates (t, s). Recall that (t, s) is the location of a point rotated by the angular displacement of the source–detector array. The expressions

$$t = x \cos \beta + y \sin \beta \qquad s = -x \sin \beta + y \cos \beta \qquad (166)$$

$$x = r \cos \phi \qquad y = r \sin \phi, \qquad (167)$$

lead to

$$p' = \frac{D_{SO} t}{D_{SO} - s} \qquad U(x, y, \beta) = \frac{D_{SO} - s}{D_{SO}}. \qquad (168)$$

The fan beam reconstruction algorithm is now written as

$$g(t, s) = \frac{1}{2} \int_0^{2\pi} \frac{D_{SO}^2}{(D_{SO} - s)^2} \int_{-\infty}^{\infty} R_\beta(p) h\left(\frac{D_{SO} t}{D_{SO} - s} - p\right) \frac{D_{SO}}{\sqrt{D_{SO}^2 + p^2}} \, dp \, d\beta. \qquad (169)$$

In a cone beam reconstruction it is necessary to tilt the fan out of the plane of rotation; thus the size of the fan and the coordinate system of the reconstructed point change. As shown in Fig. 3.37 a new coordinate system $(\tilde{t}, \tilde{s})$ is defined that represents the location of the reconstructed point with respect to the tilted fan. Because of the changing fan size both the source distance, D_{SO}, and the angular differential, β, change. The new source distance is given by

$$D_{SO}'^2 = D_{SO}^2 + \zeta^2 \qquad (170)$$

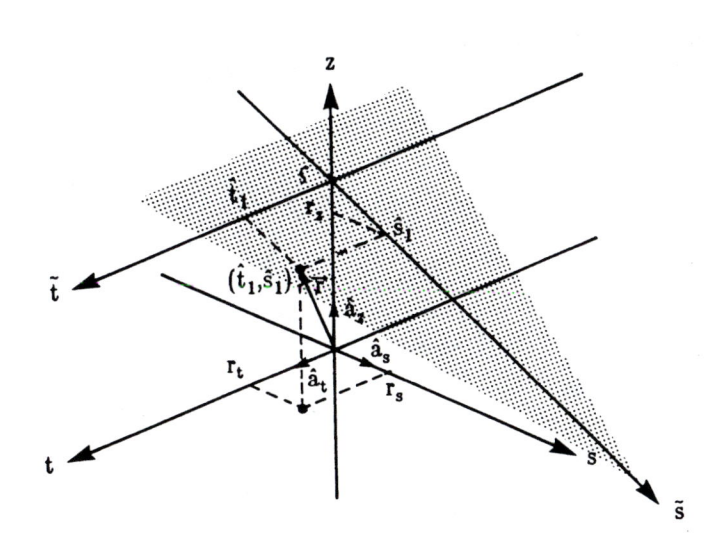

Fig. 3.37: *The $(\tilde{t}, \tilde{s})$ coordinate system represents a point in the object with respect to a tilted fan beam. (From [Kak86].)*

ALGORITHMS FOR RECONSTRUCTION WITH NONDIFFRACTING SOURCES

where ζ is the height of the fan above the center of the plane of rotation. In addition, the increment of angular rotation $d\beta'$ becomes

$$D_{SO}\, d\beta = D'_{SO}\, d\beta' \qquad d\beta' = \frac{d\beta\, D_{SO}}{\sqrt{D_{SO}^2 + \zeta^2}}. \qquad (171)$$

Substituting these new variables, D'_{SO} for D_{SO} and $d\beta'$ for $d\beta$, and writing the projection data as $R_{\beta'}(p, \zeta)$, (169) becomes

$$g(\tilde{t}, \tilde{s}) = \frac{1}{2}\int_0^{2\pi} \frac{D'^2_{SO}}{(D'_{SO} - \tilde{s})^2}$$

$$\cdot \int_{-\infty}^{\infty} R_{\beta'}(p, \zeta) h\left(\frac{D'_{SO}\tilde{t}}{D'_{SO} - \tilde{s}} - p\right) \frac{D'_{SO}}{\sqrt{D'^2_{SO} + p^2}}\, dp\, d\beta'. \qquad (172)$$

To return the reconstruction to the original (t, s, z) coordinate system we substitute

$$\tilde{t} = t, \qquad \frac{\tilde{s}}{D'_{SO}} = \frac{s}{D_{SO}}, \qquad \frac{\zeta}{D_{SO}} = \frac{z}{D_{SO} - s} \qquad (173)$$

and (170) and (171) to find

$$g(t, s) = \frac{1}{2}\int_0^{2\pi} \frac{D^2_{SO}}{(D_{SO} - s)^2}$$

$$\cdot \int_{-\infty}^{\infty} R_{\beta}(p, \zeta) h\left(\frac{D_{SO}t}{D_{SO} - s} - p\right) \frac{D_{SO}}{\sqrt{D^2_{SO} + \zeta^2 + p^2}}\, dp\, d\beta. \qquad (174)$$

The cone beam reconstruction algorithm can be broken into the following three steps:

Step 1:
  Multiply the projection data, $R_{\beta}(p, \zeta)$, by the function $(D_{SO}/\sqrt{D^2_{SO} + \zeta^2 + p^2})$ to find $R'_{\beta}(p, \zeta)$:

$$R'_{\beta}(p, \zeta) = \frac{D_{SO}}{\sqrt{D^2_{SO} + \zeta^2 + p^2}} R_{\beta}(p, \zeta). \qquad (175)$$

Step 2:
  Convolve the weighted projection $R'_{\beta}(p, \zeta)$ with $h(p)/2$ by multiplying their Fourier transforms with respect to p. Note this convolution is done independently for each elevation, ζ. The result, $Q_{\beta}(p, \zeta)$, is written

$$Q_{\beta}(p, \zeta) = R'_{\beta}(p, \zeta) * \frac{1}{2} h(p). \qquad (176)$$

Step 3:
  Finally, each weighted projection is backprojected over the three-

dimensional reconstruction grid:

$$g(t, s, z) = \int_0^{2\pi} \frac{D_{SO}^2}{(D_{SO}-s)^2} Q_\beta \left(\frac{D_{SO}t}{D_{SO}-s}, \frac{D_{SO}z}{D_{SO}-s} \right) d\beta. \quad (177)$$

The two arguments of the weighted projection, Q_β, represent the transformation of a point in the object into the coordinate system of the tilted fan shown in Fig. 3.37.

Only those points of the object that are illuminated from all directions can be properly reconstructed. In a cone beam system this region is a sphere of radius $D_{SO} \sin(\Gamma_m)$ where Γ_m is half the beamwidth angle of the cone. Outside this region a point will not be included in some of the projections and thus will not be correctly reconstructed.

Figs. 3.38 and 3.39 show reconstructions at two different levels of the object described in Fig. 3.36. In each case 100 projections of 127×127 elements were simulated and both a gray scale image of the entire plane and a line plot are shown. The reconstructed planes were at $z = 0.625$ and $z = -0.25$ planes and are marked as Plane A and Plane B in Fig. 3.36.

In agreement with [Smi85], the quality of the reconstruction varies with the elevation of the plane. On the plane of rotation ($z = 0$) the cone beam algorithm is identical to a equispatial fan beam algorithm and thus the results shown in Fig. 3.38 are quite good. Farther from the central plane each point in the reconstruction is irradiated from all directions but now at an oblique angle. As shown in Fig. 3.39 there is a noticeable degradation in the reconstruction.

3.7 Bibliographic Notes

The current excitement in tomographic imaging originated with Hounsfield's invention [Hou72] of the computed tomography (CT) scanner in 1972, which was indeed a major breakthrough. His invention showed that it is possible to get high-quality cross-sectional images with an accuracy now reaching one part in a thousand in spite of the fact that the projection data do not strictly satisfy theoretical models underlying the efficiently implementable reconstruction algorithms. (In x-ray tomography, the mismatch with the assumed theoretical models is caused primarily by the polychromaticity of the radiation used. This will be discussed in Chapter 4.) His invention also showed that it is possible to process a very large number of measurements (now approaching a million) with fairly complex mathematical operations, and still get an image that is incredibly accurate. The success of x-ray CT has naturally led to research aimed at extending this mode of image formation to ultrasound and microwave sources.

The idea of filtered backprojection was first advanced by Bracewell and Riddle [Bra67] and later independently by Ramachandran and Lakshminarayanan [Ram71]. The superiority of the filtered backprojection algorithm over

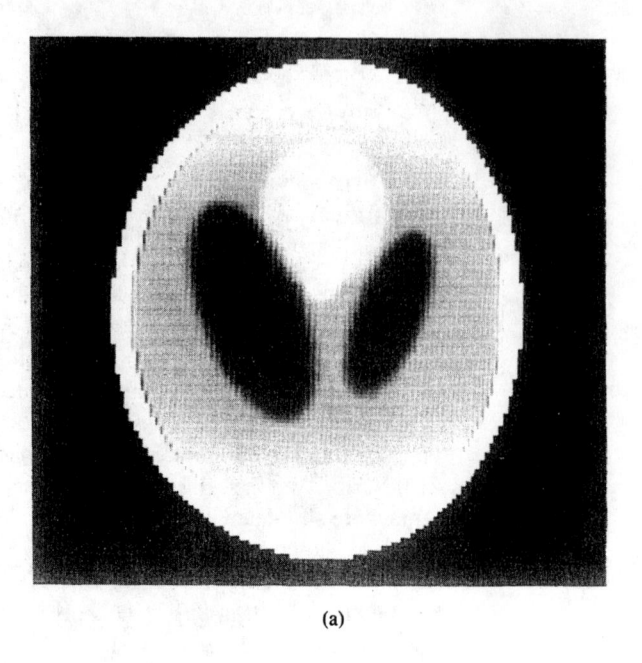

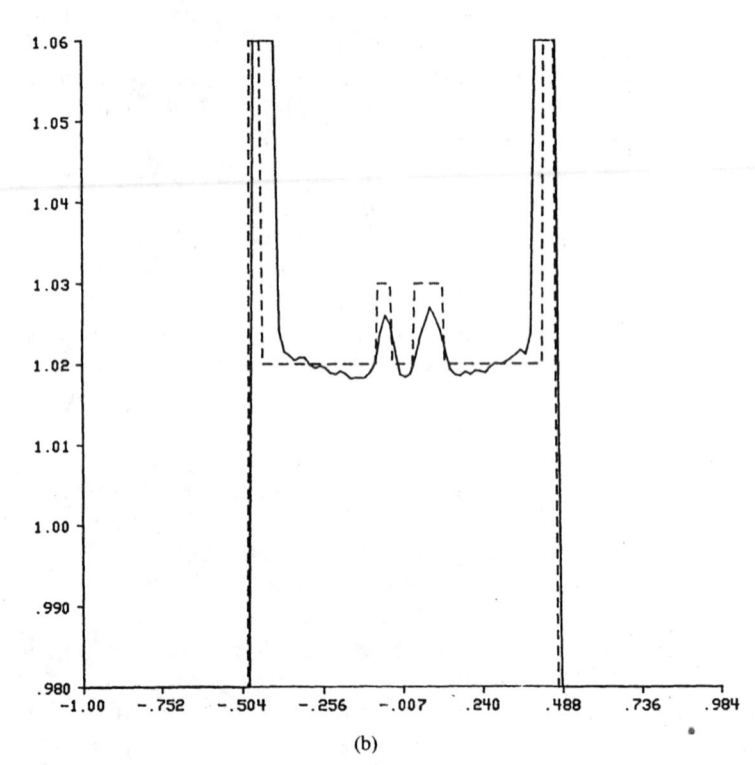

Fig. 3.38: *(a) Cone beam algorithm reconstruction of plane B in Fig. 3.36. (b) Plot of the y = −0.605 line in the reconstruction compared to the original. (From [Kak86].)*

108   COMPUTERIZED TOMOGRAPHIC IMAGING

(a)

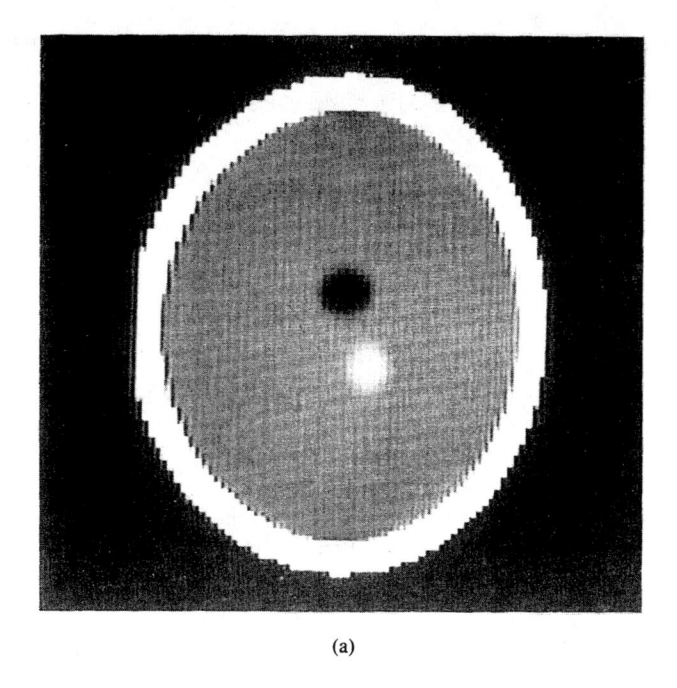

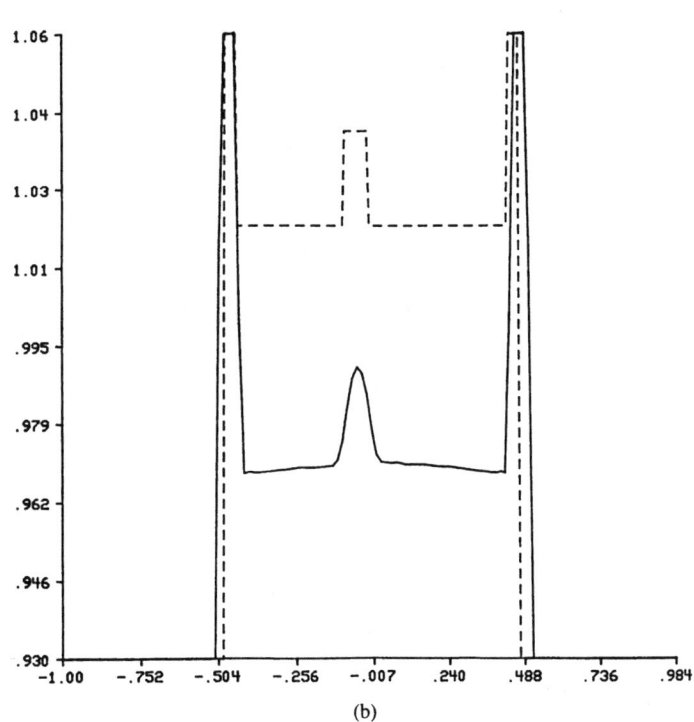

Fig. 3.39: *(a) Cone beam algorithm reconstruction of plane A in Fig. 3.36. (b) Plot of the y = −0.105 line in the reconstruction compared to the original. (From [Kak86].)*

(b)

ALGORITHMS FOR RECONSTRUCTION WITH NONDIFFRACTING SOURCES

the algebraic techniques was first demonstrated by Shepp and Logan [She74]. Its development for fan beam data was first made by Lakshminarayanan [Lak75] for the equispaced collinear detectors case and later extended by Herman and Naparstek [Her77] for the case of equiangular rays. The fan beam algorithm derivation presented here was first developed by Scudder [Scu78]. Many authors [Bab77], [Ken79], [Kwo77], [Lew79], [Tan75] have proposed variations on the filter functions of the filtered backprojection algorithms discussed in this chapter. The reader is referred particularly to [Ken79], [Lew79] for ways to speed up the filtering of the projection data by using binary approximations and/or inserting zeros in the unit sample response of the filter function. Images may also be reconstructed from fan beam data by first sorting them into parallel projection data. Fast algorithms for ray sorting of fan beam data have been developed by Wang [Wan77], Dreike and Boyd [Dre77], Peters and Lewitt [Pet77], and Dines and Kak [Din76]. The reader is referred to [Nah81] for a filtered backprojection algorithm for reconstructions from data generated by using very narrow angle fan beams that rotate *and* traverse *continuously* around the object. The reader is also referred to [Hor78], [Hor79] for algorithms for nonuniformly sampled projection data, and to [Bra67], [Lew78], [Opp75], [Sat80], [Tam81] for reconstructions from incomplete and limited projections. Full three-dimensional reconstructions have been discussed in [Chi79], [Chi80], [Smi85]. We have also not discussed the circular harmonic transform method of image reconstruction as proposed by Hansen [Han81a], [Han81b].

Tomographic imaging may also be accomplished, although less accurately, by direct Fourier inversion, instead of the filtered backprojection method presented in this chapter. This was first shown by Bracewell [Bra56] for radioastronomy, and later independently by DeRosier and Klug [DeR68] in electron microscopy and Rowley [Row69] in optical holography. Several workers who applied this method to radiography include Tretiak *et al.* [Tre69], Bates and Peters [Bat71], and Mersereau and Oppenheim [Mer74]. In order to utilize two-dimensional FFT algorithms for image formation, the direct Fourier approach calls for frequency domain interpolation from a polar grid to a rectangular grid. For some recent methods to minimize the resulting interpolation error, the reader is referred to [Sta81]. Recently Wernecke and D'Addario [Wer77] have proposed a maximum-entropy approach to direct Fourier inversion. Their procedure is especially applicable if for some reason the projection data are insufficient.

3.8 References

[Bab77]   N. Baba and K. Murata, "Filtering for image reconstruction from projections," *J. Opt. Soc. Amer.*, vol. 67, pp. 662-668, 1977.
[Bat71]   R. H. T. Bates and T. M. Peters, "Towards improvements in tomography," *New Zealand J. Sci.*, vol. 14, pp. 883-896, 1971.
[Boy83]   D. P. Boyd and M. J. Lipton, "Cardiac computed tomography," *Proc. IEEE*, vol. 71, pp. 298-307, Mar. 1983.

[Bra56] R. N. Bracewell, "Strip integration in radio astronomy," *Aust. J. Phys.*, vol. 9, pp. 198–217, 1956.

[Bra67] R. N. Bracewell and A. C. Riddle, "Inversion of fan-beam scans in radio astronomy," *Astrophys. J.*, vol. 150, pp. 427–434, Nov. 1967.

[Chi79] M. Y. Chiu, H. H. Barrett, R. G. Simpson, C. Chou, J. W. Arendt, and G. R. Gindi, "Three dimensional radiographic imaging with a restricted view angle," *J. Opt. Soc. Amer.*, vol. 69, pp. 1323–1330, Oct. 1979.

[Chi80] M. Y. Chiu, H. H. Barrett, and R. G. Simpson, "Three dimensional reconstruction from planar projections," *J. Opt. Soc. Amer.*, vol. 70, pp. 755–762, July 1980.

[Cro70] R. A. Crowther, D. J. DeRosier, and A. Klug, "The reconstruction of a three-dimensional structure from projections and its applications to electron microscopy," *Proc. Roy. Soc. London*, vol. A317, pp. 319–340, 1970.

[DeR68] D. J. DeRosier and A. Klug, "Reconstruction of three dimensional structures from electron micrographs," *Nature*, vol. 217, pp. 130–134, Jan. 1968.

[Din76] K. A. Dines and A. C. Kak, "Measurement and reconstruction of ultrasonic parameters for diagnostic imaging," Research Rep. TR-EE 77-4, School of Electrical Engineering, Purdue Univ., Lafayette, IN, Dec. 1976.

[Dre77] P. Dreike and D. P. Boyd, "Convolution reconstruction of fan-beam reconstructions," *Comp. Graph. Image Proc.*, vol. 5, pp. 459–469, 1977.

[Fel84] L. A. Feldkamp, L. C. Davis, and J. W. Kress, "Practical cone-beam algorithm," *J. Opt. Soc. Amer.*, vol. 1, pp. 612–619, June 1984.

[Ham77] R. W. Hamming, *Digital Filters*. Englewood Cliffs, NJ: Prentice-Hall, 1977.

[Han81a] E. W. Hansen, "Theory of circular image reconstruction," *J. Opt. Soc. Amer.*, vol. 71, pp. 304–308, Mar. 1981.

[Han81b] ——, "Circular harmonic image reconstruction: Experiments," *Appl. Opt.*, vol. 20, pp. 2266–2274, July 1981.

[Her77] G. T. Herman and A. Naparstek, "Fast image reconstruction based on a Radon inversion formula appropriate for rapidly collected data," *SIAM J. Appl. Math.*, vol. 33, pp. 511–533, Nov. 1977.

[Hor78] B. K. P. Horn, "Density reconstruction using arbitrary ray sampling schemes," *Proc. IEEE*, vol. 66, pp. 551–562, May 1978.

[Hor79] ——, "Fan-beam reconstruction methods," *Proc. IEEE*, vol. 67, pp. 1616–1623, 1979.

[Hou72] G. N. Hounsfield, "A method of and apparatus for examination of a body by radiation such as x-ray or gamma radiation," Patent Specification 1283915, The Patent Office, 1972.

[Jak76] C. V. Jakowatz, Jr. and A. C. Kak, "Computerized tomography using x-rays and ultrasound," Research Rep. TR-EE 76-26, School of Electrical Engineering, Purdue Univ., Lafayette, IN, 1976.

[Kak79] A. C. Kak, "Computerized tomography with x-ray emission and ultrasound sources," *Proc. IEEE*, vol. 67, pp. 1245–1272, 1979.

[Kak85] ——, "Tomographic imaging with diffracting and non-diffracting sources," in *Array Signal Processing*, S. Haykin, Ed. Englewood Cliffs, NJ: Prentice-Hall, 1985.

[Kak86] A. C. Kak and B. Roberts, "Image reconstruction from projections," in *Handbook of Pattern Recognition and Image Processing*, T. Y. Young and K. S. Fu, Eds. New York, NY: Academic Press, 1986.

[Kea78] P. N. Keating, "More accurate interpolation using discrete Fourier transforms," *IEEE Trans. Acoust. Speech Signal Processing*, vol. ASSP-26, pp. 368–369, 1978.

[Ken79] S. K. Kenue and J. F. Greenleaf, "Efficient convolution kernels for computerized tomography," *Ultrason. Imaging*, vol. 1, pp. 232–244, 1979.

[Kwo77] Y. S. Kwoh, I. S. Reed, and T. K. Truong, "A generalized $|w|$-filter for 3-D reconstruction," *IEEE Trans. Nucl. Sci.*, vol. NS-24, pp. 1990–1998, 1977.

[Lak75] A. V. Lakshminarayanan, "Reconstruction from divergent ray data," Tech. Rep. 92, Dept. of Computer Science, State Univ. of New York at Buffalo, 1975.

[Lew78] R. M. Lewitt and R. H. T. Bates, "Image reconstruction from projections," *Optik*, vol. 50, pp. 19–33 (Part I), pp. 85–109 (Part II), pp. 189–204 (Part III), pp. 269–278 (Part IV), 1978.

[Lew79] R. M. Lewitt, "Ultra-fast convolution approximation for computerized tomography," *IEEE Trans. Nucl. Sci.*, vol. NS-26, pp. 2678–2681, 1979.

[Mer74] R. M. Mersereau and A. V. Oppenheim, "Digital reconstruction of multidimensional signals from their projections," *Proc. IEEE*, vol. 62, pp. 1319–1338, 1974.

[Nah81] D. Nahamoo, C. R. Crawford, and A. C. Kak, "Design constraints and reconstruction algorithms for transverse-continuous-rotate CT scanners," *IEEE Trans. Biomed. Eng.*, vol. BME-28, pp. 79–97, 1981.

[Nap80] A. Naparstek, "Short-scan fan-beam algorithms for CT," *IEEE Trans. Nucl. Sci.*, vol. NS-27, 1980.

[Opp75] B. E. Oppenheim, "Reconstruction tomography from incomplete projections," in *Reconstruction Tomography in Diagnostic Radiology and Nuclear Medicine*, M. M. Ter Pogossian et al., Eds. Baltimore, MD: University Park Press, 1975.

[Pan83] S. X. Pan and A. C. Kak, "A computational study of reconstruction algorithms for diffraction tomography: Interpolation vs. filtered-backpropagation," *IEEE Trans. Acoust. Speech Signal Processing*, vol. ASSP-31, pp. 1262–1275, Oct. 1983.

[Par82a] D. L. Parker, "Optimal short-scan convolution reconstruction for fanbeam CT," *Med. Phys.*, vol. 9, pp. 254–257, Mar./Apr. 1982.

[Par82b] ——, "Optimization of short scan convolution reconstruction for fan-beam CT," in *Proc. International Workshop on Physics and Engineering in Medical Imaging*, Mar. 1982, pp. 199–202.

[Pet77] T. M. Peters and R. M. Lewitt, "Computed tomography with fan-beam geometry," *J. Comput. Assist. Tomog.*, vol. 1, pp. 429–436, 1977.

[Ram71] G. N. Ramachandran and A. V. Lakshminarayanan, "Three dimensional reconstructions from radiographs and electron micrographs: Application of convolution instead of Fourier transforms," *Proc. Nat. Acad. Sci.*, vol. 68, pp. 2236–2240, 1971.

[Rob83] R. A. Robb, E. A. Hoffman, L. J. Sinak, L. D. Harris, and E. L. Ritman, "High-speed three-dimensional x-ray computed tomography: The dynamic spatial reconstructor," *Proc. IEEE*, vol. 71, pp. 308–319, Mar. 1983.

[Ros82] A. Rosenfeld and A. C. Kak, *Digital Picture Processing*, 2nd ed. New York, NY: Academic Press, 1982.

[Row69] P. D. Rowley, "Quantitative interpretation of three dimensional weakly refractive phase objects using holographic interferometry," *J. Opt. Soc. Amer.*, vol. 59, pp. 1496–1498, Nov. 1969.

[Sat80] T. Sato, S. J. Norton, M. Linzer, O. Ikeda, and M. Hirama, "Tomographic image reconstruction from limited projections using iterative revisions in image and transform spaces," *Appl. Opt.*, vol. 20, pp. 395–399, Feb. 1980.

[Sch73] R. W. Schafer and L. R. Rabiner, "A digital signal processing approach to interpolation," *Proc. IEEE*, vol. 61, pp. 692–702, 1973.

[Scu78] H. J. Scudder, "Introduction to computer aided tomography," *Proc. IEEE*, vol. 66, pp. 628–637, June 1978.

[She74] L. A. Shepp and B. F. Logan, "The Fourier reconstruction of a head section," *IEEE Trans. Nucl. Sci.*, vol. NS-21, pp. 21–43, 1974.

[Smi85] B. D. Smith, "Image reconstruction from cone-beam projections: Necessary and sufficient conditions and reconstruction methods," *IEEE Trans. Med. Imaging*, vol. MI-4, pp. 14–25, Mar. 1985.

[Sta81] H. Stark, J. W. Woods, I. Paul, and R. Hingorani, "Direct Fourier reconstruction in computer tomography," *IEEE Trans. Acoust. Speech Signal Processing*, vol. ASSP-29, pp. 237–244, 1981.

[Tam81] K. C. Tam and V. Perez-Mendez, "Tomographical imaging with limited angle input," *J. Opt. Soc. Amer.*, vol. 71, pp. 582–592, May 1981.

[Tan75] E. Tanaka and T. A. Iinuma, "Correction functions for optimizing the reconstructed image in transverse section scan," *Phys. Med. Biol.*, vol. 20, pp. 789–798, 1975.

[Tre69] O. Tretiak, M. Eden, and M. Simon, "Internal structures for three dimensional images," in *Proc. 8th Int. Conf. on Med. Biol. Eng.*, Chicago, IL, 1969.

[Wan77] L. Wang, "Cross-section reconstruction with a fan-beam scanning geometry," *IEEE Trans. Comput.*, vol. C-26, pp. 264–268, Mar. 1977.

[Wer77] S. J. Wernecke and L. R. D'Addario, "Maximum entropy image reconstruction," *IEEE Trans. Comput.*, vol. C-26, pp. 351–364, 1977.

4 Measurement of Projection Data— The Nondiffracting Case

The mathematical algorithms for tomographic reconstructions described in Chapter 3 are based on projection data. These projections can represent, for example, the attenuation of x-rays through an object as in conventional x-ray tomography, the decay of radioactive nucleoids in the body as in emission tomography, or the refractive index variations as in ultrasonic tomography.

This chapter will discuss the measurement of projection data with energy that travels in straight lines through objects. This is always the case when a human body is illuminated with x-rays and is a close approximation to what happens when ultrasonic tomography is used for the imaging of soft biological tissues (e.g., the female breast).

Projection data, by their very nature, are a result of interaction between the radiation used for imaging and the substance of which the object is composed. To a first approximation, such interactions can be modeled as measuring integrals of some characteristic of the object. A simple example of this is the attenuation a beam of x-rays undergoes as it travels through an object. A line integral of x-ray attenuation, as we will show in this chapter, is the log of the ratio of monochromatic x-ray photons that enter the object to those that leave.

A second example of projection data being equal to line integrals is the propagation of a sound wave as it travels through an object. For a narrow beam of sound, the total time it takes to travel through an object is a line integral because it is the summation of the time it takes to travel through each small part of the object.

In both the x-ray and the ultrasound cases, the measured data correspond only approximately to a line integral. The attenuation of an x-ray beam is dependent on the energy of each photon and since the x-rays used for imaging normally contain a range of energies the total attenuation is a more complicated sum of the attenuation at each point along the line. In the ultrasound case, the errors are caused by the fact that sound waves almost never travel through an object in a straight line and thus the measured time corresponds to some unknown curved path through the object. Fortunately, for many important practical applications, approximation of these curved paths by straight lines is acceptable.

In this chapter we will discuss a number of different types of tomography, each with a different approach to the measurement of projection data. An excellent review of these and many other applications of CT imaging is provided in [Bat83]. The physical limitations of each type of tomography to be discussed here are also presented in [Mac83].

4.1 X-Ray Tomography

Since in x-ray tomography the projections consist of line integrals of the attenuation coefficient, it is important to appreciate the nature of this parameter. Consider that we have a parallel beam of x-ray photons propagating through a homogeneous slab of some material as shown in Fig. 4.1. Since we have assumed that the photons are traveling along paths parallel to each other, there is no loss of beam intensity due to beam divergence. However, the beam does attenuate due to photons either being absorbed by the atoms of the material, or being scattered away from their original directions of travel.

For the range of photon energies most commonly encountered for diagnostic imaging (from 20 to 150 keV), the mechanisms responsible for these two contributions to attenuation are the photoelectric and the Compton effects, respectively. Photoelectric absorption consists of an x-ray photon imparting all its energy to a tightly bound inner electron in an atom. The electron uses some of this acquired energy to overcome the binding energy within its shell, the rest appearing as the kinetic energy of the thus freed electron. The Compton scattering, on the other hand, consists of the interaction of the x-ray photon with either a free electron, or one that is only loosely bound in one of the outer shells of an atom. As a result of this interaction, the x-ray photon is deflected from its original direction of travel with some loss of energy, which is gained by the electron.

Both the photoelectric and the Compton effects are energy dependent. This means that the probability of a given photon being lost from the original beam due to either absorption or scatter is a function of the energy of that photon. Photoelectric absorption is much more energy dependent than the Compton scatter effect—we will discuss this point in greater detail in the next section.

4.1.1 Monochromatic X-Ray Projections

Consider an incremental thickness of the slab shown in Fig. 4.1. We will assume that N monochromatic photons cross the lower boundary of this layer during some arbitrary measurement time interval and that only $N + \Delta N$ emerge from the top side (the numerical value of ΔN will obviously be negative), these $N + \Delta N$ photons being unaffected by either absorption or scatter and therefore propagating in their original direction of travel. *If all the photons possess the same energy,* then physical considerations that we will not go into dictate that ΔN satisfy the following relationship [Ter67]:

$$\frac{\Delta N}{N} \cdot \frac{1}{\Delta x} = -\tau - \sigma \qquad (1)$$

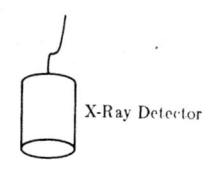

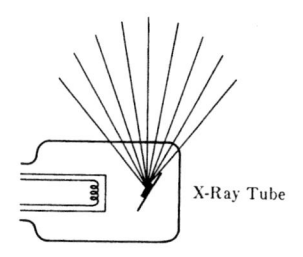

Fig. 4.1: *An x-ray tube is shown here illuminating a homogeneous material with a beam of x-rays. The beam is measured on the far side of the object to determine the attenuation of the object.*

where τ and σ represent the photon loss rates (on a per unit distance basis) due to the photoelectric and the Compton effects, respectively. For our purposes we will at this time lump these two together and represent the above equation as

$$\frac{\Delta N}{N} \cdot \frac{1}{\Delta x} = -\mu. \qquad (2)$$

In the limit, as Δx goes to zero we obtain the differential equation

$$\frac{1}{N} dN = -\mu \, dx \qquad (3)$$

which can be solved by integrating across the thickness of the slab

$$\int_{N_0}^{N} \frac{dN}{N} = -\mu \int_{0}^{x} dx \qquad (4)$$

where N_0 is the number of photons that enter the object. The number of photons as a function of the position within the slab is then given by

$$\ln N - \ln N_0 = -\mu x \qquad (5)$$

or

$$N(x) = N_0 e^{-\mu x}. \qquad (6)$$

The constant μ is called the attenuation coefficient of the material. Here we assumed that μ is constant over the interval of integration.

Now consider the experiment illustrated in Fig. 4.2, where we have shown

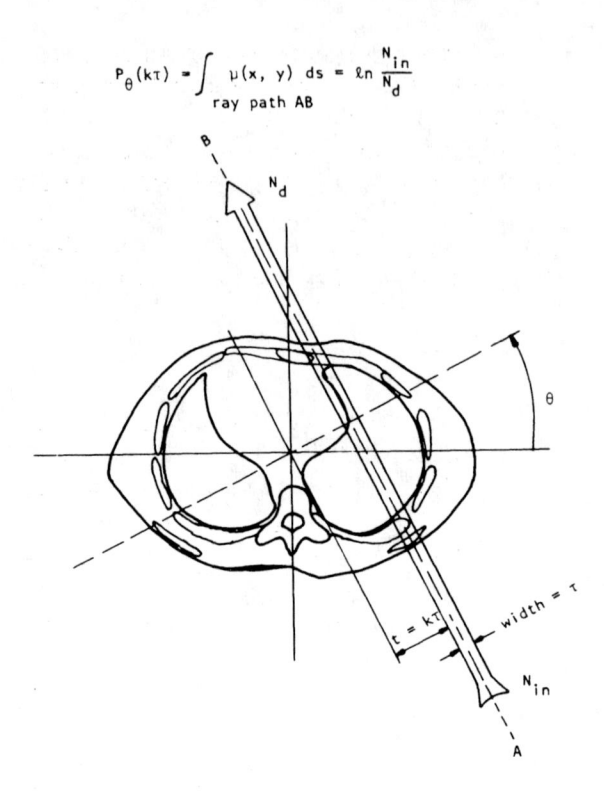

$$P_\theta(k\tau) = \int_{\text{ray path AB}} \mu(x, y)\, ds = \ln \frac{N_{in}}{N_d}$$

Fig. 4.2: *A parallel beam of x-rays is shown propagating through a cross section of the human body. (From [Kak79].)*

a cross section of the human body being illuminated by a single beam of x-rays. If we confine our attention to the cross-sectional plane drawn in the figure, we may now consider μ to be a function of two space coordinates, x and y, and therefore denote the attenuation coefficient by $\mu(x, y)$. Let N_{in} be the total number of photons that enter the object (within the time interval of experimental measurement) through the beam from side A. And let N_d be the total number of photons exiting (within the same time interval) through the beam on side B. When the width, τ, of the beam is sufficiently small, reasoning similar to what was used for the one-dimensional case now leads to the following relationship between the numbers N_d and N_{in} [Hal74], [Ter67]:

$$N_d = N_{in} \exp\left[-\int_{\text{ray}} \mu(x, y)\, ds\right] \tag{7}$$

or, equivalently,

$$\int_{\text{ray}} \mu(x, y)\, ds = \ln \frac{N_{in}}{N_d} \tag{8}$$

where ds is an element of length and where the integration is carried out along line AB shown in the figure. The left-hand side precisely constitutes a ray integral for a projection. Therefore, measurements like $\ln (N_{in}/N_d)$ taken for different rays at different angles may be used to generate projection data for the function $\mu(x, y)$. *We would like to reiterate that this is strictly true only under the assumption that the x-ray beam consists of monoenergetic photons.* This assumption is necessary because the linear attenuation coefficient is, in general, a function of photon energy. Other assumptions needed for this result include: detectors that are insensitive to scatter (see Section 4.1.4), a very narrow beam so there are no partial volume effects, and a very small aperture (see Chapter 5).

4.1.2 Measurement of Projection Data with Polychromatic Sources

In practice, the x-ray sources used for medical imaging do not produce monoenergetic photons. (Although by using the notion of beam hardening explained later, one could filter the x-ray beam to produce x-ray photons of almost the same energy. However, this would greatly reduce the number of photons available for the purpose of imaging, and the resulting degradation in the signal-to-noise ratio would be unacceptable for practically all purposes.) Fig. 4.3 shows an example of an experimentally measured x-ray tube spectrum taken from Epp and Weiss [Epp66] for an anode voltage of 105 kvp. When the energy in a beam of x-rays is not monoenergetic, (7) does not hold, and must be replaced by

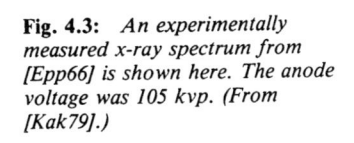

$$N_d = \int S_{in}(E) \exp\left[-\int \mu(x, y, E) \, ds\right] dE \qquad (9)$$

Fig. 4.3: *An experimentally measured x-ray spectrum from [Epp66] is shown here. The anode voltage was 105 kvp. (From [Kak79].)*

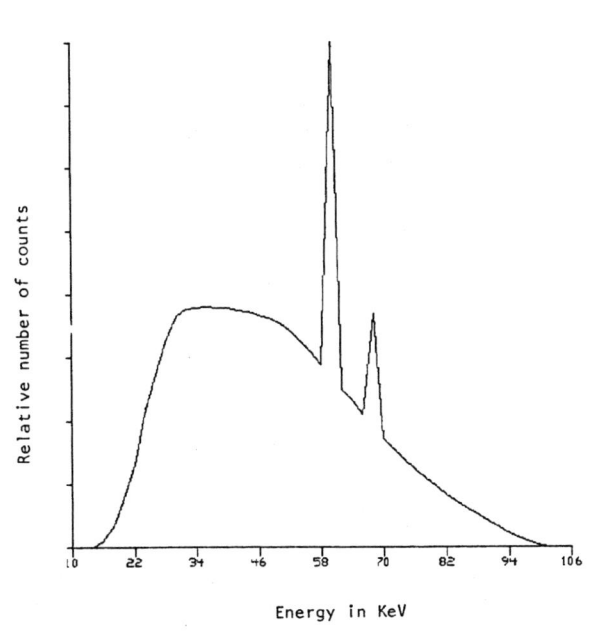

where $S_{in}(E)$ represents the incident photon number density (also called energy spectral density of the incident photons). $S_{in}(E)\,dE$ is the total number of incident photons in the energy range E and $E + dE$. This equation incorporates the fact that the linear attenuation coefficient, μ, at a point (x, y) is also a function of energy. The reader may note that if we were to measure the energy spectrum of exiting photons (on side B in Fig. 4.2) it would be given by

$$S_{exit}(E) = S_{in}(E) \exp\left[-\int \mu(x, y, E)\,ds\right]. \tag{10}$$

In discussing polychromatic x-ray photons one has to bear in mind that there are basically three different types of detectors [McC75]. The output of a detector may be proportional to the total number of photons incident on it, or it may be proportional to total photon energy, or it may respond to energy deposition per unit mass. Most counting-type detectors are of the first type, most scintillation-type detectors are of the second type, and most ionization detectors are of the third type. In determining the output of a detector one must also take into account the dependence of detector sensitivity on photon energy. In this work we will assume for the sake of simplicity that the detector sensitivity is constant over the energy range of interest.

In the energy ranges used for diagnostic examinations the linear attenuation coefficient for many tissues decreases with energy. For a propagating polychromatic x-ray beam this causes the low energy photons to be preferentially absorbed, so that the remaining beam becomes proportionately richer in high energy photons. In other words, the mean energy associated with the exit spectrum, $S_{exit}(E)$, is higher than that associated with the incident spectrum, $S_{in}(E)$. This phenomenon is called *beam hardening*.

Given the fact that x-ray sources in CT scanning are polychromatic and that the attenuation coefficient is energy dependent, the following question arises: What parameter does an x-ray CT scanner reconstruct? To answer this question McCullough [McC74], [McC75] has introduced the notion of *effective energy of a CT scanner*. It is defined as that monochromatic energy at which a given material will exhibit the same attenuation coefficient as is measured by the scanner. McCullough *et al.* [McC74] showed empirically that for the original EMI head scanner the effective energy was 72 keV when the x-ray tube was operated at 120 kV. (See [Mil78] for a practical procedure for determining the effective energy of a CT scanner.) The concept of effective energy is valid only under the condition that the exit spectra are the same for all the rays used in the measurement of projection data. (*When the exit spectra are not the same, the result is the appearance of beam hardening artifacts discussed in the next subsection.*) It follows from the work of McCullough [McC75] that it is a good assumption that the measured attenuation coefficient $\mu_{measured}$ at a point in a cross section is related to the actual attenuation coefficient $\mu(E)$ at that point by

$$\mu_{measured} \approx \frac{\int \mu(E) S_{exit}(E)\, dE}{\int S_{exit}(E)\, dE}. \tag{11}$$

This expression applies only when the output of the detectors is proportional to the total *number* of photons incident on them. McCullough has given similar expressions when detectors measure total photon *energy* and when they respond to total *energy deposition/unit mass*. Effective energy of a scanner depends not only on the x-ray tube spectrum but also on the nature of photon detection.

Although it is customary to say that a CT scanner calculates the linear attenuation coefficient of tissue (at some effective energy), the numbers actually put out by the computer attached to the scanner are integers that usually range in values from -1000 to 3000. These integers have been given the name Hounsfield units and are denoted by HU. The relationship between the linear attenuation coefficient and the corresponding Hounsfield unit is

$$H = \frac{\mu - \mu_{water}}{\mu_{water}} \times 1000 \tag{12}$$

where μ_{water} is the attenuation coefficient of water and the values of both μ and μ_{water} are taken at the effective energy of the scanner. The value $H = 0$ corresponds to water; and the value $H = -1000$ corresponds to $\mu = 0$, which is assumed to be the attenuation coefficient of air. Clearly, if a scanner were perfectly calibrated it would give a value of zero for water and -1000 for air. Under actual operating conditions this is rarely the case. However, if the assumption of linearity between the measured Hounsfield units and the actual value of the attenuation coefficient (at the effective energy of the scanner) is valid, one may use the following relationship to convert the measured number H_m into the ideal number H:

$$H = \frac{H_m - H_{m,\,water}}{H_{m,\,water} - H_{m,\,air}} \times 1000 \tag{13}$$

where $H_{m,\,water}$ and $H_{m,\,air}$ are, respectively, the measured Hounsfield units for water and air. [This relationship may easily be derived by assuming that $\mu = aH_m + b$, calculating a and b in terms of $H_{m,\,water}$, $H_{m,\,air}$, and μ_{water}, and then using (12).]

Brooks [Bro77a] has used (11) to show that the Hounsfield unit H at a point in a CT image may be expressed as

$$H = \frac{H_c + H_p Q}{1 + Q} \tag{14}$$

where H_c and H_p are the Compton and photoelectric coefficients of the material being measured, expressed in Hounsfield units. The parameter Q, called the spectral factor, depends only upon the x-ray spectrum used and may be obtained by performing a scan on a calibrating material. A noteworthy feature of H_c and H_p is that *they are both energy independent.* Equation (14) leads to the important result that if two different CT images are reconstructed using two different incident spectra (resulting in two different values of Q), from the resulting two measured Hounsfield units for a given point in the cross section, one may obtain some degree of chemical identification of the material at that point from H_c and H_p. Instead of performing two different scans, one may also perform only one scan with split detectors for this purpose [Bro78a].

4.1.3 Polychromaticity Artifacts in X-Ray CT

Beam hardening artifacts, whose cause was discussed above, are most noticeable in the CT images of the head, and involve two different types of distortions. Many investigators [Bro76], [DiC78], [Gad75], [McD77] have shown that beam hardening causes an elevation in CT numbers for tissues close to the skull bone. To illustrate this artifact we have presented in Fig. 4.4 a computer simulation reconstruction of a water phantom inside a skull. The projection data were generated on the computer using the 105-kvp x-ray tube spectrum (Fig. 4.3) of Epp and Weiss [Epp66]. The energy dependence of the attenuation coefficients of the skull bone was taken from an ICRU report [ICR64] and that of water was taken from Phelps *et al.* [Phe75]. Reconstruction from these data was done using the filtered backprojection algorithm (Chapter 3) with 101 projections and 101 parallel rays in each projection.

Note the "whitening" effect near the skull in Fig. 4.4(a). This is more quantitatively illustrated in Fig. 4.4(b) where the elevation of the reconstructed values near the skull bone is quite evident. (When CT imaging was in its infancy, this whitening effect was mistaken for gray matter of the cerebral cortex.) For comparison, we have also shown in Fig. 4.4(b) the reconstruction values along a line through the center of the phantom obtained when the projection data were generated for monochromatic x-rays.

The other artifact caused by polychromaticity is the appearance of streaks and flares in the vicinity of thick bones and between bones [Due78], [Jos78], [Kij78]. (Note that streaks can also be caused by aliasing [Bro78b], [Cra78].) This artifact is illustrated in Fig. 4.5. The phantom used was a skull with water and five circular bones inside. Polychromatic projection data were generated, as before, using the 105-kvp x-ray spectrum. The reconstruction using these data is shown in Fig. 4.5(a) with the same number of rays and projections as before. Note the wide dark streaks between the bones inside the skull. Compare this image with the reconstruction shown in Fig. 4.5(b) for the case when x-rays are monochromatic. In x-ray CT of the head, similar dark and wide streaks appear in those cross sections that include the petrous bones, and are sometimes called the *interpetrous lucency artifact.*

(a)

(b)

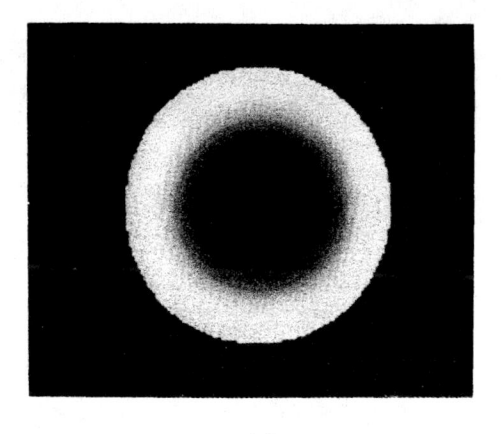

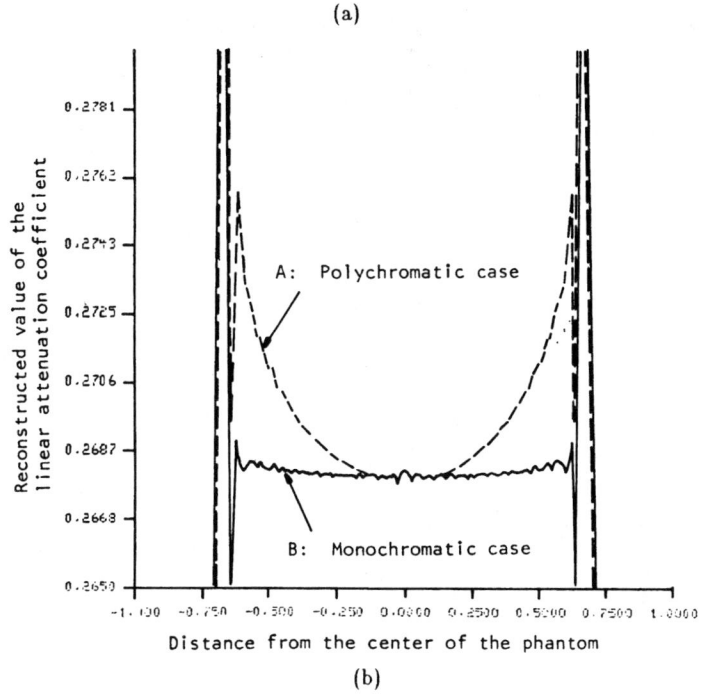

Fig. 4.4: *This reconstruction shows the effect of polychromaticity artifacts in a simulated skull. (a) shows the reconstructed image using the spectrum in Fig. 4.3, while (b) is the center line of the reconstruction for both the polychromatic and monochromatic cases. (From [Kak79].)*

Various schemes have been suggested for making these artifacts less apparent. These fall into three categories: 1) preprocessing of projection data, 2) postprocessing of the reconstructed image, and 3) dual-energy imaging.

Preprocessing techniques are based on the following rationale: If the assumption of the photons being monoenergetic were indeed valid, a ray integral would then be given by (8). For a homogeneous absorber of attenuation coefficient μ, this implies

$$\mu \ell = \ln \frac{N_{\text{in}}}{N_d} \tag{15}$$

Fig. 4.5: *Hard objects such as bones also can cause streaks in the reconstructed image. (a) Reconstruction from polychromatic projection data of a phantom that consists of a skull with five circular bones inside. The rest of the "tissue" inside the skull is water. The wide dark streaks are caused by the polychromaticity of x-rays. The polychromatic projections were simulated using the spectrum in Fig. 4.3. (b) Reconstruction of the same phantom as in (a) using projections generated with monochromatic x-rays. The variations in the gray levels outside the bone areas within the skull are less than 0.1% of the mean value. The image was displayed with a narrow window to bring out these variations. Note the absence of streaks shown in (a). (From [Kak79].)*

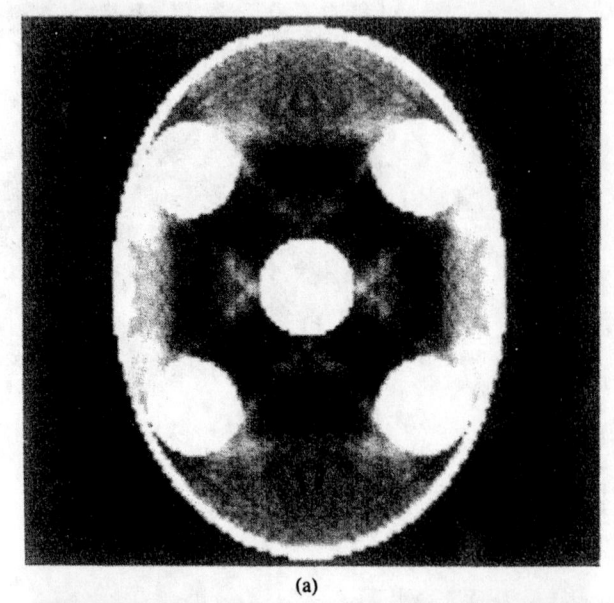

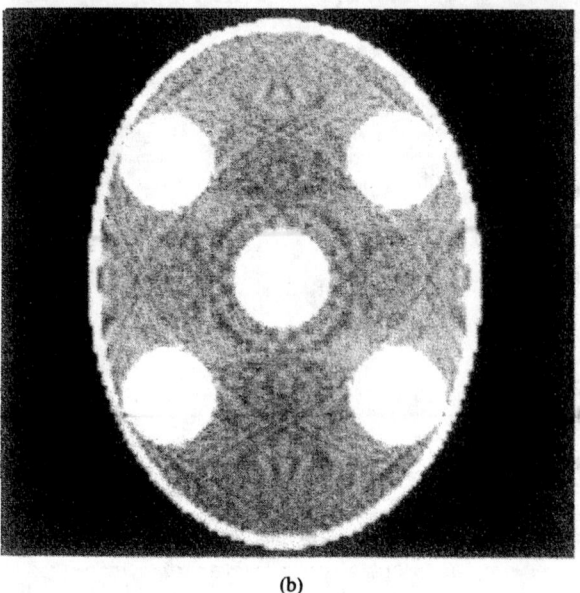

(a)

(b)

where ℓ is the thickness of the absorber. This equation says that under ideal conditions the experimental measurement ln (N_{in}/N_d) should be linearly proportional to the absorber thickness. This is depicted in Fig. 4.6. However, under actual conditions a result like the solid curve in the figure is obtained. Most preprocessing corrections simply specify the selection of an "appropriate" absorber and then experimentally obtain the solid curve in Fig. 4.6.

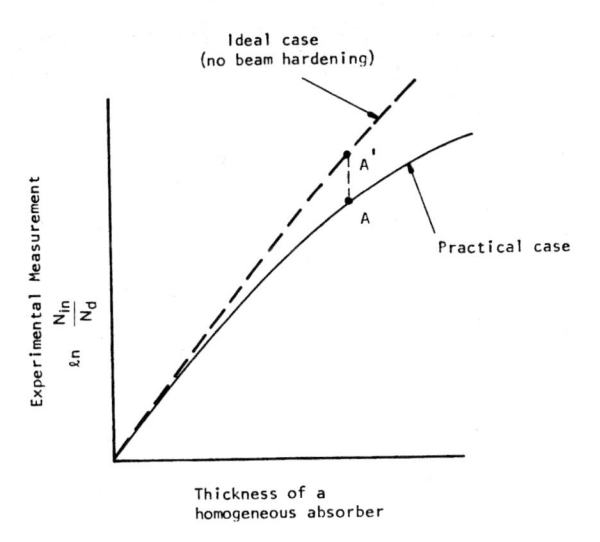

Fig. 4.6: *The solid curve shows that the experimental measurement of a ray integral depends nonlinearly on the thickness of a homogeneous absorber. (Adapted from [Kak79].)*

Thus, should a ray integral be measured at A, it is simply increased to A' for tomographic reconstruction. This procedure has the advantage of very rapid implementation and works well for soft-tissue cross sections because differences in the composition of various soft tissues are minimal (they are all approximately water-like from the standpoint of x-ray attenuation). For preprocessing corrections see [Bro76], [McD75], [McD77], and for a technique that combines preprocessing with image deconvolution see [Cha78].

Preprocessing techniques usually fail when bone is present in a cross section. In such cases it is possible to postprocess the CT image to improve the reconstruction. In the iterative scheme one first does a reconstruction (usually incorporating the linearization correction mentioned above) from the projection data. This reconstruction is then thresholded to get an image that shows only the bone areas. This thresholded image is then "forward-projected" to determine the contribution made by bone to each ray integral in each projection. On the basis of this contribution a correction is applied to each ray integral. The resulting projection data are then backprojected again to form another estimate of the object. Joseph and Spital [Jos78] and Kijewski and Bjarngard [Kij78] have obtained very impressive results with this technique. A fast reprojection technique is described in [Cra86].

The dual-energy technique proposed by Alvarez and Macovski [Alv76a], [Due78] is theoretically the most elegant approach to eliminating the beam hardening artifacts. Their approach is based on modeling the energy dependence of the linear attenuation coefficient by

$$\mu(x, y, E) = a_1(x, y)g(E) + a_2(x, y)f_{KN}(E). \tag{16}$$

The part $a_1(x, y)g(E)$ describes the contribution made by photoelectric absorption to the attenuation at point (x, y); $a_1(x, y)$ incorporates the material parameters at (x, y) and $g(E)$ expresses the (material independent) energy dependence of this contribution. The function $g(E)$ is given by

$$g(E) = \frac{1}{E^3}. \qquad (17)$$

(See also Brooks and DiChiro [Bro77b]. They have concluded that $g(E) = E^{-2.8}$.) The second part of (16) given by $a_2(x, y)f_{KN}(E)$ gives the Compton scatter contribution to the attenuation. Again $a_2(x, y)$ depends upon the material properties, whereas $f_{KN}(E)$, the Klein–Nishina function, describes the (material independent) energy dependence of this contribution. The function $f_{KN}(E)$ is given by

$$f_{KN}(\alpha) = \frac{1+\alpha}{\alpha^2} \left[\frac{2(1+\alpha)}{1+2\alpha} - \frac{1}{\alpha} \ln(1+2\alpha) \right]$$
$$+ \frac{1}{2\alpha} \ln(1+2\alpha) - \frac{(1+3\alpha)}{(1+2\alpha)^2} \qquad (18)$$

with $\alpha = E/510.975$. The energy E is in kilo-electron volts.

The importance of (16) lies in the fact that all the energy dependence has been incorporated in the known and material independent functions $g(E)$ and $f_{KN}(E)$. Substituting this equation in (9) we get

$$N_d = \int S_0(E) \exp\left[-(A_1 g(E) + A_2 f_{KN}(E))\right] dE \qquad (19)$$

where

$$A_1 = \int_{\text{ray path}} a_1(x, y) \, ds \qquad (20)$$

and

$$A_2 = \int_{\text{ray path}} a_2(x, y) \, ds. \qquad (21)$$

A_1 and A_2 are, clearly, ray integrals for the functions $a_1(x, y)$ and $a_2(x, y)$. Now if we could somehow determine A_1 and A_2 for each ray, from this information the functions $a_1(x, y)$ and $a_2(x, y)$ could be separately reconstructed. And, once we know $a_1(x, y)$ and $a_2(x, y)$, using (16) *an attenuation coefficient tomogram could be presented at any energy, free from beam hardening artifacts.*

A few words about the determination of A_1 and A_2: Note that it is the intensity N_d that is measured by the detector. Now suppose instead of making one measurement we make two measurements for each ray path for two different source spectra. Let us call these measurements I_1 and I_2; then

$$I_1(A_1, A_2) = \int S_1(E) \exp\left[-(A_1 g(E) + A_2 f_{KN}(E))\right] dE \qquad (22)$$

and

$$I_2(A_1, A_2) = \int S_2(E) \exp\left[-(A_1 g(E) + A_2 f_{KN}(E))\right] dE \qquad (23)$$

which gives us two (integral) equations for the two unknowns A_1 and A_2. The two source spectra, $S_1(E)$ and $S_2(E)$, may for example be obtained by simply changing the tube voltage on the x-ray source or adding filtration to the incident beam. This, however, requires that two scans be made for each tomogram. In principle, one can obtain equivalent results from a single scan with split detectors [Bro78a] or by changing the tube voltage so that alternating projections are at different voltages. Alvarez and Macovski [Alv76b] have shown that statistical fluctuations in $a_1(x, y)$ and $a_2(x, y)$ caused by the measurement errors in I_1 and I_2 are small compared to the differences of these quantities for body tissues.

4.1.4 Scatter

X-ray scatter leads to another type of error in the measurement of a projection. Recall that an x-ray beam traveling through an object can be attenuated by photoelectric absorption or by scattering. Photoelectric absorption is energy dependent and leads to beam hardening as was discussed in the previous section. On the other hand, attenuation by scattering occurs because some of the original energy in the beam is deflected onto a new path. The scatter angle is random but generally more x-rays are scattered in the forward direction.

The only way to prevent scatter from leading to projection errors is to build detectors that are perfectly collimated. Thus any x-rays that aren't traveling in a straight line between the source and the detector are rejected. A perfectly collimated detector is especially difficult to build in a *fourth-generation*, fixed-detector scanner (to be discussed in Section 4.1.5). In this type of machine the detectors must be able to measure x-rays from a very large angle as the source rotates around the object.

X-ray scatter leads to artifacts in reconstruction because the effect changes with each projection. While the intensity of scattered x-rays is approximately constant for different rotations of the object, the intensity of the primary beam (at the detector) is not. Once the x-rays have passed through the collimator the detector simply sums the two intensities. For rays through the object where the primary intensity is very small, the effect of scatter will be large, while for other rays when the primary beam is large, scattered x-rays will not lead to much error. This is shown in Fig. 4.7 [Glo82], [Jos82].

For reasons mentioned above, the scattered energy causes larger errors in some projections than others. Thus instead of spreading the error energy over the entire image, there is a directional dependence that leads to streaks in reconstruction. This is shown in the reconstructions of Fig. 4.8.

Correcting for scatter is relatively easy compared to beam hardening. While it is possible to estimate the scatter intensity by mounting detectors

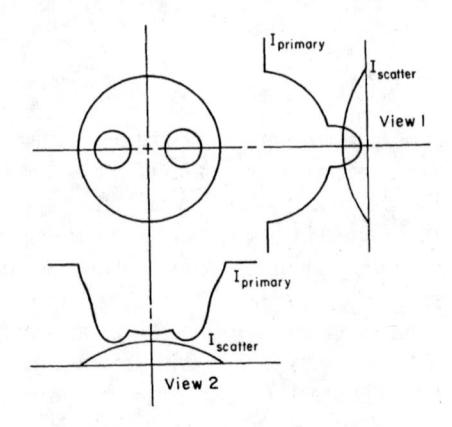

Fig. 4.7: *The effect of scatter on two different projections is shown here. For the projections where the intensity of the primary beam is high the scatter makes little difference. When the intensity of the scattered beam is high compared to the primary beam then large (relative) errors are seen.*

slightly out of the imaging plane, good results have been obtained by assuming a constant scatter intensity over the entire projection [Glo82].

4.1.5 Different Methods for Scanning

There are two scan configurations that lead to rapid data collection. These are i) fan beam rotational type (usually called the rotate-rotate or the third generation) and ii) fixed detector ring with a rotating source type (usually called the rotate-fixed or the fourth generation). As we will see later, both of these schemes use fan beam reconstruction concepts. While the reconstruction algorithms for a parallel beam machine are simpler, the time to scan with an x-ray source across an object and then rotate the entire source–detector arrangement for the next scan is usually too long. The time for scanning across the object can be reduced by using an array of sources, but only at great cost. Thus almost all CT machines in production today use a fan beam configuration.

In a (third-generation) fan beam rotation machine, a fan beam of x-rays is used to illuminate a multidetector array as shown in Fig. 4.9. Both the source and the detector array are mounted on a yoke which rotates continuously around the patient over 360°. Data collection time for such scanners ranges from 1 to 20 seconds. In this time more than 1000 projections may be taken. If the projections are taken "on the fly" there is a rotational smearing present in the data; however, it is usually so small that its effects are not noticeable in the final image. Most such scanners use fan beams with fan angles ranging from 30 to 60°. The detector bank usually has 500 to 700 or more detectors, and images are reconstructed on 256 × 256, 320 × 320, or 512 × 512 matrices.

There are two types of x-ray detectors commonly used: solid state and xenon gas ionization detectors. Three xenon ionization detectors, which are often used in third-generation scanners, are shown in Fig. 4.10. Each

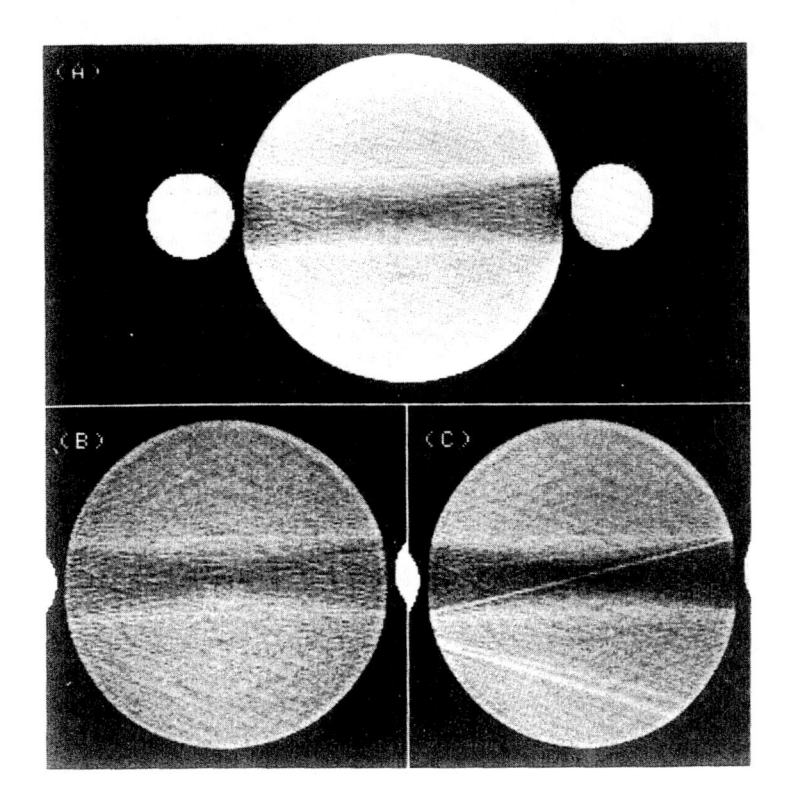

Fig. 4.8: *Reconstructions are shown from an x-ray phantom with 15-cm-diameter water and two 4-cm Teflon rods. (A) Without 120-kvp correction; (B) same with polynomial beam hardening correction; and (C) 120-kvp/80-kvp dual-energy reconstruction. Note that the artifacts remain after polychromaticity correction. (Reprinted with permission from [Glo82].)*

Fig. 4.9: *In a third-generation fan beam x-ray tomography machine a point source of x-rays and a detector array are rotated continuously around the patient. (From [Kak79].)*

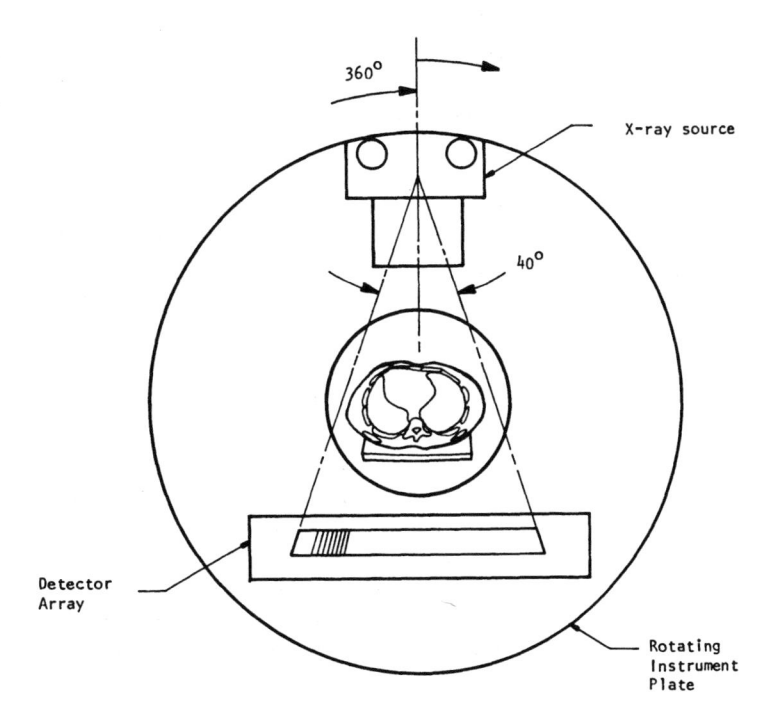

MEASUREMENT OF PROJECTION DATA 127

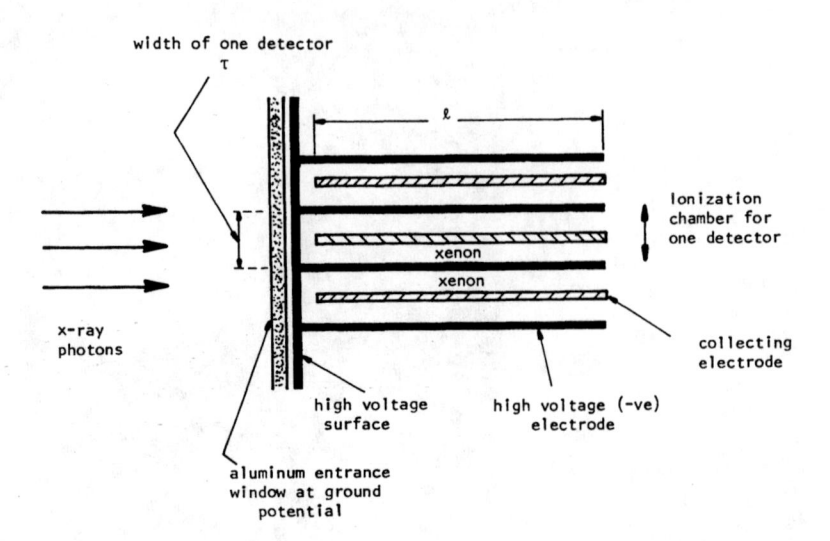

Fig. 4.10: *A xenon gas detector is often used to measure the number of x-ray photons that pass through the object. (From [Kak79].)*

detector consists of a central collecting electrode with a high voltage strip on each side. X-ray photons that enter a detector chamber cause ionizations with high probability (which depends upon the length, ℓ, of the detector and the pressure of the gas). The resulting current through the electrodes is a measure of the incident x-ray intensity. In one commercial scanner, the collector plates are made of copper and the high voltage strips of tantalum. In the same scanner, the length ℓ (shown in Fig. 4.10) is 8 cm, the voltage applied between the electrodes 170 V, and the pressure of the gas 10 atm. The overall efficiency of this particular detector is around 60%. The primary advantages of xenon gas detectors are that they can be packed closely and that they are inexpensive. The entrance width, τ, in Fig. 4.10 may be as small as 1 mm.

Yaffee *et al.* [Yaf77] have discussed in detail the energy absorption efficiency, the linearity of response, and the sensitivity to scattered and off-focus radiation for xenon gas detectors. Williams [Wil78] has discussed their use in commercial CT systems.

In a fixed-detector and rotating-source scanner (fourth generation) a large number of detectors are mounted on a fixed ring as shown in Fig. 4.11. Inside this ring is an x-ray tube that continually rotates around the patient. During this rotation the output of the detector integrators facing the tube is sampled every few milliseconds. All such samples for any one detector constitute what is known as a *detector-vertex* fan. (The fan beam data thus collected from a fourth-generation machine are similar to third-generation fan beam data.) Since the detectors are placed at fixed equiangular intervals around a ring, the data collected by sampling a detector are approximately equiangular, but not exactly so because the source and the detector rings must have different radii. Generally, interpolation is used to convert these data into a more precise equiangular fan for reconstruction using the algorithms in Chapter 3.

Note that the detectors do not have to be packed closely (more on this at the

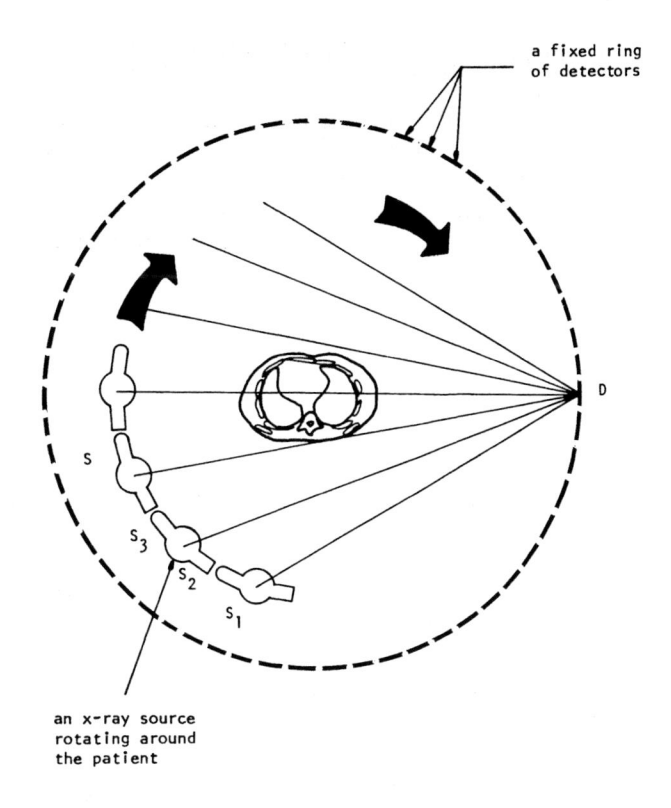

Fig. 4.11: *In a fourth-generation scanner an x-ray source rotates continuously around the patient. A stationary ring of detectors completely surrounds the patient. (From [Kak79].)*

end of this section). This observation together with the fact that the detectors are spread all around on a ring allows the use of scintillation detectors as opposed to ionization gas chambers. Most scintillation detectors currently in use are made of sodium iodide, bismuth germanate, or cesium iodide crystals coupled to photo-diodes. (See [Der77a] for a comparison of sodium iodide and bismuth germanate.) The crystal used for fabricating a scintillation detector serves two purposes. First, it traps most of the x-ray photons which strike the crystal, with a degree of efficiency which depends upon the photon energy and the size of the crystal. The x-ray photons then undergo photoelectric absorption (or Compton scatter with subsequent photoelectric absorption) resulting in the production of secondary electrons. The second function of the crystal is that of a phosphor—a solid which can transform the kinetic energy of the secondary electrons into flashes of light. The geometrical design and the encapsulation of the crystal are such that most of these flashes of light leave the crystal through a side where they can be detected by a photomultiplier tube or a solid state photo-diode.

A commercial scanner of the fourth-generation type uses 1088 cesium iodide detectors and in each detector fan 1356 samples are taken. This particular system differs from the one depicted in Fig. 4.9 in one respect: the x-ray source rotates around the patient *outside* the detector ring. This makes it necessary to nutate the detector ring so that measurements like those shown in the figure may be made [Haq78].

An important difference exists between the third- and the fourth-generation configurations. The data in a third-generation scanner are limited essentially in the number of rays in each projection, although there is no limit on the number of projections themselves; one can have only as many rays in each projection as the number of detectors in the detector array. On the other hand, the data collected in a fourth-generation scanner are limited in the number of projections that may be generated, while there is no limit on the number of rays in each projection.[1] (It is now known that for good-quality reconstructions the number of projections should be comparable to the number of rays in each projection. See Chapter 5.)

In a fan beam rotating detector (third-generation) scanner, if one detector is defective the same ray in every projection gets recorded incorrectly. Such correlated errors in all the projections form ring artifacts [She77]. On the other hand, when one detector fails in a fixed detector ring type (fourth-generation) scanner, it implies a loss or partial recording of one complete projection; when a large number of projections are measured, a loss of one projection usually does not noticeably degrade the quality of a reconstruction [Shu77]. The reverse is true for changes in the x-ray source. In a third-generation machine, the entire projection is scaled and the reconstruction is not greatly affected; while in fourth-generation scanners source instabilities lead to ring artifacts. Reconstructions comparing the effects of one bad ray in all projections to one bad projection are shown in Fig. 4.12.

The very nature of the construction of a gas ionization detector in a third-generation scanner lends them a certain degree of collimation which is a protection against receiving scatter radiation. On the other hand, the detectors in a fourth-generation scanner cannot be collimated since they must be capable of receiving photons from a large number of directions as the x-ray tube is rotating around the patient. This makes fixed ring detectors more vulnerable to scattered radiation.

When conventional CT scanners are used to image the heart, the reconstruction is blurred because of the heart's motion during the data collection time. The scanners in production today take at least a full second to collect the data needed for a reconstruction but a number of modifications have been proposed to the standard fan beam machines so that satisfactory images can be made [Lip83], [Mar82].

Certainly the simplest approach is to measure projection data for several complete rotations of the source and then use only those projections that occur during the same instant of the cardiac cycle. This is called *gated CT* and is usually accomplished by recording the patient's EKG as each projection is

---

[1] Although one may generate a very large number of rays by taking a large number of samples in each projection, "useful information" would be limited by the width of the focal spot on the x-ray tube and by the size of the detector aperture.

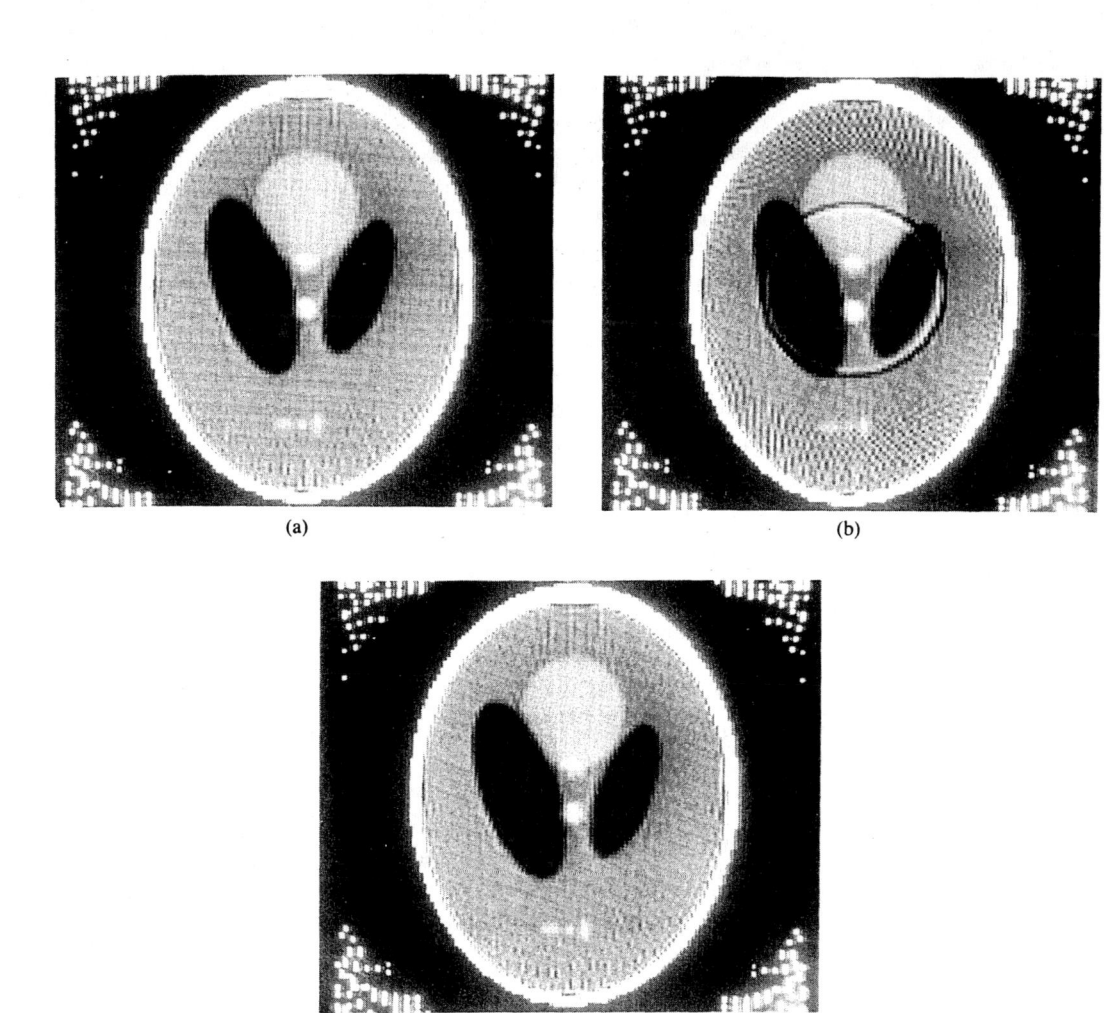

Fig. 4.12: *Three reconstructions are shown here to demonstrate the ring artifact due to a bad detector in a third-generation (rotating detector) scanner. (a) shows a standard reconstruction with 128 projections and 128 rays. (b) shows a ring artifact due to scaling detector 80 in all projections by 0.995. (c) shows the effect of scaling all rays in projection 80 by 0.995.*

measured. A full set of projection data for any desired portion of the EKG cycle is estimated by selecting all those projections that occur at or near the right time and then using interpolation to estimate those projections where no data are available. More details of this procedure can be found in [McK81].

Notwithstanding interpolation, missing projections are a shortcoming of the gated CT approach. In addition, for angiographic imaging, where it is necessary to measure the flow of a contrast medium through the body, the movement is not periodic and the techniques of gated CT do not apply. Two new hardware solutions have been proposed to overcome these problems—in both schemes the aim is to generate all the necessary projections in a time interval that is sufficiently short so that within the time interval the object may be assumed to be in a constant state. In the Dynamic Spatial Reconstructor (DSR) described by Robb *et al.* in [Rob83], 14 x-ray sources and 14 large circular fluorescent screens are used to measure a full set (112 views) of projections in a time interval of 0.127 second. In addition, since the x-ray intensity is measured on a fluorescent screen in two dimensions (and then recorded using video cameras), the reconstructions can be done in three dimensions.

A second approach described by Boyd and Lipton [Boy83], [Pes85], and implemented by Imatron, uses an electron beam that is scanned around a circular anode. The circular anode surrounds the patient and the beam striking this target ring generates an x-ray beam that is then measured on the far side of the patient using a fixed array of detectors. Since the location of the x-ray source is determined completely by the deflection of the electron beam and the deflection is controlled electronically, an entire scan can be made in 0.05 second.

4.1.6 Applications

Certainly, x-ray tomography has found its biggest use in the medical industry. Fig. 4.13 shows an example of the fine detail that has made this type of imaging so popular. This image of a human head corresponds to an axial plane and the subject's eyes, nose, and ear lobes are clearly visible. The

Fig. 4.13: *This figure shows a typical x-ray tomographic image produced with a third-generation machine. (Courtesy of Carl Crawford of the General Electric Medical Systems Division in Milwaukee, WI.)*

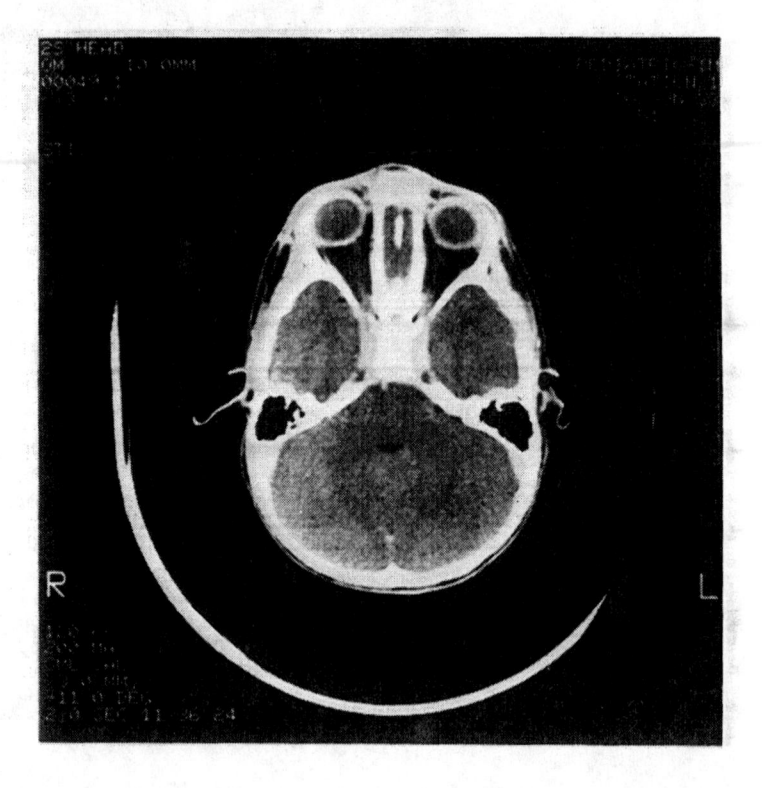

reader is referred to [Axe83] and a number of medical journals, including the *Journal of Computerized Tomography,* for additional medical applications.

Computerized tomography has also been applied to nondestructive testing (NDT) of materials and industrial objects. The rocket motor in Fig. 4.14 was examined by the Air Force-Aerojet Advanced Computed Tomography System I (AF/ACTS-I)[2] and its reconstruction is shown in Fig. 4.15. In the reconstruction, the outer ring is a PVC pipe used to support the motor, a grounding wire shows in the upper left as a small circular object, and the large mass with the star-shaped void represents solid fuel propellant. Several anomalies in the propellant are indicated with square boxes.

Fig. 4.14: *A conventional photograph is shown here of a solid fuel rocket motor studied by the Aerojet Corporation. (Courtesy of Jim Berry and Gary Cawood of Aerojet Strategic Propulsion Company.)*

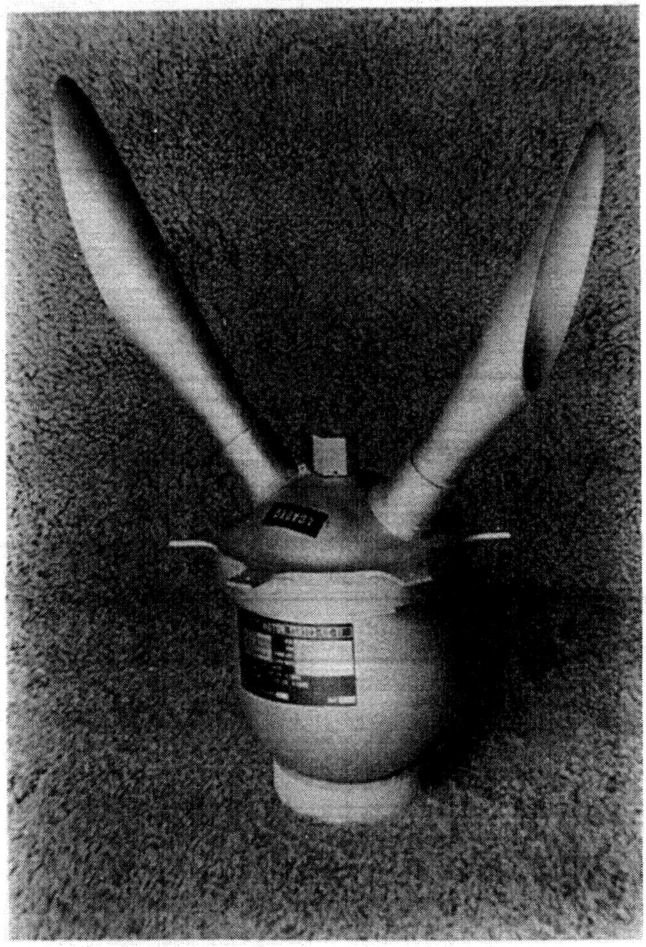

[2] This project was sponsored by Air Force Wright Aeronautical Laboratories, Air Force Materials Laboratory, Air Force Systems Command, United States Air Force, Wright-Patterson AFB, OH.

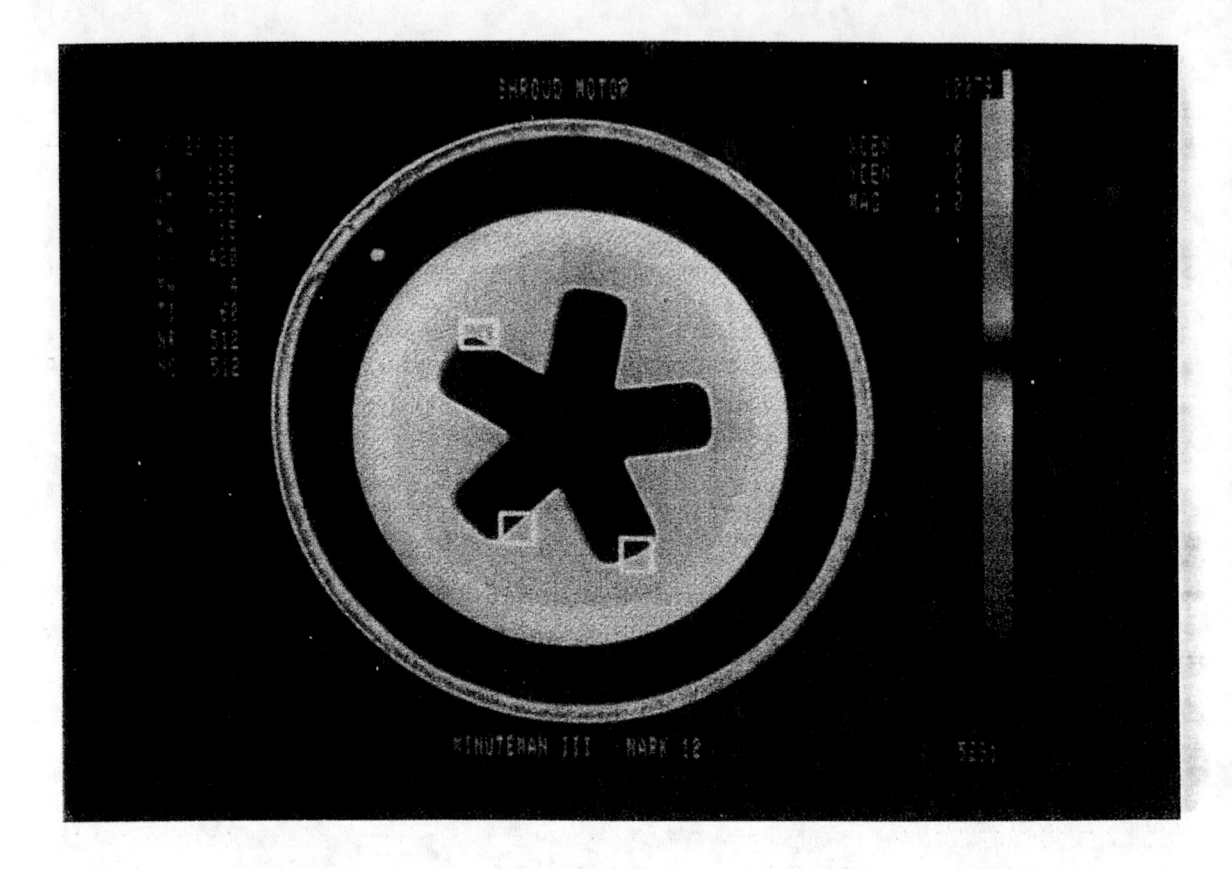

Fig. 4.15: *A cross section of the motor in Fig. 4.14 is shown here. The white squares indicate flaws in the rocket propellant. (Courtesy of Aerojet Strategic Propulsion Company.)*

An Optical Society of America meeting on Industrial Applications of Computerized Tomography described a number of unique applications of CT [OSA85]. These include imaging of core samples from oil wells [Wan85], quality assurance [All85], [Hef85], [Per85], and noninvasive measurement of fluid flow [Sny85] and flame temperature [Uck85].

4.2 Emission Computed Tomography

In conventional x-ray tomography, physicians use the attenuation coefficient of tissue to infer diagnostic information about the patient. Emission CT, on the other hand, uses the decay of radioactive isotopes to image the distribution of the isotope as a function of time. These isotopes may be administered to the patient in the form of radiopharmaceuticals either by injection or by inhalation. Thus, for example, by administering a radioactive isotope by inhalation, emission CT can be used to trace the path of the isotope through the lungs and the rest of the body.

Radioactive isotopes are characterized by the emission of gamma-ray photons or positrons, both products of nuclear decay. (Note that gamma-ray photons are indistinguishable from x-ray photons; different terms are used simply to indicate their origin.) The concentration of such an isotope in any cross section changes with time due to radioactive decay, flow, and biochemical kinetics within the body. This implies that all the data for one cross-sectional image must be collected in a time interval that is short compared to the time constant associated with the changing concentration. But then this aspect also gives emission CT its greatest potential and utility in diagnostic medicine, because now by analyzing the images taken at different times for the same cross section we can determine the functional state of various organs in a patient's body.

Emission CT is of two types: single photon emission CT and positron emission CT. The word *single* in the former refers to the product of the radioactive decay, a single photon, while in positron emission CT the decay produces a single positron. After traveling a short distance the positron comes to rest and combines with an electron. The annihilation of the emitted positron results in *two* oppositely traveling gamma-ray photons. We will first discuss CT imaging of (single) gamma-ray photon emitters.

4.2.1 Single Photon Emission Tomography

Fig. 4.16 shows a cross section of a body with a distributed source emitting gamma-ray photons. For the purpose of imaging, any very small, nevertheless macroscopic, element of this source may be considered to be an isotropic source of gamma-rays. The number of gamma-ray photons emitted per second by such an element is proportional to the concentration of the source at that point. Assume that the collimator in front of the detector has infinite collimation, which means it accepts only those photons that travel toward it in the parallel ray-bundle R_1R_2. (Infinite collimation, in practice, would imply

Fig. 4.16: *In single photon emission tomography a distributed source of gamma-rays is imaged using a collimated detector. (From [Kak79].)*

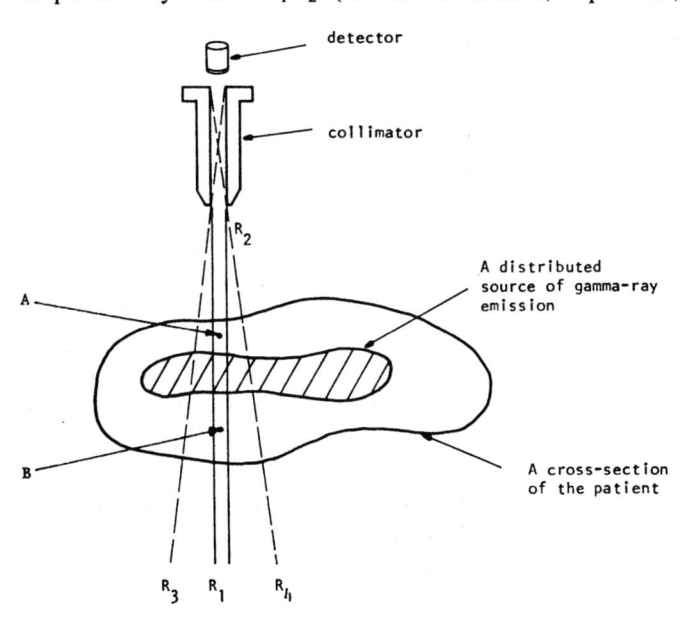

an infinitely long time to make a statistically meaningful observation.) Then clearly the total number of photons recorded by the detector in a "statistically meaningful" time interval is proportional to the total concentration of the emitter along the line defined by R_1R_2. In other words, it is a ray integral as defined in Chapter 3. By moving the detector-collimator assembly to an adjacent position laterally, one may determine this integral for another ray parallel to R_1R_2. After one such scan is completed, generating one projection, one may either rotate the patient or the detector-collimator assembly and generate other projections. Under ideal conditions it should be possible to generate the projection data required for the usual reconstruction algorithms.

Figs. 4.17 and 4.18 show, respectively, axial and sagittal SPECT images of a head. The axial images are normal CT reconstructions at different cross-sectional locations, while the images of Fig. 4.18 were found by reformatting the original reconstructed images into four sagittal views. The reconstructions are 64 × 64 images representing the concentration of an amphetamine tagged with iodine-123. The measured data for these reconstructions consisted of 128 projections (over 360°) each with 64 rays.

As the reader might have noticed already, the images in Figs. 4.17 and 4.18 look blurry compared to the x-ray CT images as exemplified by the reconstructions in Fig. 4.13. To get better resolution in emission CT, one might consider using more detectors to provide finer sampling of each projection; unfortunately, that would mean fewer events per detector and thus a diminished signal-to-noise ratio at each detector. One could consider increasing the dosage of the radioactive isotope to enhance the signal-to-noise ratio, but that is limited by what the body can safely absorb. The length of

Fig. 4.17: *Axial SPECT images showing the concentration of iodine-123 at four cross-sectional planes are shown here. The 64 × 64 reconstructions were made by measuring 128 projections each with 64 rays. (The images were produced on a General Electric 4000T/Star and are courtesy of Grant Gullberg of General Electric in Milwaukee, WI.)*

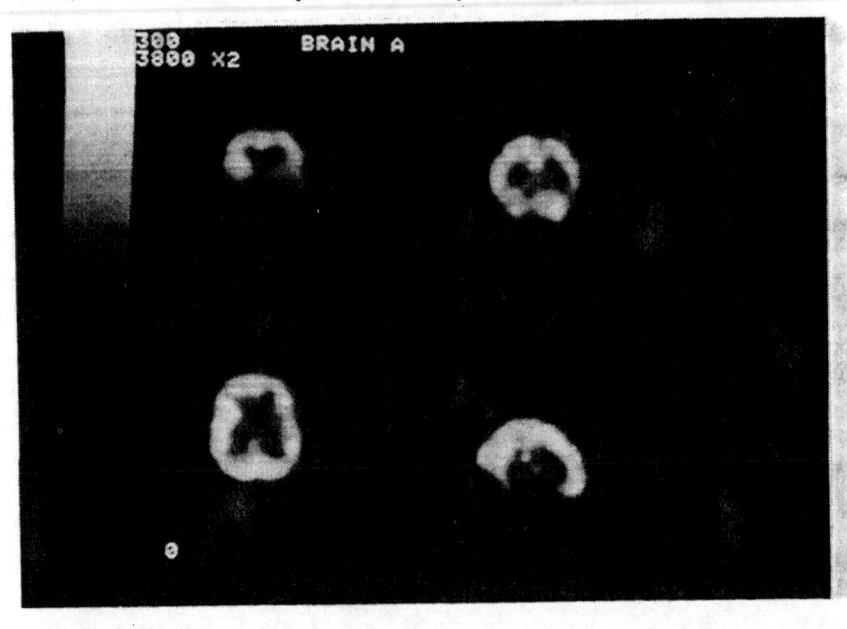

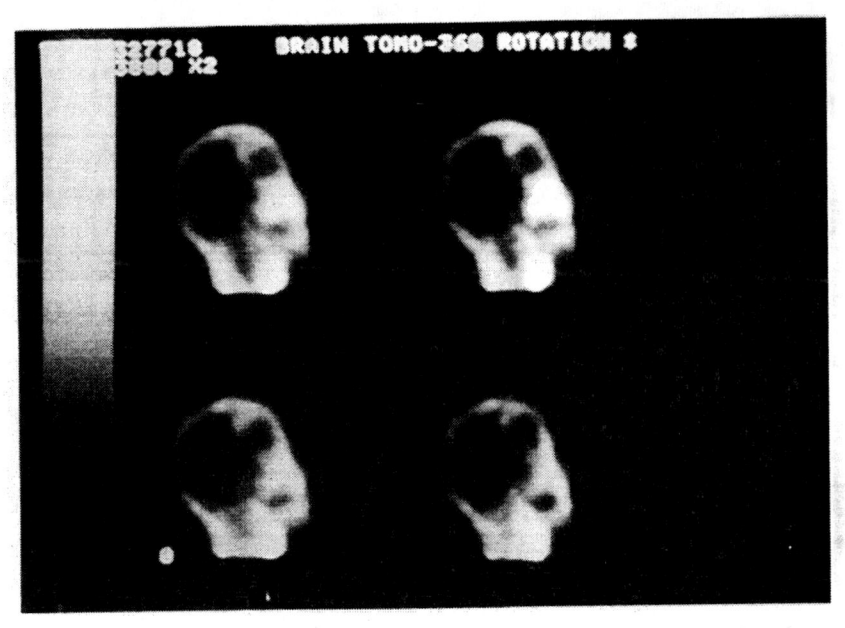

Fig. 4.18: *The reconstructed data in Fig. 4.17 were reformatted to produce the four sagittal images shown here. (The images were produced on a General Electric 4000T/Star and are courtesy of Grant Gullberg of General Electric in Milwaukee, WI.)*

time over which the events are integrated could also be prolonged for an increased signal-to-noise ratio, but usually that is constrained by body motion [Bro81].

A serious difficulty with tomographic imaging of a gamma-ray emitting source is caused by the attenuation that photons suffer during their travel from the emitting nuclei to the detector.[3] The extent of this attenuation depends upon both the photon energy and the nature of the tissue. Consider two elemental sources of equal strength at points A and B in Fig. 4.16: because of attenuation the detector will find the source at A stronger than the one at B. The effect of attenuation is illustrated in Fig. 4.19, which shows reconstructions of a disk phantom for three different values of the attenuation: $\mu = 0.05$, 0.11, and 0.15 cm^{-1}, obtained by using three different media in the phantom. The original disk phantom is also shown for comparison. (These reconstructions were done using 360° of projection data.)

A number of different approaches for attenuation compensation have been developed. These will now be briefly discussed in the following section.

4.2.2 Attenuation Compensation for Single Photon Emission CT

Consider the case where gamma-ray emission is taking place in a medium that can everywhere be characterized by a constant linear attenuation

---

[3] There is also the difficulty caused by the fact that for a collimator the parallel beam R_1R_2 in Fig. 4.16 is only an idealization. The detector in that figure will accept photons from a point source anywhere within the volume $R_3R_2R_4$. Also, in this volume the response of the detector will decrease as an isotropic source is moved away from it. However, such nonuniformities are not large enough to cause serious distortions in the reconstructions. This was first shown by Budinger [Bud74]. See also [Gus78].

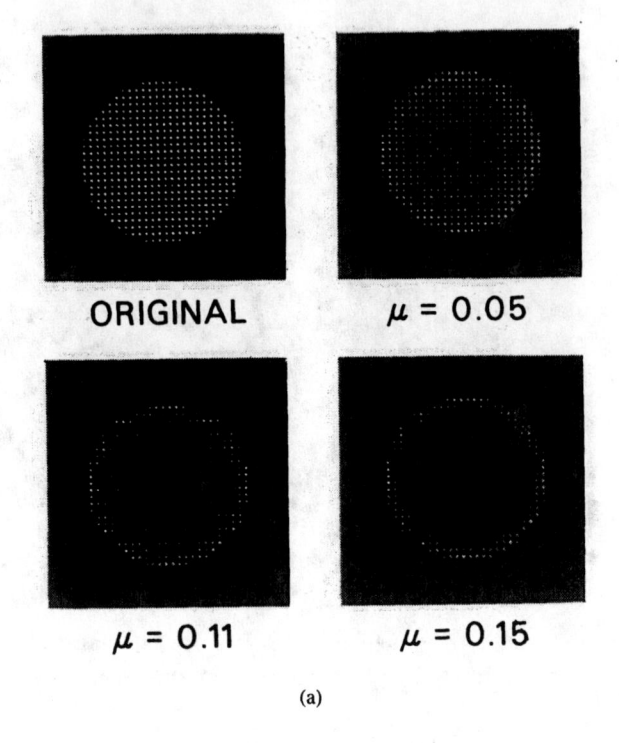

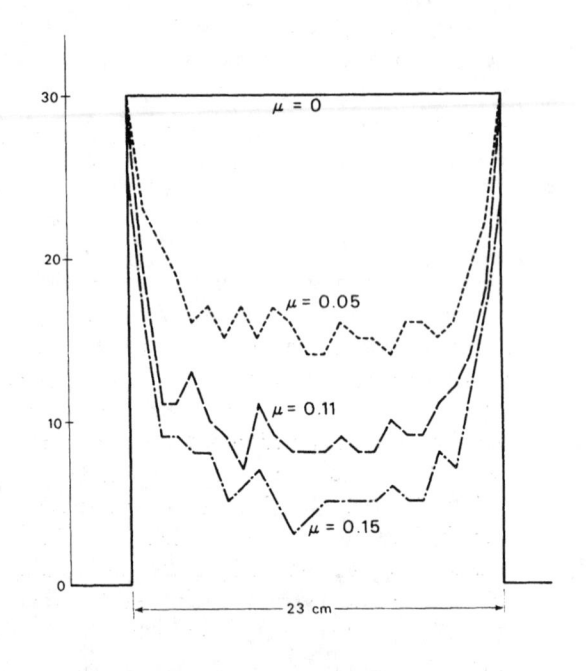

Fig. 4.19: *Four reconstructions of a gamma-ray emitting disk phantom are shown in (a) for different values of attenuation. (b) shows a quantitative comparison of the reconstructed values on the center line. (Courtesy of T. Budinger.)*

coefficient. Let $\rho(x, y)$ denote the source distribution in a desired cross section. In the absence of any attenuation the projection data $P_\theta(t)$ are given from Chapter 3 by

$$P_\theta(t) = \iint \rho(x, y)\delta(x \cos \theta + y \sin \theta - t) \, dx \, dy. \tag{24}$$

However, in the presence of attenuation this relationship must be modified to include an exponential attenuation term, $e^{-\mu(d-s)}$, where, as shown in Fig. 4.20, $s = -x \sin \theta + y \cos \theta$ and $d = d(t, \theta)$ is the distance from the line CC' to the edge of the object. Thus the ray integral actually measured is given by

$$P_\theta(t) = \iint \rho(x, y) \exp[-\mu(d-s)]\delta(x \cos \theta + y \sin \theta - t) \, dx \, dy. \tag{25}$$

For convex objects the distance d, which is a function of x, y, and θ, can be determined from the external shape of the object. We can now write

$$S_\theta(t) = P_\theta(t) \exp[\mu d] = \iint \rho(x, y) \exp[-\mu(x \sin \theta - y \cos \theta)]$$
$$\cdot \delta(x \cos \theta + y \sin \theta - t) \, dx \, dy. \tag{26}$$

The function $S_\theta(t)$ has been given the name *exponential Radon transform*. In [Tre80], Tretiak and Metz have shown that

$$\hat{\rho}(r, \phi) = \int_0^{2\pi} \left[\int_{-\infty}^{\infty} S_\theta(r \cos(\theta - \phi) - t) h(t) \, dt \right] \exp[\mu r \sin(\theta - \phi)] \, d\theta \tag{27}$$

is an attenuation compensated reconstruction of $\rho(x, y)$ provided the convolving function $h(t)$ is chosen such that the point spread function of the system given by

$$b(r, \phi) = \int_0^{2\pi} h(r \cos(\theta - \phi)) \exp[\mu r \sin(\theta - \phi)] \, d\theta \tag{28}$$

fits some desired point spread function (ideally a delta function but in practice a low pass filtered version of a delta function). Note that because the integration in (28) is over one period of the integrand (considered as a function of θ), the function $b(r, \phi)$ is independent of ϕ which makes it radially symmetric. Good numerical approximations to $h(t)$ are presented in [Tre80]. In [Tre80] Tretiak and Metz have provided analytical solutions for $h(t)$. Note that (27) possesses a filtered backprojection implementation very similar to that described in Chapter 3. Each modified projection $S_\theta(t)$ is first convolved with the function $h(t)$; the resulting filtered projections are then backprojected as discussed before. For each θ the backprojected contribution at a given pixel is multiplied by the exponential weight $e^{\mu r \sin(\theta - \phi)}$.

Budinger and his associates have done considerable work on incorporating

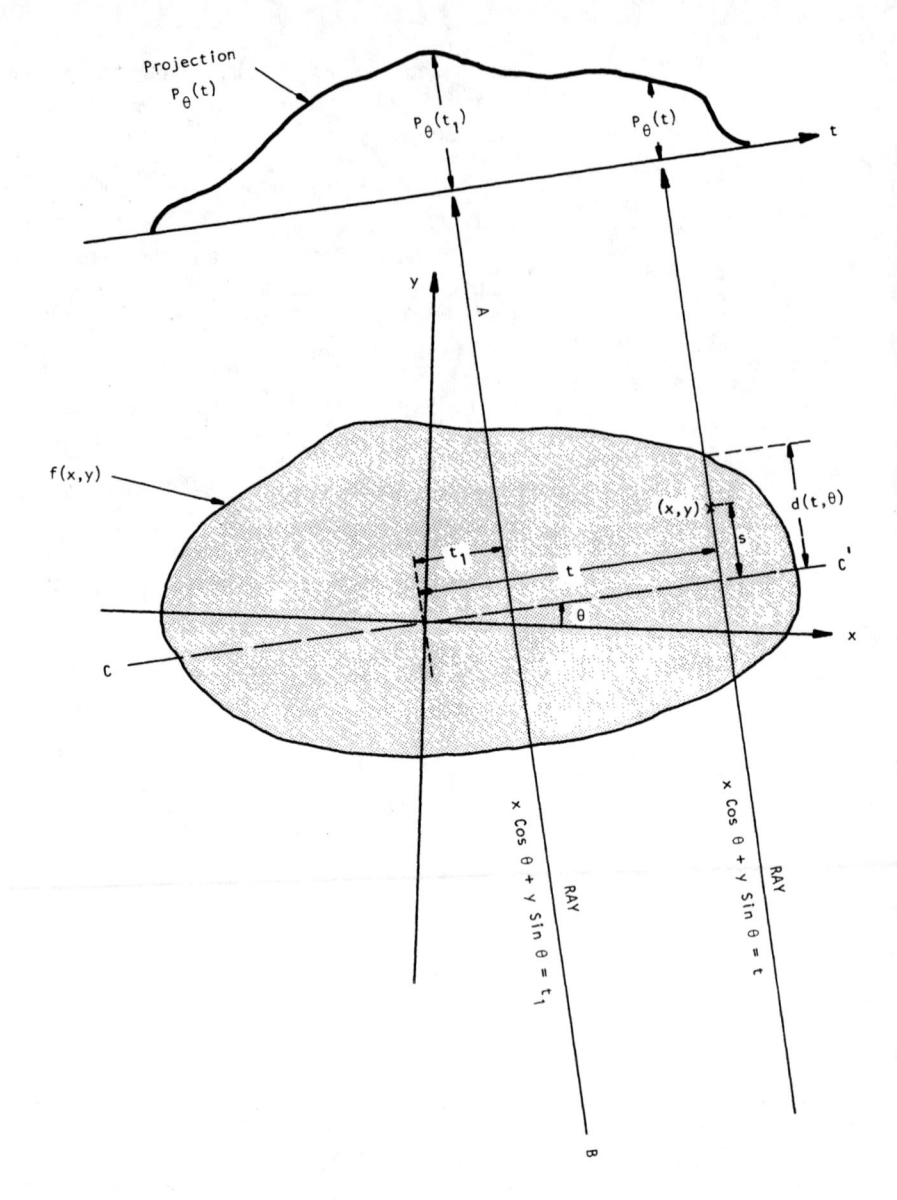

Fig. 4.20: *Several parameters for attenuation correction are shown here. (From [Kak79].)*

attenuation compensation in their iterative least squares reconstruction techniques [Bud76]. In these procedures one approximates an image to be reconstructed by a grid as shown in Fig. 4.21 and an assumption is made that the concentration of the nuclide is constant within each grid block, the concentration in block m being denoted by $\rho(m)$. In the absence of attenuation, the projection measured at a sampling point t_k with projection angle θ_j is given by

$$P_\theta(t_k) = \sum_m \rho(m) f_k^\theta(m) \qquad (29)$$

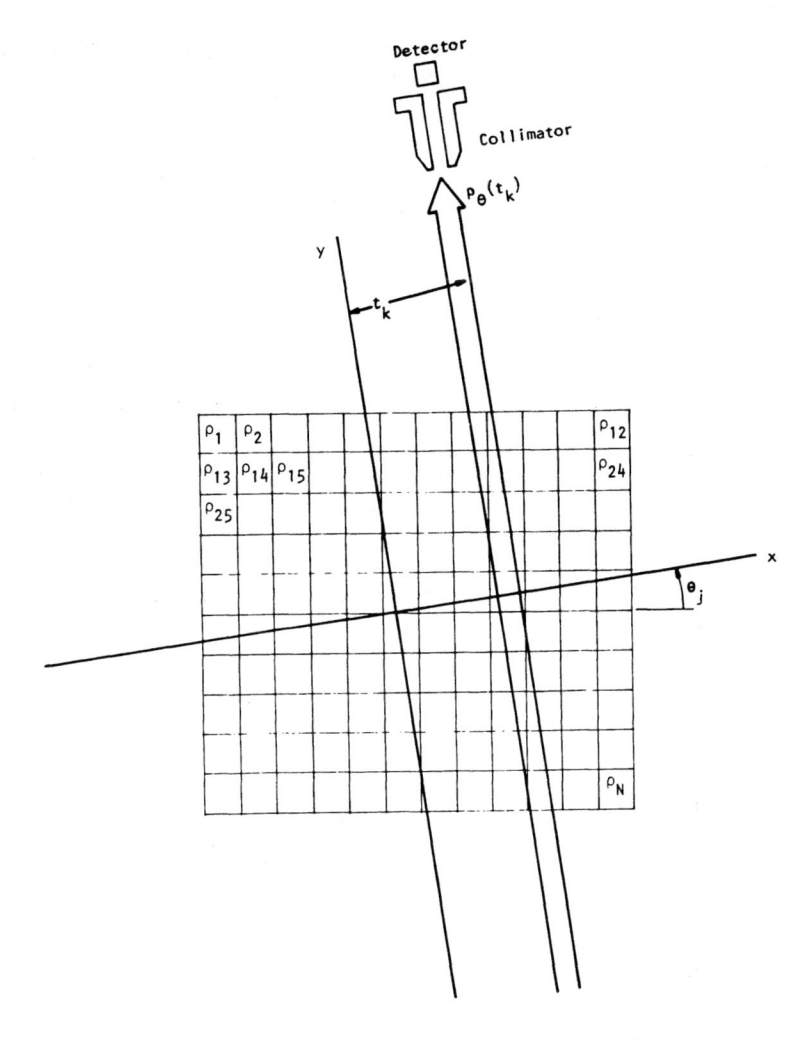

Fig. 4.21: *This figure shows the grid representation for a source distribution. The concentration of the source is assumed to be constant in each grid square. (From [Kak79].)*

where $f_k^\theta(m)$ is a geometrical factor equal to that fraction of the mth block that is intercepted by the kth ray in the view at angle θ. (The above equation may be solved by a variety of iterative techniques [Ben70], [Goi72], [Her71].)

Once the problem of image reconstruction is set up as in (29), one may introduce attenuation compensation by simply modifying the geometrical factors as shown here:

$$P_\theta(t_k) = \sum_{m=1}^{N} \rho(m) f_k^\theta(m) \exp[-\mu \ell_m^\theta] \qquad (30)$$

where ℓ_m^θ is the distance from the center of the mth cell to the edge of the reconstruction domain in the view θ. The above equations could be solved, as any set of simultaneous equations, for the unknowns $\rho(n)$.

MEASUREMENT OF PROJECTION DATA

Unfortunately, this rationale is flawed: In actual practice the attenuating path length for the mth cell does not extend all the way to the detector or, for that matter, even to the end of the reconstruction domain. For each cell and for a given ray passing that cell it only extends to the end of the object along that ray. To incorporate this knowledge in attenuation compensation, Budinger and Gullberg [Bud76] have used an iterative least squares approach. They first reconstruct the emitter concentration ignoring the attenuation. This reconstruction is used to determine the boundaries of the object by using an edge detection algorithm. With this information the attenuation factors $\exp(-\mu \ell_m^\theta)$ can now be calculated where ℓ_m^θ is now the distance from the mth pixel to the edge of the object along a line $\theta + 90°$. The source concentration is then calculated using the least squares approach. This method, therefore, requires two reconstructions. Also required is a large storage file for the coefficients ℓ_m^θ.

For other approaches to attenuation compensation the reader is referred to [Bel79], [Cha79a], [Cha79b], [Hsi76].

4.2.3 Positron Emission Tomography

With positron emission tomography (PET), we want to determine the concentration and location of a positron emitting compound in a desired cross section of the human body. Perhaps the most remarkable feature of a positron emitter, at least from the standpoint of tomographic imaging, is the fact that an emitted positron can't exist in nature for any length of time. When brought to rest, it interacts with an electron and, as a result, *their masses are annihilated,* creating two photons of 511 keV each. [Note that the mass of an electron (or positron) at rest is equivalent to an energy of approximately 511 keV.] These two photons are called annihilation gamma-ray photons and are emitted at very nearly 180° from one another (Fig. 4.22). It is also important to note that the annihilation of a positron occurs with high probability only after it has been brought to rest. Note that, on the average, 1-MeV and 5-

Fig. 4.22: *In positron emission tomography the decay of a positron/electron pair is detected by a pair of photons. Since the photons are released in opposite directions it is possible to determine which ray it came from and measure a projection. (From [Kak79].)*

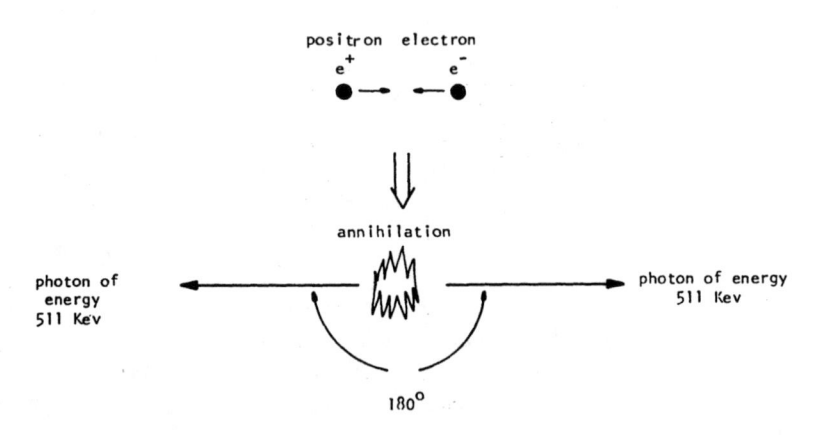

MeV positrons traverse 4 mm and 2.5 cm, respectively, in water before annihilation. Therefore, for accurate localization it is important that the emitted positrons have as little kinetic energy as possible. Usually, in practice, this desirable property for a positron emitting compound has to be balanced against the competing property that in a nuclear decay if the positron emission process is to dominate over other competing processes, such as electron capture decay, the decay energy must be sufficiently large and, hence, lead to large positron kinetic energy.

The fact that the annihilation of a positron leads to two gamma-ray photons traveling in opposite directions forms the basis of a unique way of detecting positrons. Coincident detection by two physically separated detectors of two gamma-ray photons locates a positron emitting nucleus on a line joining the two detectors. Clearly, a few words about coincident detection are in order. Recall that in emission work, each photon is detected separately and therefore treated as a distinct entity (hence the name "event" for the arrival of a photon). Now suppose the detectors D_1 and D_2 in Fig. 4.23(a) record two photons simultaneously (i.e., in coincidence) that would indicate a positron annihilation on the line joining AA'. We have used the phrase "simultaneous detection" here in spite of the fact that the distances SA and SA' may not be equal. The "coincidence resolving time" of circuits that check for whether the two photons have arrived simultaneously is usually on the order of 10 to 25 ns—a sufficiently long interval of time to make path difference considerations unimportant. This means that if the two annihilation photons arrive at the two detectors within this time interval, they are considered to be in coincidence.

Positron devices have one great advantage over single photon devices discussed in the preceding subsection, that is, electronic collimation. This is

Fig. 4.23: *A pair of detectors and a coincidence testing circuit are used to determine the location of a positron emission. Arrival of coincident photons at the detectors D_1 and D_2 implies that there was a positron emission somewhere on the line AA'. This is known as electronic collimation. (From [Kak79].)*

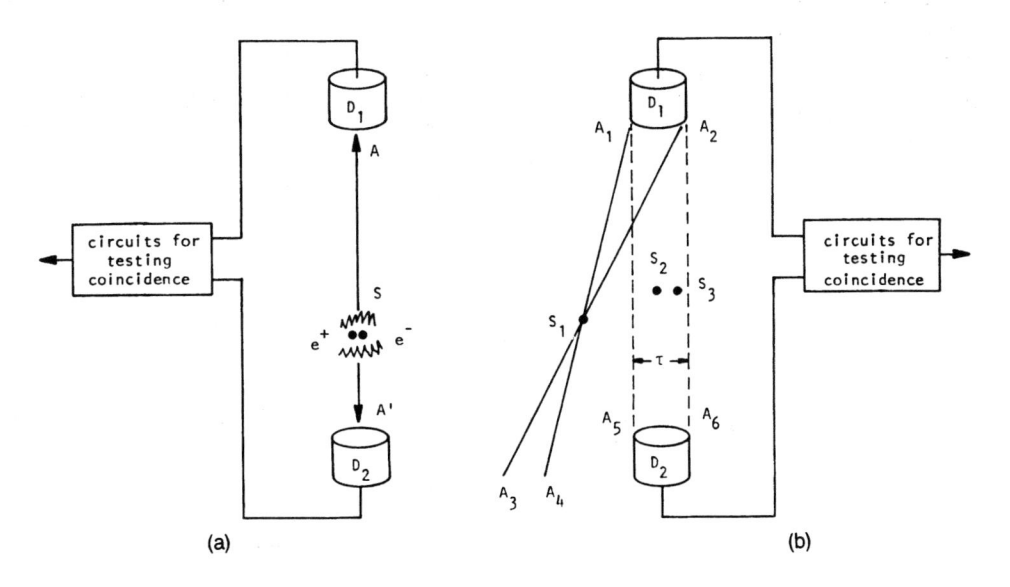

illustrated by Fig. 4.23(b). Let us say we have a small volume of a positron emitting source at location S_1 in the figure. For all the annihilation photons emitted into the conical volume $A_2S_1A_2$, their counterparts will be emitted into the volume A_3SA_4 so as to miss the detector D_2 completely. Clearly then, with coincident detection, the source S_1 will *not* be detected at all with this detector pair. On the other hand, the source located at S_2 will be detected. Note that, by the same token, if the same small source is located at S_3 it will be detected with a slightly reduced intensity (therefore, sensitivity) because of its off-center location. (This effect contributes to spatial variance of the point spread function of positron devices.) In order to appreciate this electronic collimation the reader should bear in mind that if we had used the detectors D_1 and D_2 as ordinary (meaning noncoincident) gamma-ray detectors (with no collimation), we wouldn't have been able to differentiate between the sources at locations S_1 and S_2 in the figure. The property of electronic collimation discussed here was first pointed out in 1951 by Wrenn *et al.*, [Wre51] who also pointed out how it might be somewhat influenced by background scatter.

It is easy to see how the projection data for positron emission CT might be generated. In Fig. 4.23 if we ignore variations in the useful solid angle subtended at the detectors by various point sources within $A_1A_2A_5A_6$ (and, also, if for a moment we ignore attenuation), then it is clear that the total number of coincident counts by detectors D_1 and D_2 is proportional to the integral of the concentration of the positron emitting compound over the volume $A_1A_2A_5A_6$. This by definition is a ray integral in a projection, provided the width τ shown in the figure is sufficiently small.

This principle has been incorporated in the many positron scanners. As an example, the detector arrangement in the positron system (PETT) developed originally at Washington University by TerPogossian and his associates [Hof76] is shown in Fig. 4.24(a). The system uses six detector banks, containing eight scintillation detectors each. Each detector is operated in coincidence with all the detectors in the opposite bank. For finer sampling of the projection data and also to generate more views, the entire detector gantry is rotated around the patient in 3° increments over an arc of 60°, and for each angular position the gantry is also translated over a distance of 5 cm in 1-cm increments. A multislice version of this scanner is described in [Ter78a] and [Mul78]. These scanners have formed the basis for the development of Ortec ECAT [Phe78]. Many other scanners [Boh78], [Cho76], [Cho77], [Der77b], [Ter78b], [Yam77] use a ring detector system, a schematic of which is shown in Fig. 4.24(b). Derenzo [Der77a] has given a detailed comparison of sodium iodide and bismuth germanate crystals for such ring detector systems. The reader will notice that the detector configuration in a positron ring system is identical to that used in the fixed-detector x-ray CT scanners described in Section 4.1. Therefore, by placing a rotating x-ray source inside the ring in Fig. 4.24(b) one can have a dual-purpose scanner, as proposed by Cho [Cho78]. The reader is also referred to [Car78a] for a characterization of the

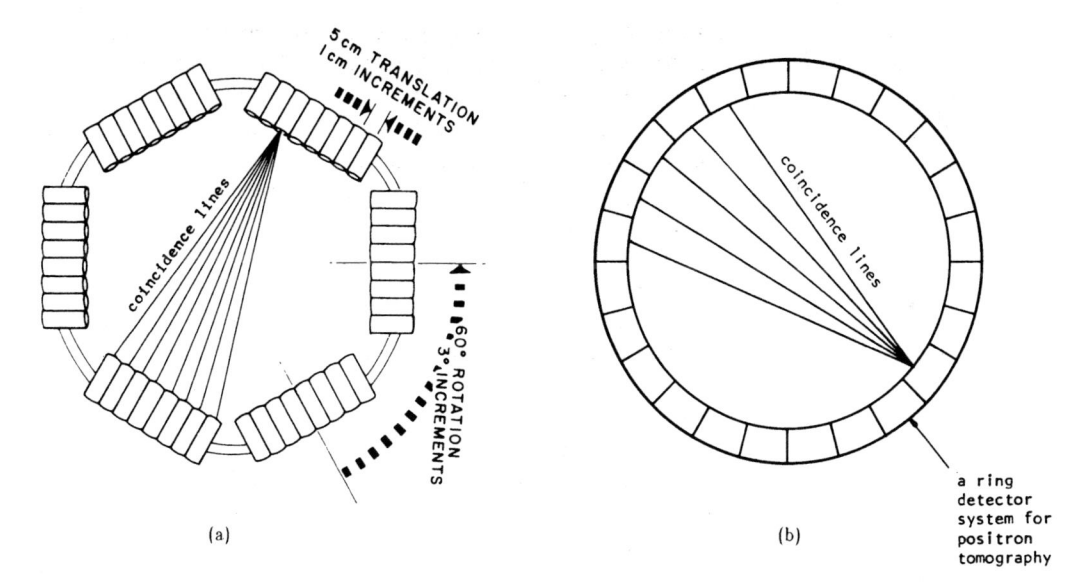

Fig. 4.24: (a) Detector arrangement in the PETT III CAT. (b) A ring detector system for positron cameras. Each detector in the ring works in coincidence with a number of the other detectors. (From [Kak79].)

performance of positron imaging systems and to [Bud77] for a comparison of positron tomography with single photon gamma-ray tomography. While our discussion here has focused on reconstructing two-dimensional distributions of positron concentration (from the one-dimensional projection data), by using planar arrays for recording coincidences there have also been attempts at direct reconstruction of the three-dimensional distribution of positrons [Chu77], [Tam78].

4.2.4 Attenuation Compensation for Positron Tomography

Two major engineering advantages of positron tomography over single photon emission tomography are: 1) the electronic collimation already discussed, 2) easier attenuation compensation.[4] We will now show why attenuation compensation is easier in positron tomography.

Let's say that the detectors D_1 and D_2 in Fig. 4.25 are being used to measure one ray in a projection and let's also assume that there is a source of positron emitters located at the point S. Suppose for a particular positron annihilation, the two annihilation gamma-ray photons labeled γ_1 and γ_2 in the figure are released toward D_1 and D_2, respectively. The *probability* of γ_1 reaching detector D_1 is given by

$$\exp\left[-\int_L^{L_1} \mu(x)\,dx\right] \qquad (31)$$

---

[4] On the other hand, one of the disadvantages of positron emission CT in relation to single gamma-ray emission CT is that the dose of radiation delivered to a patient from the administration of a positron emitting compound (radionuclide) includes, in addition to the contribution from the annihilation radiation, that contributed by the kinetic energy of positrons.

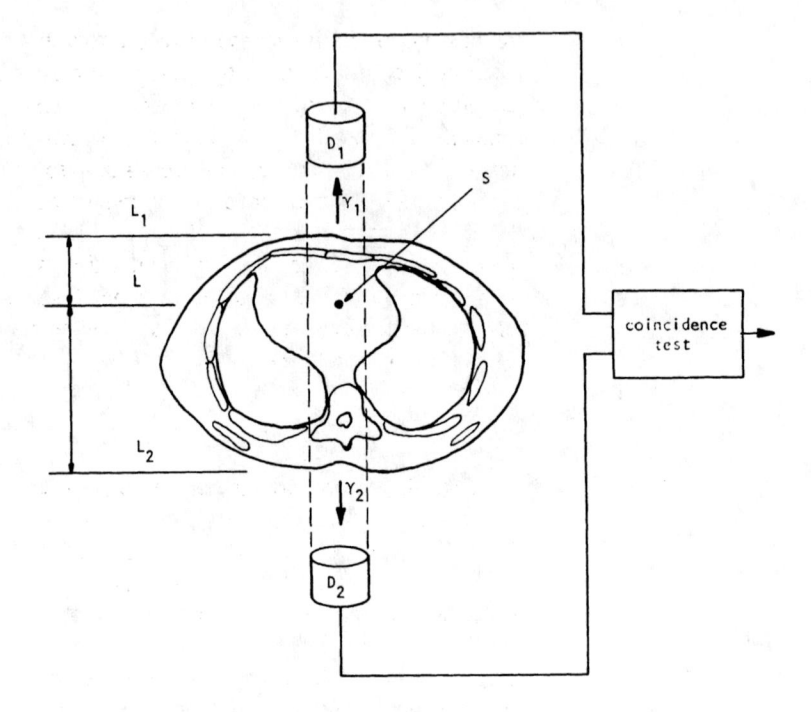

Fig. 4.25: *A photon emitted at S and traveling toward the D_1 detector is attenuated over a distance of $L_1 - L$, while a photon traveling toward the D_2 detector undergoes an attenuation proportional to $L - L_2$. (From [Kak79].)*

where $\mu(x)$ is the attenuation coefficient at 511 keV as a function of distance along the line joining the two detectors. Similarly, the probability of the photon γ_2 reaching the detector D_2 is given by

$$\exp\left[-\int_{L_2}^{L} \mu(x)\,dx\right]. \tag{32}$$

Then the probability that this particular annihilation will be recorded by the detectors is given by the product of the above two probabilities

$$\exp\left[-\int_{L}^{L_1} \mu(x)\,dx\right] \cdot \exp\left[-\int_{L_2}^{L} \mu(x)\,dx\right] \tag{33}$$

which is equal to

$$\exp\left[-\int_{L_2}^{L_1} \mu(x)\,dx\right]. \tag{34}$$

This is a most remarkable result because, first, this attenuation factor is the same no matter where positron annihilation occurs on the line joining D_1 and D_2, and, second, the factor above is exactly the attenuation that a beam of monoenergetic photons at 511 keV would undergo in propagating from L_1 at one side to L_2 at the other. Therefore, one can readily compensate for attenuation by first doing a transmission study (one does not have to do a reconstruction in this study) to record total transmission loss for each ray in each projection. Then, in the positron emission study, the data for each ray can simply be attenuation compensated when corrected (by division) by this transmission loss factor. This method of attenuation compensation has been used in the PETT and other [Bro78] positron emission scanners.

There are other approaches to attenuation compensation in positron CT [Cho77]. For example, at 511-keV photon energy, a human head may be modeled as possessing constant attenuation (which is approximately equal to that of water). If in a head study the head is surrounded by a water bath, the attenuation factor given by (34) may now be easily calculated from the shape of the water bath [Eri76].

4.3 Ultrasonic Computed Tomography

When diffraction effects can be ignored, ultrasound CT is very similar to x-ray tomography. In both cases a transmitter illuminates the object and a line integral of the attenuation can be estimated by measuring the energy on the far side of the object. Ultrasound differs from x-rays because the propagation speed is much lower and thus it is possible to measure the exact pressure of the wave as a function of time. From the pressure waveform it is possible, for example, to measure not only the attenuation of the pressure field but also the delay in the signal induced by the object. From these two measurements it is possible to estimate the attenuation coefficient and the refractive index of the object. The first such tomograms were made by Greenleaf *et al.* [Gre74], [Gre75], followed by Carson *et al.* [Car76], Jackowatz and Kak [Jak76], and Glover and Sharp [Glo77].

Before we discuss ultrasonic tomography any further it should be borne in mind that the conventional method of using pulse-echo ultrasound to form images is also tomographic—in the sense that it is cross-sectional. In other words, in a conventional pulse-echo B-scan image (see Chapter 8), tissue structures aren't superimposed upon each other. One may, therefore, ask: Why computerized ultrasonic tomography? The answer lies in the fact that with pulse-echo systems we can only see tissue interfaces, although, on account of scattering, there are some returns from within the bulk of the tissue. [Work is now progressing on methods of correlating (quantitatively) these scattered returns with the local properties of tissue [Fla83], [Kuc84]. This correlation is made difficult by the fact that the scattered returns are modified every time they pass through an interface; hence the interest in computed ultrasonic tomography as an alternative strategy for quantitative imaging with sound.]

From the discussion in a previous chapter on algorithms, it is clear that in computerized tomography it is essential to know the path that a ray traverses from the source to the detector. In x-ray and emission tomography these paths are straight lines (within limits of the detector collimators), but this isn't always the case for ultrasound tomography. When an ultrasonic beam propagates through tissue, it undergoes a deflection at every interface between tissues of different refractive indices. Carson *et al.* [Car77] have discussed some of the distortions introduced in a CT image by hard tissues such as bone. (For a computer simulation study of these distortions, see [Far78].) It has been suggested [Joh75] that perhaps we could correct for refraction by using the following iterative scheme: we could first reconstruct a refractive index tomogram ignoring refraction; rays could then be digitally traced through this tomogram indicating the propagation paths; these curved paths could then be used for a subsequent reconstruction, and the process repeated. Another possible approach is to use inverse scattering solutions to the problem [Iwa75], [Mue80]. Both of these approaches will be discussed in later chapters. The problem of tomographic imaging of hard tissues with ultrasound remains unsolved.

In this section we will assume that we are only dealing with soft-tissue structures. (The refraction effects are much smaller now and can generally be ignored.) An important application of this case is ultrasonic tumor detection in the female breast [Car78b], [Gre78], [Gre81], [Sch84].

Our review here will only deal with transmission ultrasound. Recently it has been shown theoretically that it is also possible to achieve (computed) tomographic imaging with reflected ultrasound [Nor79a], [Nor79b]. Clinical verification of this new technique has yet to be carried out. (See Chapter 8 for more information.)

4.3.1 Fundamental Considerations

Like the x-ray case, first consider ultrasonic waves propagating from a transmitting transducer through a single layer of tissue and measured by a receiver on the far side of the tissue, as diagrammed in Fig. 4.26(a). Because ultrasonic waves in the range 1 to 10 MHz are highly attenuated by air, the tissue layer is immersed in water or another fluid. Water serves to couple the energy of the transducer into the object and provides a good refractive index match with the tissue. Ignoring the effects of refraction, here we will model the received waveform by considering only the direct path (or ray) between the two transducers.

If an electrical signal, $x(t)$, is applied to the transmitting transducer as shown in Fig. 4.26(a), a number of effects can be identified that determine the electrical signal produced by the receiving transducer. We can write an expression for the received signal, $y(t)$, by considering each of these effects in the frequency domain. Thus the Fourier transform of the received signal, $Y(f)$, is given by a simple multiplication of the following factors:

1) the transmitter transfer function relating the electrical signal to the resulting pressure wave, $H_1(f)$;
2) the attenuation, $e^{-\alpha_w(f)\ell_{w_1}}$, and phase change, $e^{-j\beta_w(f)\ell_{w_1}}$, caused by the water on the near side of the tissue;

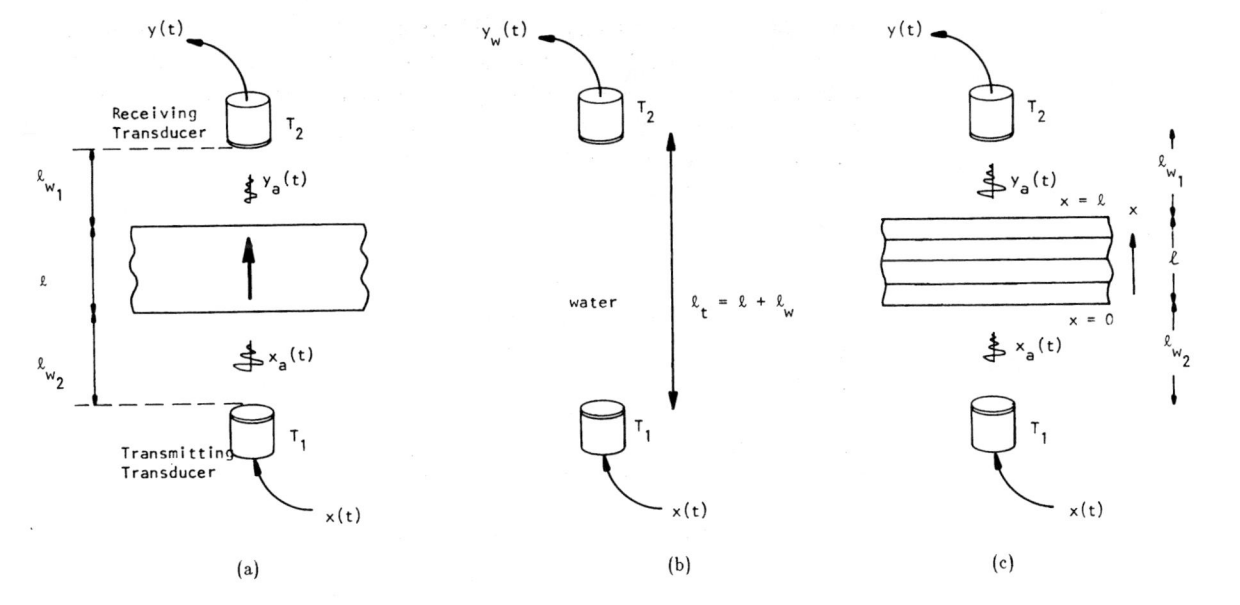

Fig. 4.26: *As an ultrasonic beam travels between two transducers (a) it undergoes a phase shift in water over a distance of ℓ_{w_1} and ℓ_{w_2}, and both a phase shift and an attenuation due to the object. In (b) the beam undergoes a phase shift as it goes through the water and in (c) the beam travels through both the water and a multilayered object. (From [Kak79].)*

3) the transmittance of the front surface of the tissue or the percentage of energy in the water that is coupled into the tissue, τ_1;

4) the attenuation, $e^{-\alpha(f)\ell}$, and phase change, $e^{-j\beta(f)\ell}$, caused by the layer of tissue;

5) the transmittance of the rear surface of the tissue or the percentage of energy in the tissue that is coupled into the water, τ_2;

6) the attenuation, $e^{\alpha_w(f)\ell_{w_2}}$, and phase change, $e^{-j\beta_w(f)\ell_{w_2}}$, caused by the water on the far side of the tissue;

7) the receiver transfer function relating a pressure wave to the resulting electrical signal, $H_2(f)$.

We will assume the center frequency of the transducers is high enough so that beam divergence may be neglected. (If the center frequency is too low, the transmitted wavefront will diverge excessively as it propagates toward the receiver; the resulting loss of signal would then have to be compensated for by another factor.) With these assumptions the Fourier transform $Y(f)$ of the received signal $y(t)$ is related to $X(f)$, the Fourier transform of the signal $x(t)$, as follows [Din76], [Kak78]:

$$Y(f) = X(f)H_1(f)H_2(f)A_\tau$$
$$\cdot \exp\left[-[\alpha(f)+j\beta(f)]\ell\right]\exp\left[-[\alpha_w(f)+j\beta_w(f)]\ell_w\right] \quad (35)$$

where

$$\ell_w = \ell_{w_1} + \ell_{w_2} \quad (36)$$

ℓ_{w_1} and ℓ_{w_2} being water path lengths on two sides of the tissue layer and ℓ

being the thickness of the tissue. $\alpha(f)$ and $\beta(f)$ are the attenuation and phase coefficients, respectively, of the tissue layer; $\alpha_w(f)$ and $\beta_w(f)$ are the corresponding coefficients for the water medium; $H_1(f)$ and $H_2(f)$ are, respectively, the transfer functions of the transducers T_1 and T_2. In the above equation A_τ is given by

$$A_\tau = \tau_1 \cdot \tau_2 \tag{37}$$

where τ_1 and τ_2 are, respectively, the transmittances of the front and the back faces of the layer.

In order not to concern ourselves with the transducer properties, as depicted by functions $H_1(f)$ and $H_2(f)$, we will always normalize the received signal $y(t)$ by the direct water path signal $y_w(t)$; see Fig. 4.26(b). Clearly,

$$Y_w(f) = X(f)H_1(f)H_2(f) \exp\left[-[\alpha_w(f)+j\beta_w(f)](\ell+\ell_w)\right] \tag{38}$$

where $Y_w(f)$ is the Fourier transform of $y_w(t)$. Therefore, from (35) and (38)

$$Y(f) = Y_w(f)A_\tau \exp\left[-[(\alpha(f)-\alpha_w(f))\ell + j(\beta(f)-\beta_w(f))\ell]\right]. \tag{39}$$

In most cases, the attenuation coefficient of water is much smaller than that of tissue [Din79b] and may simply be neglected. Therefore,

$$Y(f) = Y_w(f)A_\tau \exp\left[-[\alpha(f)\ell + j(\beta(f)-\beta_w(f))\ell]\right]. \tag{40}$$

Extending this rationale to multilayered objects such as the one shown in Fig. 4.26(c), we get for the Fourier transform $Y(f)$ of the received signal:

$$Y(f) = X(f)H_1(f)H_2(f)A_\tau \exp\left[-\int_0^\ell [\alpha(x,f)+j\beta(x,f)]\,dx\right]$$
$$\cdot \exp\left[-j\beta_w(f)\ell_w\right] \tag{41}$$

where $A_\tau = \tau_1\tau_2\tau_3\cdots\tau_N$ (τ_i being the transmittance at the ith interface) and where $\alpha(f)$ and $\beta(f)$ have been replaced by $\alpha(x,f)$ and $\beta(x,f)$ since, now, they are functions of position along the path of propagation. This equation corresponds to (35) for the single layer case. Combining it with (37) and again ignoring the attenuation of water, we get

$$Y(f) = A_\tau Y_w(f) \exp\left[-\int_0^\ell \alpha(x,f)\,dx\right]$$
$$\cdot \exp\left[-j2\pi f \int_0^\ell (1/V(x)-1/V_w)\,dx\right] \tag{42}$$

where we have ignored dispersion in each layer (it is very small for soft tissues [Wel77]) and expressed $\beta(x,f)$ and $\beta_w(f)$ as $2\pi f/V(x)$ and $2\pi f/V_w$, respectively. $V(x)$ and V_w are propagation velocities in the layer at x, and water, respectively. Now let $y'_w(t)$ denote the inverse transform of

$$y'_w(t) = A_\tau Y_w(f) \exp\left[-\int_0^t \alpha(x, f)\, dx\right]. \tag{43}$$

We may consider $y'_w(t)$ to be an "attenuated" water path signal. This is the hypothetical signal that would be received if it underwent the same loss as the actual signal going through tissue. By the shift property, the relationship depicted in (42) may be expressed as

$$y(t) = y'_w(t - T_d) \tag{44}$$

where

$$T_d = \frac{1}{V_w} \int_0^t [n(x) - 1]\, dx \tag{45}$$

with the refractive index $n(x)$ given by

$$n(x) = \frac{V_w}{V(x)}. \tag{46}$$

The relationship among the signals $x(t)$, $y_w(t)$, $y'_w(t)$, and $y(t)$ is also depicted in Fig. 4.27.

As implied by our discussion on refraction, in the actual tomographic imaging of soft biological tissues the assumptions made above regarding the propagation of a sound beam are only approximately satisfied. In propagating through a complex tissue structure, the interfaces encountered are usually not perpendicular to the beam. However, since the refractive index variations in soft tissues are usually less than 5% the beam bending effects are usually not that serious; especially so at the resolution with which the projection data are currently measured. But minor geometrical distortions are still introduced. For example, when the projection data are taken with a simple scan–rotate configuration, a round disk-like soft-tissue phantom with a refractive index less than one would appear larger by about 3 to 5% as a result of such distortion.

4.3.2 Ultrasonic Refractive Index Tomography

Here the aim is to make cross-sectional images for the refractive index coefficient of soft tissue. From the discussion in the preceding section, for a ray like AB in Fig. 4.28

$$\int_A^B [1 - n(x, y)]\, ds = -V_w T_d. \tag{47}$$

Therefore, a measurement of T_d gives us a ray integral for the function

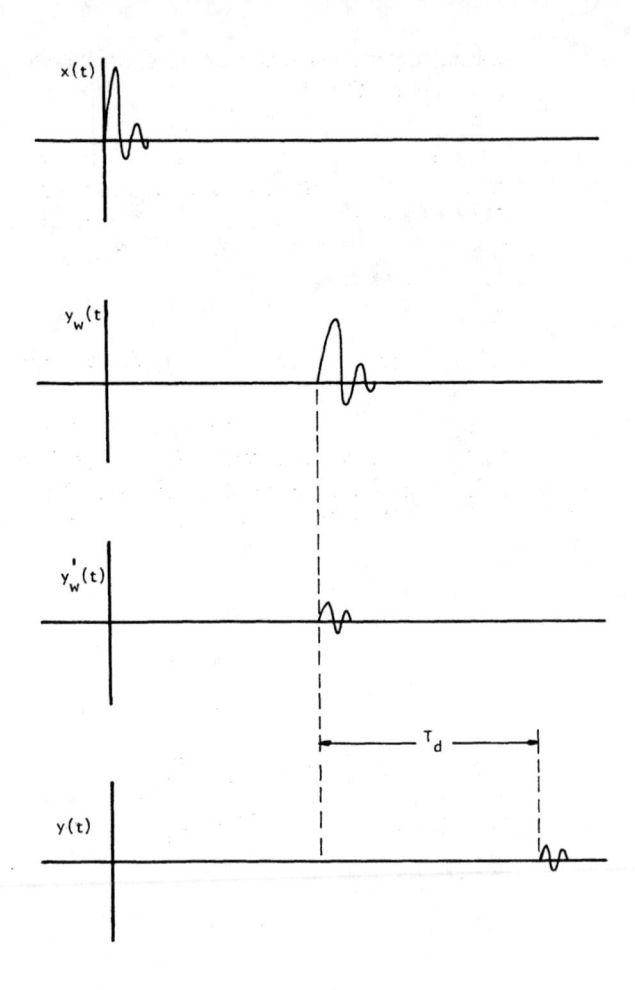

Fig. 4.27: *The phase shift and the attenuation of an ultrasonic signal, $x(t)$, as it travels through water, $y_w(t)$, and is attenuated, $y'_w(t)$, and then phase shifted by the object, $y(t)$, are shown here. (From [Kak79].)*

$(1 - n(x, y))$, and hence, from such measurements we may reconstruct $1 - n(x, y)$ (or $n(x, y)$). Note that one usually makes the image for $1 - n(x, y)$ rather than $n(x, y)$ itself. This is to ensure that in the reconstructed image the numerical values reconstructed for background are zero, since the refractive index of water is 1. In (47) T_d is positive if the transit time through the tissue structure is longer than the transit time through the direct water path. Usually the opposite is the case, since most tissues are faster than water. Therefore, most often T_d is negative making the right-hand side of the above equation positive.

Measuring the time of flight (TOF) of an ultrasonic pulse is generally done by thresholding the received signal and measuring the time between the source excitation and the first time the received signal is larger than the threshold. Since acoustic energy travels at 1500 m/s in water, the TOF measured is on the order of 100 μs and is easily measured with fairly straightforward digital hardware. More details of this process and preprocessing algorithms that can be used to clean up the projection data are described in [Cra82].

A refractive index reconstruction made for a Formalin-fixed dog's heart is shown in Fig. 4.29.[5] After this and other experiments reported in this section, the heart was cut at the level chosen; the cut section is shown in Fig. 4.30. The reconstruction shown here was made with only 18 measured projections (which were then extrapolated to 72; see [Din76]) and 56 rays in each projection.

4.3.3 Ultrasonic Attenuation Tomography

Here one seeks to construct cross-sectional images of soft-tissue structures for the attenuation coefficient. Let $\alpha(x, y, f)$ be the attenuation coefficient as a function of frequency at a point (x, y) in a cross-sectional plane. Since $\alpha(x, y, f)$ is a function of frequency, strictly speaking one may make the tomogram at only one chosen frequency. This can be done by using pulsed CW[6] transmission through tissue [Mil77] since in pulsed CW signals most of the energy is concentrated around a single frequency. Another approach to the problem is to recognize that in soft tissues

$$\alpha(x, y, f) = \alpha_0(x, y)|f| \qquad (48)$$

is a good approximation in the low MHz range. Clearly now, instead of reconstructing the attenuation coefficient $\alpha(x, y, f)$ one can reconstruct the parameter $\alpha_0(x, y)$. To the extent the above approximation applies, $\alpha_0(x, y)$ completely characterizes the attenuation properties of the soft tissue at location (x, y).

In order to obtain a tomogram for $\alpha_0(x, y)$, we need projection data with each ray being given by

$$\int_{\text{ray}} \alpha_0(x, y) \, ds. \qquad (49)$$

The path of integration could, for example, be the ray AB in Fig. 4.28. We will call the above integral the integrated attenuation coefficient, although it must be multiplied by a frequency in order to get $\int \alpha(x, y, f) \, ds$ at that frequency.

A number of different techniques for measuring the integrated attenuation coefficient using broadband pulsed ultrasound are presented in [Kak78]. In

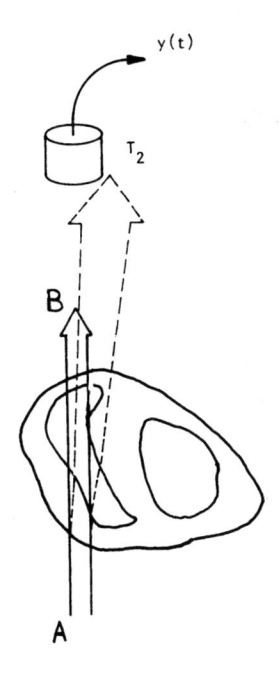

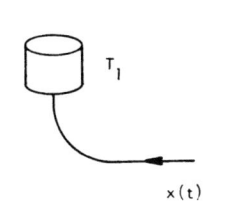

Fig. 4.28: *In ultrasound refractive index tomography the time it takes for an ultrasound pulse to travel between points A and B is measured. (From [Kak79].)*

---

[5] The reconstructions of a dog's heart presented here are not meant to imply the suitability of computerized ultrasonic tomography for *in vivo* cardiovascular imaging. Air in the lungs and refraction due to the surrounding rib cage would preclude that as a practical possibility. *Ultrasonic tomography of the female breast for tumor detection would be an ideal candidate for such techniques.* The reconstructions presented were done on dogs' hearts because of their easy availability.

[6] CW is an abbreviation for continuous wave. Pulsed CW means that the signal is a few cycles of a continuous sinusoid.

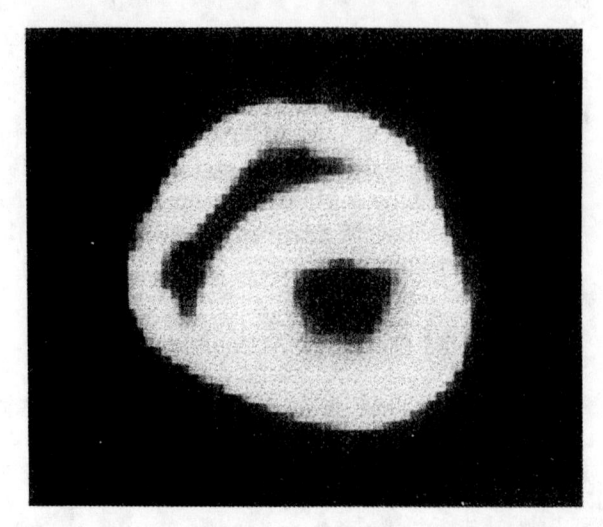

Fig. 4.29: *A refractive index reconstruction of the dog's heart. (From [Kak79].)*

Fig. 4.30: *After data collection the dog's heart was cut at the level for which reconstructions were made. (From [Kak79].)*

what follows we will list some of these techniques with brief descriptions and show reconstructions obtained by using them.

i) Energy-Ratio Method: It has been shown in [Kak78] that

$$\int_{\text{ray}} \alpha_0(x, y) \, ds = \frac{1}{2(f_2 - f_1)} \ln \left| \frac{E_1}{E_2} \right| \qquad (50)$$

where E_1 and E_2 are, respectively, weighted energies in frequency bands $(f_1 - \Omega, f_1 + \Omega)$ and $(f_2 - \Omega, f_2 + \Omega)$ of the transfer functions of the tissue structure along the desired ray. The transfer function, $H(f)$, is defined by

$$H(f) = \frac{Y_a(f)}{X_a(f)} \qquad (51)$$

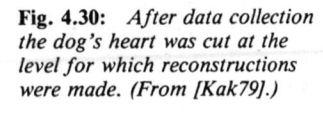

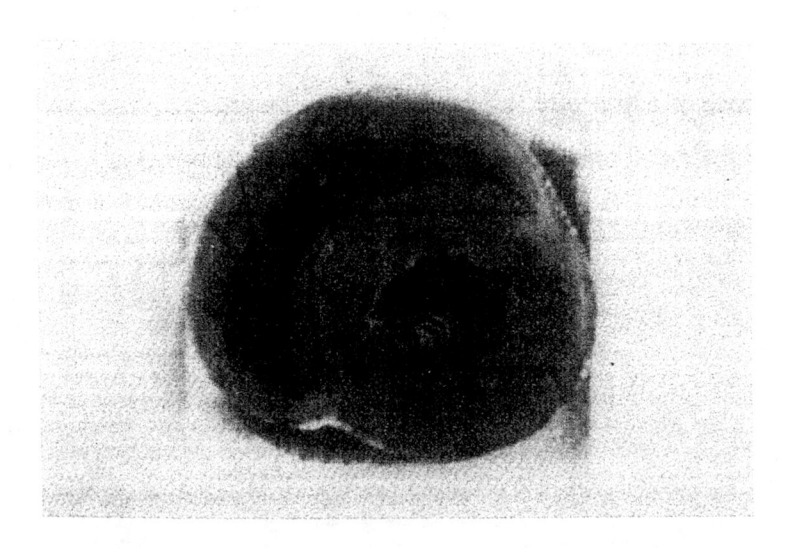

154 COMPUTERIZED TOMOGRAPHIC IMAGING

where $Y_a(f)$ and $X_a(f)$ are Fourier transforms of the signals $y_a(t)$ and $x_a(t)$, respectively (Fig. 4.26(c)). One can show that in terms of the experimentally measured signals $y(t)$ and $y_w(t)$ [Din79b]:

$$|H(f)| = \left| \frac{Y(f)}{Y_w(f)} \right| . \qquad (52)$$

In terms of the function $H(f)$, E_1 and E_2 required in (50) are given by (Fig. 4.31):

$$E_1 = 2 \int_{f_1-\Omega}^{f_1+\Omega} |X(f-f_1)|^2 |H(f)|^2 \, df \qquad (53)$$

and

$$E_2 = 2 \int_{f_2-\Omega}^{f_2+\Omega} |X(f-f_2)|^2 |H(f)|^2 \, df \qquad (54)$$

where $X(f)$ is any arbitrary weighting function. The weighting function can be used to emphasize those frequencies at which there is more confidence in the calculation of $H(f)$.

A major advantage of the energy-ratio method is that the calculation of the integrated attenuation coefficient doesn't depend upon the knowledge of transmittances (as incorporated in the factor A_r). To the extent this calculation doesn't depend on the magnitude of the received signal (but only on its spectral composition) this method should also be somewhat insensitive to the partial loss of signal caused by beam refraction. The extent of this "insensitivity" is not yet known.

A reconstruction using this method is shown in Fig. 4.32.

ii) *Division of Transforms Followed by Averaging Method:* Let $H_a(f)$

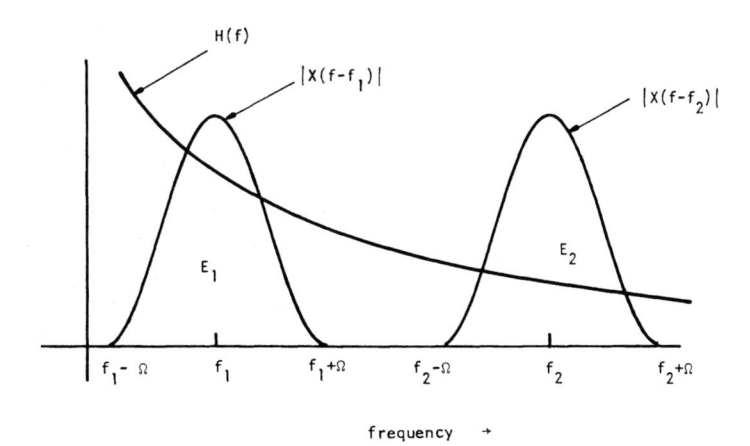

Fig. 4.31: $H(f)$ *is the transfer function of the tissue structure. The weighted integrals of* $|H(f)|^2$ *over the two intervals shown give* E_1 *and* E_2. *(From [Kak79].)*

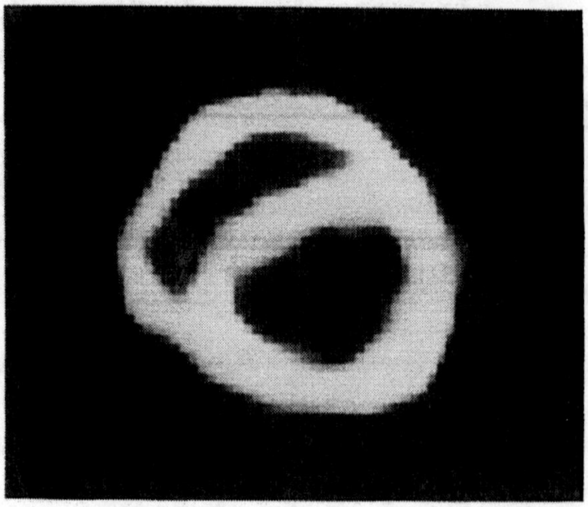

Fig. 4.32: *An attenuation reconstruction of the dog's heart by the energy-ratio method. (From [Kak79].)*

denote

$$H_A(f) = -\ln |H(f)| = -\ln \left| \frac{Y(f)}{Y_w(f)} \right|. \tag{55}$$

Now let $F(f_1, f_2, \Omega_1, \Omega_2)$ denote the following:

$$F(f_1, f_2, \Omega_1, \Omega_2) = \frac{1}{2\Omega_2} \int_{f_2-\Omega_2}^{f_2+\Omega_2} H_A(f) \, df - \frac{1}{2\Omega} \int_{f_1-\Omega_1}^{f_1+\Omega_1} H_A(f) \, df. \tag{56}$$

Then one can show that

$$\text{projection data} = \int_{\text{ray}} \alpha_0(x, y) \, ds = F. \tag{57}$$

Again, the method is independent of the value of transmittances at tissue–tissue and tissue–medium interfaces. The method may also possess some immunity to noise because of the integration in (56). In Fig. 4.33 a reconstruction for the dog's heart is shown using this method. The level chosen was the same as that for the refractive index tomogram.

iii) Frequency-Shift Method: From the standpoint of data processing the above two methods suffer from a disadvantage. In order to use them one must determine the transfer function $H(f)$ from the recorded waveform $y(t)$ for each ray and $y_w(t)$. This requires that for each ray the entire time signal $y(t)$ be digitized and recorded, and this may take anywhere from 100 to 300 samples depending upon the maximum frequency (above the noise level) in the acoustic pulse produced by the transmitting transducer. This is in marked contrast to the case of x-ray tomography where for each ray one records only *one number,* i.e., the *total* number of photons arriving at the detector during the measurement time interval.

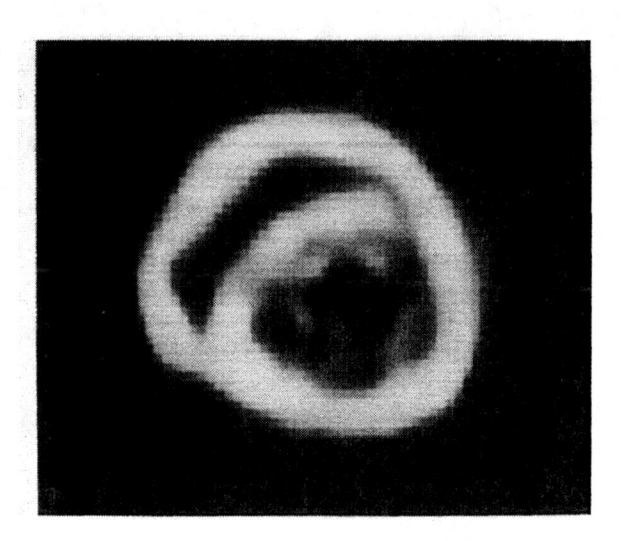

Fig. 4.33: *An attenuation reconstruction of the dog's heart obtained from the averages of the function $H_A(f)$. (From [Kak79].)*

In the frequency-shift method the integrated attenuated coefficient is measured by measuring the center frequencies of the direct water path signal $y_w(t)$ and the signal received after transmission through tissue, $y(t)$. The relationship is [Din79b]

$$\int_{\text{ray}} \alpha_0(x, y) \, ds = \frac{f_0 - f_r}{2\sigma^2}. \tag{58}$$

where f_0 is the frequency at which $Y_w(f)$ is a maximum and f_r is that at which $Y(f)$ is a maximum; σ^2 is a measure of the width of the power spectrum of $y_w(t)$.

For a precise implementation this method also requires that the entire waveform $y(t)$ be recorded for each ray. However, we are speculating that it might be possible to construct some simple circuit that could be attached to the receiving transducer the output of which would directly be f_r [Nap81]. (Such a circuit could estimate, perhaps suboptimally, the frequency f_r from the zeros and locations of maxima and minima of the waveforms.) The center frequency f_0 needs to be determined only once for an experiment so it shouldn't pose any logistical problems.

In Fig. 4.34 we have shown a reconstruction using this method. The reconstruction was made from the same data that were recorded for the preceding two experiments.

4.3.4 Applications

A clinical study discussing the use of ultrasound tomography for the diagnosis of breast abnormalities was described by Schreiman *et al.* in [Sch84]. In this study the information from refractive index images was combined with that from attenuation images and compared against mammo-

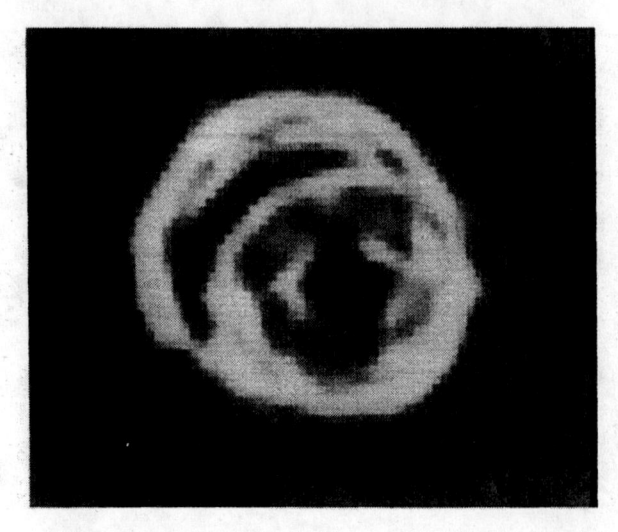

Fig. 4.34: *An attenuation reconstruction obtained by using the frequency-shift method. (From [Kak79].)*

grams. In addition, the design of a program to automatically diagnose breast tomograms based on the attenuation constant and the index of refraction near the lesion was described.

The mammograms and ultrasound tomographic images in Figs. 4.35 and 4.36, respectively, show a small spiculated cancer in the upper outer quadrant of a right breast. The tomographic reconstructions shown in Fig. 4.36 were based on the measurement of 60 parallel projections each with 200 rays. For each ray the time of arrival and the signal level of a 5-MHz ultrasound signal were measured and stored on tape for off-line processing. The total data collection time was 5 minutes.

In this study the attenuation and refractive index images were based on a full wave rectified and low pass filtered version of the measured ultrasonic pressure wave. The time delay caused by the object was measured by timing the instant when the filtered signal first crossed a threshold. This gives a direct estimate of the time delay, T_d, as described in Section 4.3.2. On the other hand, the attenuation of the signal was measured by integrating the first two microseconds of the filtered signal. While this method doesn't take into account the frequency dependence of the attenuation coefficient, it does have the overriding advantage that its hardware implementation is very simple and fast.

4.4 Magnetic Resonance Imaging[7]

No book describing tomographic imaging would be complete without a discussion of (nuclear) magnetic resonance imaging (MRI). While the principles of nuclear magnetic resonance have been well known since the

---

[7] We appreciate the help of Kevin King of General Electric's Medical Systems Group and Greg Kirk of Resonex, Inc. in preparing this material.

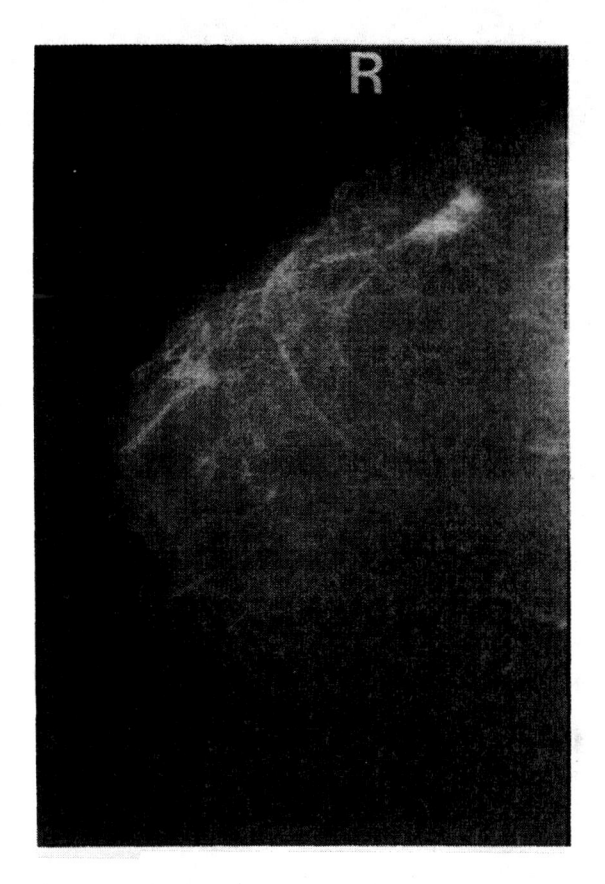

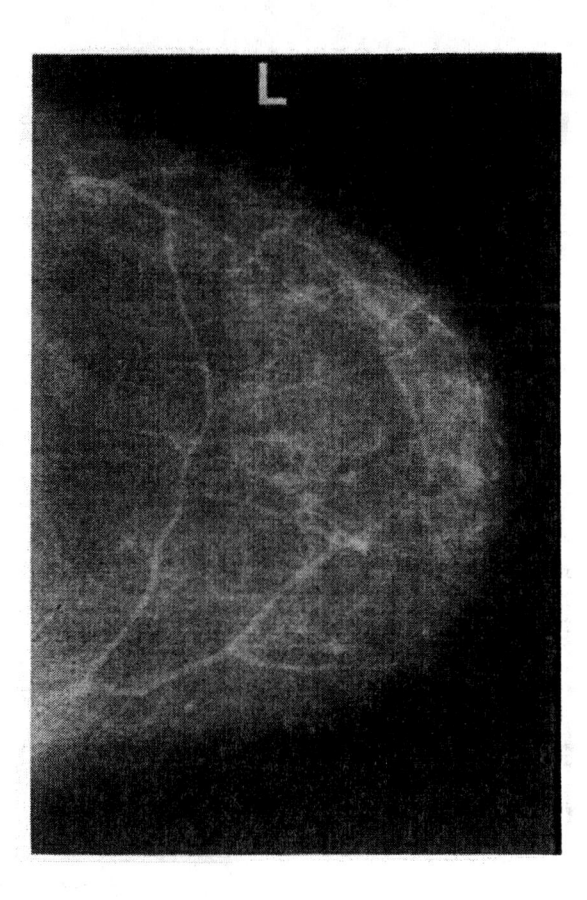

Fig. 4.35: *The x-ray mammograms of these female breasts show a small spiculated cancer in the upper outer quadrant of the right breast. (Courtesy of Jim Greenleaf of the Mayo Clinic in Rochester, MN.)*

1950s, only since 1972 has it been used for imaging. In the sense that the images produced represent a cross section of the object, MRI is a tomographic technique. Two head images obtained using MRI are shown in Fig. 4.37.

The fundamentals of chemistry and physics required to derive MRI are beyond the scope of this book. A rigorous derivation requires the use of quantum mechanics, but since acceptable models of the process can be built using classical mechanics, this will be the approach used here. For more information the reader is referred to excellent accounts of the theory in [Man82], [Mac83], [Cho82], [Hin83], [Pyk82].

Magnetic resonance imaging is based on the measurement of radio frequency electromagnetic waves as a spinning nucleus returns to its equilibrium state. Any nucleus with an odd number of particles (protons and neutrons) has a magnetic moment, and, when the atom is placed in a strong magnetic field, the moment of the nucleus tends to line up with the field. If the atom is then excited by another magnetic field it emits a radio frequency signal as the nucleus returns to its equilibrium position. Since the frequency of the signal is dependent on not only the type of atom but also the magnetic

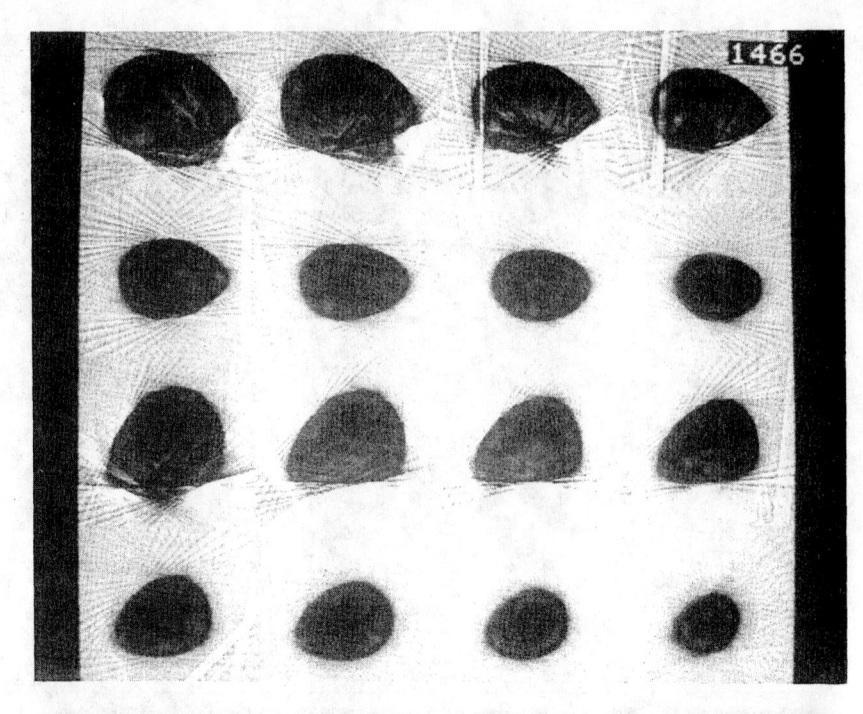

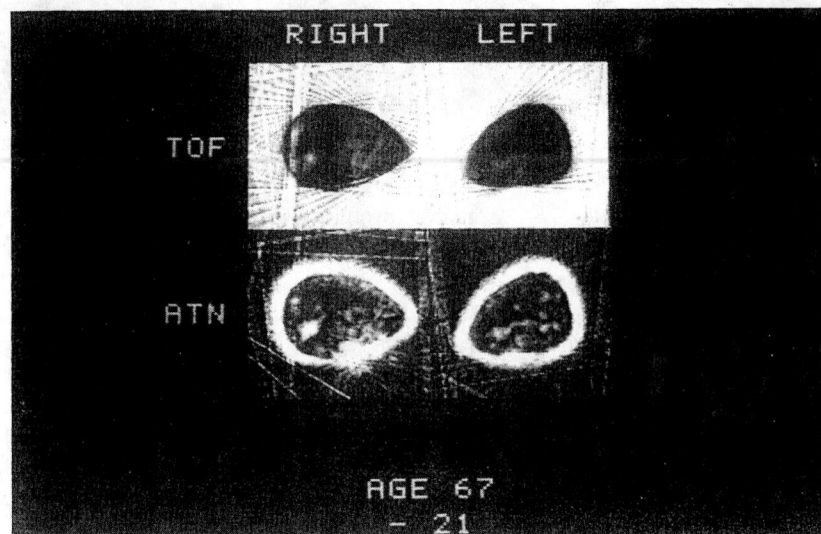

Fig. 4.36: *The time of flight (TOF) images on top and the combined TOF and attenuation (ATN) images on the bottom show the small cancer. (Reprinted with permission from [Sch84].)*

fields present, the position and type of each nucleus can be detected by appropriate signal processing.

Two of the more interesting atoms for MRI are hydrogen and phosphorus. The hydrogen atom is found most often bound into a water molecule while phosphorus is an important link in the transfer of energy in biological

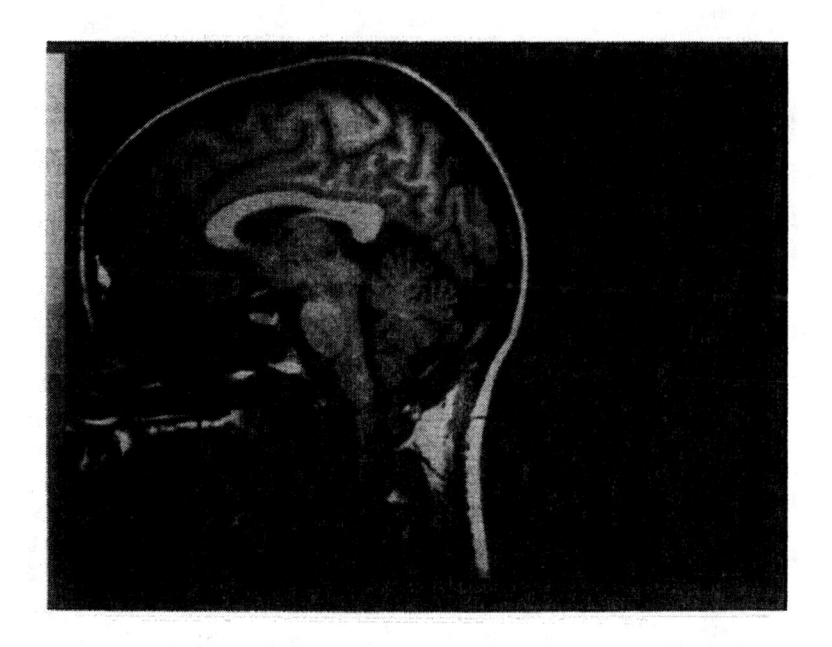

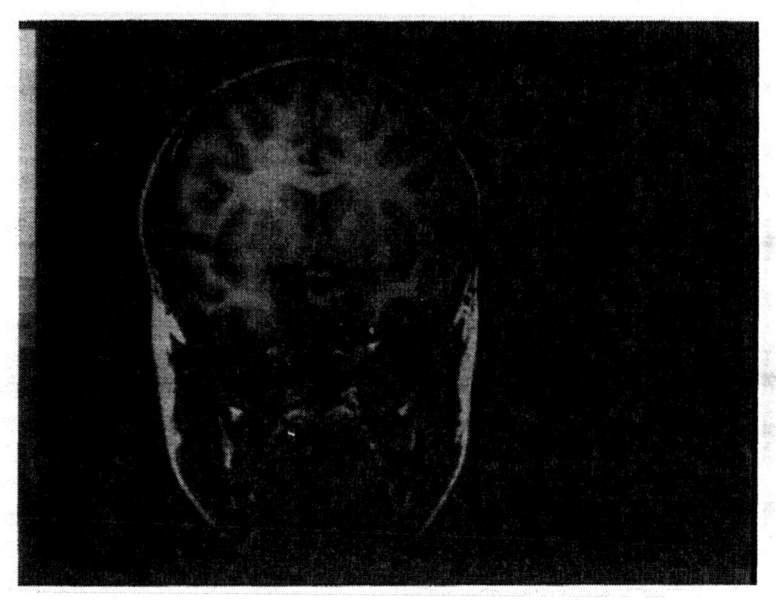

Fig. 4.37: *These two images demonstrate the contrast and resolution obtainable using MRI. They were obtained using a 1.5-Tesla Signa® system at General Electric's MR Development Center. (Courtesy of General Electric's Medical Systems Group.)*

systems. Both of these atoms have an odd number of nucleons and thus act like a spinning magnetic dipole when placed into a strong field.

When a spinning magnetic moment is placed in a strong magnetic field and perturbed it processes much like a spinning top or gyroscope. The frequency of precession is determined by the magnitude of the external field and the type and chemical binding of the atom. The precession frequency is known as the

Larmor frequency and is given by

$$\omega = \gamma H \tag{59}$$

where H is the magnitude of the local magnetic field and γ is known as the gyromagnetic constant. The gyromagnetic constant, although primarily a function of the type of nucleus, also changes slightly due to the chemical elements surrounding the nucleus. These small changes in the gyromagnetic constant are known as chemical shifts and are used in NMR spectroscopy to identify the compounds in a sample. In MRI, on the other hand, a spatially varying field is used to code each position with a unique resonating frequency. Image reconstruction is done using this information.

Recalling that a magnetic field has both a magnitude and direction at a point in three space, (x, y, z), the field is described by the vector quantity $\vec{H}(x, y, z)$. When necessary we will use the orthogonal unit vectors $\hat{x}$, $\hat{y}$, and $\hat{z}$ to represent the three axes. Conventionally, the z-axis is aligned along the axis of the static magnetic field used to align the magnetic moments. The static magnetic field is then described by $\vec{H}_0 = H_0 \hat{z}$.

A radio frequency magnetic wave in the (x, y)-plane and at the Larmor frequency, $\omega_0 = \gamma H_0$, is used to perturb the magnetic moments from their equilibrium position. The degree of tipping or precession that occurs is dependent on the strength of the field and the length of the pulse. Using the classical mechanics model a sinusoidal field of magnitude H_1 that lasts t_p seconds will cause the magnetic moment to precess through an angle given by

$$\theta = \gamma H_1 t_p. \tag{60}$$

The actual transmitted field, $\vec{H}_1(x, y, z)$, is given by

$$\vec{H}_1(x, y, z) = 2H_1 \cos \omega_0 t \, \hat{x}. \tag{61}$$

Generally, H_1 and t_p are varied so that the moment will be flipped either 90 or 180°. By flipping the moments 90° the maximum signal is obtained as the system returns to equilibrium while 180° flips are often used to change the sign of the phase (with respect to the $H_{\hat{1}}$-axis) of the moment.

It is important to note that only those nuclei where the magnitude of the local field is H_0 will flip according to (60). Those nuclei with a local magnetic field near H_0 will flip to a small degree while those nuclei with a local field far from H_0 will not be flipped at all. This property of spinning nuclei in a magnetic field is used in MRI to restrict the active nuclei to restricted sections of the body [Man82]. Typical slice thicknesses in 1986 machines are from 3 to 10 mm.

After the radio frequency (RF) pulse is applied there are two effects that can be measured as the magnetic moment returns to its equilibrium position. They are known as the longitudinal and transverse relaxation times. The longitudinal or spin–lattice relaxation time, T_1, is the simpler of the two and represents the time it takes for the energy to dissipate and the moment to return to its equilibrium position along the $\hat{z}$-axis. In addition, after the RF pulse is applied, the spinning magnetic moments gradually become out of phase due to the effects of nearby nuclei. The time for this to occur is known as the transverse or spin-spin relaxation time, T_2. In practice, there is a third parameter called T_2^* that also takes into account the local inhomogeneities of the magnetic field. Because of physical constraints the following relationship always holds:

$$T_2^* \leq T_2 \leq T_1. \tag{62}$$

Note that T_2^* includes the effect of T_2.

The process of tipping (or even flipping) a moment and its eventual return to the equilibrium state are diagrammed in Fig. 4.38. Conventionally the magnetic moments are shown in a coordinate system that rotates at the Larmor frequency. The direction of the magnetic moment before and immediately after a 45° pulse is shown in Figs. 4.38(a) and (b). Fig. 4.38(c) diagrams the moments as they start to return to the equilibrium position and some of the moments become out of phase. The time T_2 is shorter than T_1 so the moments are totally out of phase before they return to the equilibrium position. This is shown in Fig. 4.38(d). Finally, after several T_1 intervals the moments return to their equilibrium position as shown in Fig. 4.38(e).

As the spinning moments return to their equilibrium position they generate an electromagnetic wave at the Larmor frequency. This wave is known as the free induction decay (FID) signal and can be detected using coils around the object. When the magnetic moments are in phase, as they are immediately following an RF excitation, the FID signal is proportional to both the density and the transverse component of the magnetic moments. Near time $t = 0$,

Fig. 4.38: *As an excited magnetic moment relaxes toward its equilibrium position it emits a free induction decay (FID) signal which can be thought of as the transverse component of the precessing moment. In addition, as the moment returns to its equilibrium state the longitudinal component of the magnetic field returns to the value of M_0.*

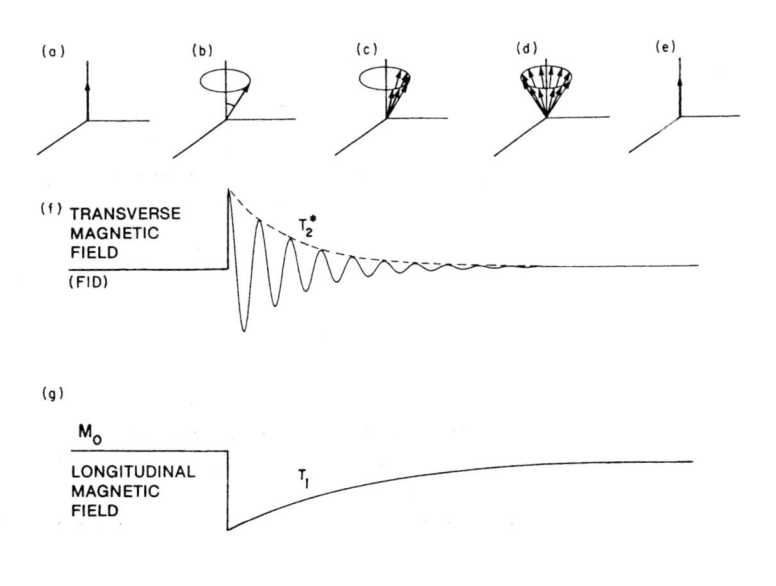

MEASUREMENT OF PROJECTION DATA   163

immediately following the end of the RF pulse, the received signal is given by

$$S(t) = \rho \sin(\theta) \cos(\omega_0 t) \qquad (63)$$

where again θ is the flip angle and ρ is the density of the magnetic moments. From this signal it is easy to verify that the largest FID signal is generated by a 90° pulse.

Both the spin-spin and the spin-lattice relaxation processes contribute to the decay of the FID signal. The FID signal after a 90° pulse can be written as

$$S(t) = \rho \cos(\omega_0 t) \exp[-t/T_2^*] \exp[-t/T_1] \qquad (64)$$

where the exponentials with respect to T_1 and T_2^* represent the attenuation of the FID signal due to the return to equilibrium (T_1) and the dephasing (T_2^*).

In tissue the typical times for T_1 and T_2 are 0.5 s and 50 ms, respectively. Thus the decay of the FID signal is dominated by the spin-spin relaxation time (T_2 and T_2^*) and the effects of the spin-lattice time (e^{-t/T_1} in the equation above) are hidden. A typical FID signal is shown in Fig. 4.38(f).

A clinician is interested in three parameters of the object: spin density, T_1 and T_2. The spin density is easiest to measure; it can be estimated from the magnitude of the FID immediately following the RF pulse. On the other hand, the T_1 and the T_2 parameters are more difficult.

To give our readers just a flavor of the algorithms used in MRI we will only discuss imaging of the spin density. More complicated pulse sequences, such as those described in [Cho82], are used to weight the image by the object's T_1 or T_2 parameters. In addition, much work is being done to discover combinations of the above parameters that make tissue characterization easier.

There are many ways to spatially encode the FID signal so that tomographic images can be formed. We will only discuss two of them here. The first measures line integrals of the object and then uses the Fourier Slice Theorem to reconstruct the object. The second approach measures the two-dimensional Fourier transform of the object directly so that a simple inverse Fourier transform can be used to estimate the object.

To restrict the imaging to a single plane a magnetic gradient

$$\Delta H_p = G_z z \qquad (65)$$

is superimposed on the background field H_0 as is shown in Fig. 4.39. If a narrow band excitation at the Larmor frequency $\omega_0 = \gamma H_0$ is then applied to the object only those nuclei near the plane $z = 0$ will be excited. For maximum response the excitation should be long enough to cause each nucleus to precess through 90°.

A projection of the object in the plane $z = 0$ is measured by applying a readout gradient of the form

$$\Delta H_r = G_x x + G_y y \qquad (66)$$

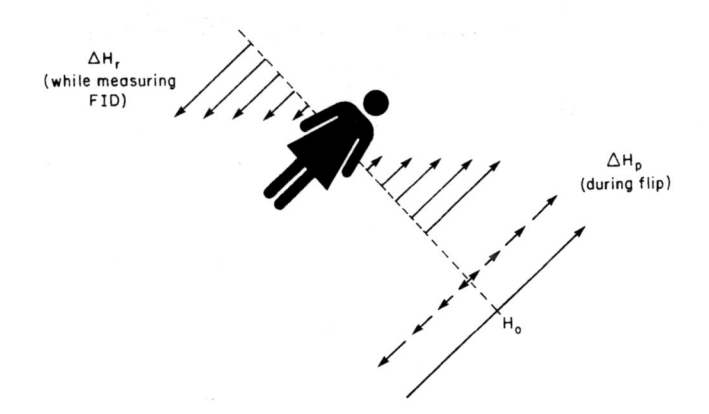

Fig. 4.39: *To measure projections of a three-dimensional object a field of strength $\Delta H_p = G_z z$ used to restrict the initial flip to a single plane. Then a readout gradient $\Delta H_r = G_x x + G_y y$ is used to measure projections of the object. In the case shown here the integrals are along lines perpendicular to the page.*

as the nuclei return to the equilibrium state. This second gradient serves to split each line integral into a separate frequency.

Consider the line

$$G_x x + G_y y = \Delta H_r = \text{constant}. \tag{67}$$

Along this line the FID signal will be at a unique frequency given by

$$\omega = -\gamma(H + \Delta H_r). \tag{68}$$

To measure a projection in the plane it is necessary to apply the readout gradient and then find the Fourier transform of the received signal. Each temporal frequency component of the FID signal will then correspond to a single line integral of the object. This is illustrated in Fig. 4.39.

A two-dimensional reconstruction of an object can be easily found by rotating the readout gradient and then using the reconstruction algorithms discussed in Chapter 3. A full three-dimensional reconstruction is easily formed by stacking the two-dimensional images.

A more common approach to magnetic resonance imaging is to use a phase encoding gradient. The gradient, applied between the excitation pulse and the readout of the FID, spatially encodes each position in the object with a phase. This leads to a very natural reconstruction scheme because data can be collected over a rectangular grid in the Fourier domain. Thus reconstructions using this method can be performed using a two-dimensional FFT instead of the Fourier backprojection usually found in computerized tomography.

One possible sequence of events is presented next. Like the projection approach described above, a magnetic gradient is applied to the object as the nuclei are excited. This restricts the imaging to a single plane where the local magnetic field and the frequency of the excitation satisfy the Larmor equation. This is shown in Fig. 4.40.

Two perpendicular gradients are used to encode each point in the plane. First a gradient, for example in the y direction or $\Delta H_p = G_y y$, is applied for T seconds. Because the frequency of precession is related to the local

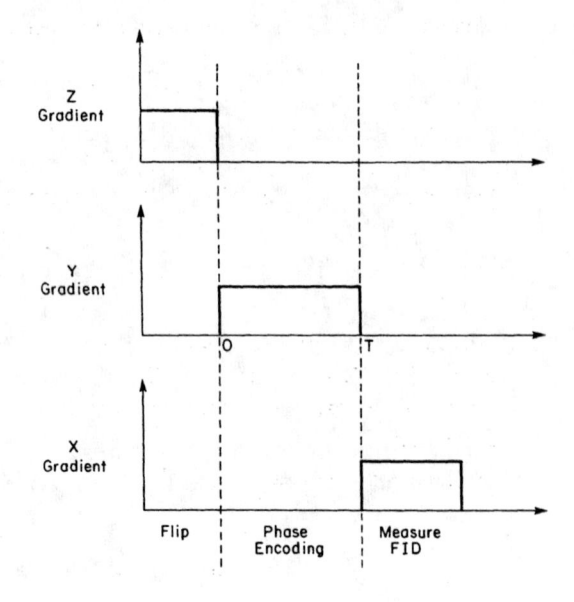

Fig. 4.40: *Three different gradients are used to measure the Fourier transform of an object using MRI. First a gradient in the z direction is used to restrict the flip to a single plane of the object. Then a second gradient, this time in y, is used to encode each line of constant y with a different phase. Finally, a third gradient, in x, is used while the FID signal is read to split each line of constant x into a different line integral.*

magnetic field, nuclei at different points in the object start spinning at different rates. After T seconds, when the phase encoding gradient is turned off, each line of constant y will have accumulated a phase given by

$$\phi = \omega t = (H_0 + \Delta H_p)\gamma T \qquad (69)$$

$$= \omega_0 T + G_y y \gamma T. \qquad (70)$$

Like the projection case the FID is measured while applying a readout gradient, this time along the x-axis or

$$\Delta H_r = G_x x. \qquad (71)$$

As before, the number of spinning nuclei along each line of constant x is now encoded by the frequency of the received signal. Unlike the previous case each position along the line is also encoded with a unique phase (see (69)). The following phase encoded line integral is measured:

$$p_{q_y}(t) = \iint \rho(x, y) \exp[jyq_y] \exp[jxq_x] \exp[j\omega_0 t] \, dx \, dy \qquad (72)$$

where $q_y = G_y \gamma T$ and $q_x = G_x \gamma t$. Note that except for the $e^{j\omega_0 t}$ term this equation is similar to the inverse Fourier transform of the data $\rho(x, y)$. To recover the phase encoded line integrals it is necessary to find the inverse Fourier transform of the data with respect to time or

$$p(w, q_y) = \frac{1}{2\pi} \int p_{q_y}(t) \exp[-jq_x w] \, dq_x. \qquad (73)$$

Finally, to recover the phase shifted projections it is necessary to shift the

166   COMPUTERIZED TOMOGRAPHIC IMAGING

frequency of $p(w, q_y)$ by the Larmor frequency, ω_0, or

$$\rho(x, q_y) = p(w - \omega_0, q_y). \tag{74}$$

A complete reconstruction is formed by stepping the phase encoding gradient, G_y, through N steps between G_{MAX} and $-G_{MAX}$ and measuring the phase encoded line integrals $p_{q_y}(t)$. To prevent aliasing it is important that

$$G_{MAX} \gamma T > \frac{\pi}{\Delta} \tag{75}$$

where the minimum feature size in the object is described by Δ. Note that in general the FID signal, $p_{q_y}(t)$, will be sampled in both q_y and t and thus the integral equations presented here will be approximated with discrete summations.

Since each line integral containing the point x, y is encoded with a different phase the spin density at any point can be recovered by inverting the integral equations. This is easily done by finding the Fourier transform of the collection of line integrals or

$$\rho(x, y) = \frac{1}{2\pi} \int p(x, q_y) \exp[-jq_y y] \, dq_y. \tag{76}$$

While a reconstruction can be done with either approach most images today are produced by direct Fourier inversion as opposed to the convolution backprojection algorithms described in Chapter 3. Two errors found in MRI machines are nonlinear gradients and a nonuniform static magnetic field. These errors affect the final reconstruction in different ways depending on the reconstruction technique.

First consider nonlinear gradients. In the direct Fourier approach only the magnitude of the gradients changes and not their direction. Thus any nonlinearities show up as a warping of the image space. As long as the gradient is monotonic the image will look sharp, although a bit distorted. On the other hand, in the projection approach the direction of the gradients is constantly changing so that each projection is warped differently. This leads to a blurring of the final reconstruction [ODo85].

The effect is similar with a nonhomogeneous static field, H_0. Since the gradient fields are simply added to the static field to determine the Larmor frequency a nonhomogeneous field can be thought of as a warping of the projection data. Since the Fourier approach doesn't change the angle of the projections, using phase changes to distinguish the different parts of the line integral, the direct Fourier approach yields sharper images.

In the simple analysis above we have ignored two important limitations on MRI. The first is the frequency spreading due to the T_2 relaxation time. In the analysis above we assumed a short enough measurement interval so that the relaxation could be considered negligible. Since the resolution in the frequency domain is linearly dependent on the measurement time the maximum possible measurement time should be used. Unfortunately the exponential attenuation of the FID signal broadens the frequency spectrum thereby determining the ultimate resolution of the magnetic resonance image.

A much more difficult problem is the data collection time. In the procedure described above each measurement is made assuming all the magnetic moments are at rest. Since the spin-lattice relaxation time is on the order of a second this implies that only a single FID can be measured per second. Since a three-dimensional image requires at least a million data points this is a severe restriction.

In practice, pulse sequences have been designed that allow more than one FID to be measured during the T_1 relaxation time. This can be done using a combination of gradients and selective gradients to only excite a single plane within the object and also using selective spin-echo pulses to measure more than one projection (or Fourier transform) within a single plane.

4.5 Bibliographic Notes

Because of the absence of any refraction or diffraction, with x-rays the problem of tomographic imaging reduces to reconstructing an image from its line integrals. A mathematical solution to the problem of reconstructing a function from its projections was given by Radon [Rad17] in 1917. More recently, some of the first investigators to examine this problem either theoretically or experimentally (and often independently) include (in a roughly chronological order): Bracewell [Bra56], Oldendorf [Old61], Cormack [Cor63], [Cor64], Kuhl and Edwards [Kuh63], DeRosier and Klug [DeR68], Tretiak et al. [Tre69], Rowley [Row69], Berry and Gibbs [Ber70], Ramachandran and Lakshminarayanan [Ram71], Bender et al. [Ben70], and Bates and Peters [Bat71]. A detailed survey of the work done in computed tomographic imaging till 1979 appears in [Kak79].

Detailed information about a number of the applications described in this book is also covered in books by Macovski [Mac83] and Herman [Her80]. For information about alternate approaches to single photon emission tomography the reader is referred to [Kno83]. A more detailed presentation of ultrasound tomography can be found in [Cra82], [Car78b]. Additional information about the physical basis of nuclear magnetic resonance can be found in a number of chemistry and physics texts including [Sha76], [Far71], [Man82], [Pyk82]. The algorithms used to reconstruct images using NMR information are described in [Cho82], [Hin83], [Man82], [Pyk82].

The reader is also referred to [Kak79], [Kak81] for a survey of medical tomographic imaging. For applications in radio astronomy, where the aim is to reconstruct the "brightness" distribution of a celestial source of radio waves from its strip integral measurements taken with special antenna beams, the reader is referred to [Bra56], [Bra67]. For electron microscopy applications, where one attempts to reconstruct the molecular structure of complex biomolecules from transmission micrograms, the reader should look to [Cro70], [Gor71]. The applications of this technique in optical interferometry, where the aim is to determine the refractive index field of an optically transparent medium, are discussed in [Ber70], [Row69], [Swe73]. The applications of tomography in earth resources imaging are presented in [Din79a], [Lyt80]. For information about a large number of industrial applications the reader is referred to [OSA85].

4.6 References

[All85] C. J. Allan, N. A. Keller, L. R. Lupton, T. Taylor, and P. D. Tonner, "Tomography: An overview of the AECL program," *Appl. Opt.*, vol. 24, pp. 4067-4075, Dec. 1, 1985.

[Alv76a] R. E. Alvarez and A. Macovski, "Energy-selective reconstructions in x-ray computerized tomography," *Phys. Med. Biol.*, vol. 21, pp. 733-744, 1976.

[Alv76b] ——, "Noise and dose in energy dependent computerized tomography," *Proc. S.P.I.E.*, vol. 96, pp. 131-137, 1976.

[Axe83] L. Axel, P. H. Arger, and R. A. Zimmerman, "Applications of computerized tomography to diagnostic radiology," *Proc. IEEE*, vol. 71, pp. 293-297, Mar. 1983.

[Bat71] R. H. T. Bates and T. M. Peters, "Towards improvements in tomography," *New Zealand J. Sci.*, vol. 14, pp. 883-896, 1971.

[Bat83] R. H. T. Bates, K. L. Garden, and T. M. Peters, "Overview of computerized tomography with emphasis on future developments," *Proc. IEEE*, vol. 71, pp. 356-372, Mar. 1983.

[Bel79] S. Bellini, M. Pianentini, and P. L. de Vinci, "Compensation of tissue absorption in emission tomography," *IEEE Trans. Acoust. Speech Signal Processing*, vol. ASSP-27, pp. 213-218, June 1979.

[Ben70] R. Bender, S. H. Bellman, and R. Gordon, "ART and the ribosome: A preliminary report on the three dimensional structure of individual ribosomes determined by an algebraic reconstruction technique," *J. Theor. Biol.*, vol. 29, pp. 483-487, 1970.

[Ber70] M. V. Berry and D. F. Gibbs, "The interpretation of optical projections," *Proc. Roy. Soc. London*, vol. A314, pp. 143-152, 1970.

[Boh78] C. Bohm, L. Eriksson, M. Bergstrom, J. Litton, R. Sundman, and M. Singh, "A computer assisted ringdetector positron camera system for reconstruction tomography of the brain," *IEEE Trans. Nucl. Sci.*, vol. NS-25, pp. 624-637, 1978.

[Boy83] D. P. Boyd and M. J. Lipton, "Cardiac computed tomography," *Proc. IEEE*, vol. 71, pp. 298-307, Mar. 1983.

[Bra56] R. N. Bracewell, "Strip integration in radio astronomy," *Aust. J. Phys.*, vol. 9, pp. 198-217, 1956.

[Bra67] R. H. Bracewell and A. C. Riddle, "Inversion of fan-beam scans in radio astronomy," *Astrophys. J.*, vol. 150, pp. 427-434, Nov. 1967.

[Bro76] R. A. Brooks and G. DiChiro, "Principles of computer assisted tomography (CAT) in radiographic and radioisotopic imaging," *Phys. Med. Biol.*, vol. 21, pp. 689-732, 1976.

[Bro77a] R. A. Brooks, "A quantitative theory of the Hounsfield unit and its application to dual energy scanning," *J. Comput. Assist. Tomog.*, vol. 1, pp. 487-493, 1977.

[Bro77b] R. A. Brooks and G. DiChiro, "Slice geometry in computer assisted tomography," *J. Comput. Assist. Tomog.*, vol. 1, pp. 191-199, 1977.

[Bro78a] ——, "Split-detector computed tomography: A preliminary report," *Radiology*, vol. 126, pp. 255-257, Jan. 1978.

[Bro78b] R. A. Brooks, G. H. Weiss, and A. J. Talbert, "A new approach to interpolation in computed tomography," *J. Comput. Assist. Tomog.*, vol. 2, pp. 577-585, Nov. 1978.

[Bro78] G. L. Brownell and S. Cochavi, "Transverse section imaging with carbon-11

[Bro81]   labeled carbon monoxide," *J. Comput. Assist. Tomog.*, vol. 2, pp. 533–538, Nov. 1978.

[Bro81]   R. A. Brooks, V. J. Sank, W. S. Friauf, S. B. Leighton, H. E. Cascio, and G. DiChiro, "Design considerations for positron emission tomography," *IEEE Trans. Biomed. Eng.*, vol. BME-28, pp. 158–177, Feb. 1981.

[Bud74]   T. F. Budinger and G. T. Gullberg, "Three dimensional reconstruction of isotope distributions," *Phys. Med. Biol.*, vol. 19, pp. 387–389, June 1974.

[Bud76]   ——, "Transverse section reconstruction of gamma-ray emitting radionuclides in patients," in *Reconstruction Tomography in Diagnostic Radiology and Nuclear Medicine*, M. M. TerPogossian et al., Eds. Baltimore, MD: University Park Press, 1976.

[Bud77]   T. F. Budinger, S. E. Derenzo, G. T. Gullberg, W. L. Greenberg, and R. H. Huesman, "Emission computer assisted tomography with single photon and positron annihilation photon emitters," *J. Comput. Assist. Tomog.*, vol. 1, pp. 131–145, 1977.

[Car76]   P. L. Carson, T. V. Oughton, and W. R. Hendee, "Ultrasound transaxial tomography by reconstruction," in *Ultrasound in Medicine II*, D. N. White and R. W. Barnes, Eds. New York, NY: Plenum Press, 1976, pp. 391–400.

[Car77]   P. L. Carson, T. V. Oughton, W. R. Hendee, and A. S. Ahuja, "Imaging soft tissue through bone with ultrasound transmission tomography by reconstruction," *Med. Phys.*, vol. 4, pp. 302–309, July/Aug. 1977.

[Car78a]   L. R. Carroll, "Design and performance characteristics of a production model positron imaging system," *IEEE Trans. Nucl. Sci.*, vol. NS-25, pp. 606–614, Feb. 1978.

[Car78b]   P. L. Carson, D. E. Dick, G. A. Thieme, M. L. Dick, E. J. Bayly, T. V. Oughton, G. L. Dubuque, and H. P. Bay, "Initial investigation of computed tomography for breast imaging with focussed ultrasound beams," in *Ultrasound in Medicine*, D. White and E. A. Lyons, Eds. New York, NY: Plenum Press, 1978, pp. 319–322.

[Cha78]   R. C. Chase and J. A. Stein, "An improved image algorithm for CT scanners," *Med. Phys.*, vol. 5, pp. 497–499, Dec. 1978.

[Cha79a]   L. T. Chang, "A method for attenuation correction in radionuclide computed tomography," *IEEE Trans. Nucl. Sci.*, vol. NS-25, pp. 638–643, Feb. 1979.

[Cha79b]   ——, "Attenuation correction and incomplete projection in single photon emission computed tomography," *IEEE Trans. Nucl. Sci.*, vol. 26, no. 2, pp. 2780–2789, Apr. 1979.

[Cho76]   Z. H. Cho, L. Eriksson, and J. Chan, "A circular ring transverse axial positron camera," in *Reconstruction Tomography in Diagnostic Radiology and Medicine*, M. M. TerPogossian et al., Eds. Baltimore, MD: University Park Press, 1976, pp. 393–421.

[Cho77]   Z. H. Cho, M. B. Cohen, M. Singh, L. Eriksson, J. Chan, N. MacDonald, and L. Spolter, "Performance and evaluation of the circular ring transverse axial positron camera," *IEEE Trans. Nucl. Sci.*, vol. NS-24, pp. 532–543, 1977.

[Cho78]   Z. H. Cho, O. Nalcioglu, and M. R. Furukhi, "Analysis of a cylindrical hybrid positron camera with bismuth germanate (BGO) scintillation crystals," *IEEE Trans. Nucl. Sci.*, vol. NS-25, pp. 952–963, Apr. 1978.

[Cho82]   Z. H. Cho, H. S. Kim, H. B. Song, and J. Cumming, "Fourier transform nuclear magnetic resonance tomographic imaging," *Proc. IEEE*, vol. 70, pp. 1152–1173, Oct. 1982.

[Chu77]   G. Chu and K. C. Tam, "Three dimensional imaging in the positron camera using Fourier techniques," *Phys. Med. Biol.*, vol. 22, pp. 245–265, 1977.

[Cor63]   A. M. Cormack, "Representation of a function by its line integrals with some radiological applications," *J. Appl. Phys.*, vol. 34, pp. 2722–2727, 1963.

[Cor64]   ——, "Representation of a function by its line integrals with some radiological applications, II," *J. Appl. Phys.*, vol. 35, pp. 2908–2913, Oct. 1964.

[Cra78]   C. R. Crawford and A. C. Kak, "Aliasing artifacts in CT images," Research Rep. TR-EE 78-55, School of Electrical Engineering, Purdue Univ., Lafayette, IN, Dec. 1978.

[Cra82]   ——, "Multipath artifacts in ultrasonic transmission tomography," *Ultrason. Imaging*, vol. 4, no. 3, pp. 234–266, July 1982.

[Cra86] C. R. Crawford, "Reprojection using a parallel backprojector," *Med. Phys.*, vol. 13, pp. 480-483, July/Aug. 1986.

[Cro70] R. A. Crowther, D. J. DeRosier, and A. Klug, "The reconstruction of a three-dimensional structure from projections and its applications to electron microscopy," *Proc. Roy. Soc. London,* vol. A317, pp. 319-340, 1970.

[DeR68] D. J. DeRosier and A. Klug, "Reconstruction of three dimensional structures from electron micrographs," *Nature*, vol. 217, pp. 130-134, Jan. 1968.

[Der77a] S. E. Derenzo, "Positron ring cameras for emission computed tomography," *IEEE Trans. Nucl. Sci.*, vol. NS-24, pp. 881-885, Apr. 1977.

[Der77b] S. E. Derenzo, T. F. Budinger, J. L. Cahoon, R. H. Huesman, and H. G. Jackson, "High resolution computed tomography of positron emitters," *IEEE Trans. Nucl. Sci.*, vol. NS-24, pp. 544-558, Feb. 1977.

[DiC78] G. DiChiro, R. A. Brooks, L. Dubal, and E. Chew, "The apical artifact: Elevated attenuation values toward the apex of the skull," *J. Comput. Assist. Tomog.*, vol. 2, pp. 65-79, Jan. 1978.

[Din76] K. A. Dines and A. C. Kak, "Measurement and reconstruction of ultrasonic parameters for diagnostic imaging," Research Rep. TR-EE 77-4, School of Electrical Engineering, Purdue Univ., Lafayette, IN, Dec. 1976.

[Din79a] K. A. Dines and R. J. Lytle, "Computerized geophysical tomography," *Proc. IEEE*, vol. 67, pp. 1065-1073, 1979.

[Din79b] K. A. Dines and A. C. Kak, "Ultrasonic attenuation tomography of soft biological tissues," *Ultrason. Imaging*, vol. 1, pp. 16-33, 1979.

[Due78] A. J. Duerinckx and A. Macovski, "Polychromatic streak artifacts in computed tomography images," *J. Comput. Assist. Tomog.*, vol. 2, pp. 481-487, Sept. 1978.

[Epp66] E. R. Epp and H. Weiss, "Experimental study of the photon energy spectrum of primary diagnostic x-rays," *Phys. Med. Biol.*, vol. 11, pp. 225-238, 1966.

[Eri76] L. Erikkson and Z. H. Cho, "A simple absorption correction in positron (annihilation gamma coincidence detection) transverse axial tomography," *Phys. Med. Biol.*, vol. 21, pp. 429-433, 1976.

[Far71] T. C. Farrar and E. D. Becker, *Pulse and Fourier Transform NMR, Introduction to Theory and Methods*. New York, NY: Academic Press, 1971.

[Far78] E. J. Farrell, "Processing limitations of ultrasonic image reconstruction," in *Proc. 1978 Conf. on Pattern Recognition and Image Processing*, May 1978, pp. 8-15.

[Fla83] S. W. Flax, N. J. Pelc, G. H. Glover, F. D. Gutmann, and M. McLachlan, "Spectral characterization and attenuation measurements in ultrasound," *Ultrason. Imaging*, vol. 5, pp. 95-116, 1983.

[Gad75] M. Gado and M. Phelps, "The peripheral zone of increased density in cranial computed tomography," *Radiology*, vol. 117, pp. 71-74, 1975.

[Glo77] G. H. Glover and J. L. Sharp, "Reconstruction of ultrasound propagation speed distribution in soft tissue: Time-of-flight tomography," *IEEE Trans. Sonics Ultrason.*, vol. SU-24, pp. 229-234, July 1977.

[Glo82] G. H. Glover, "Compton scatter effects in CT reconstructions," *Med. Phys.*, vol. 9, pp. 860-867, Nov./Dec. 1982.

[Goi72] M. Goiten, "Three dimensional density reconstruction from a series of two dimensional projections," *Nucl. Instrum. Methods*, vol. 101, pp. 509-518, 1972.

[Gor71] R. Gordon and G. T. Herman, "Reconstruction of pictures from their projections," *Commun. Assoc. Comput. Mach.*, vol. 14, pp. 759-768, 1971.

[Gre74] J. F. Greenleaf, S. A. Johnson, S. L. Lee, G. T. Herman, and E. H. Wood, "Algebraic reconstruction of spatial distributions of acoustic absorption within tissue from their two dimensional acoustic projections," in *Acoustical Holography*, vol. 5, P. S. Greene, Ed. New York, NY: Plenum Press, 1974, pp. 591-603.

[Gre75] J. F. Greenleaf, S. A. Johnson, W. F. Wamoya, and F. A. Duck, "Algebraic reconstruction of spatial distributions of acoustic velocities in tissue from their time-of-flight profiles," in *Acoustical Holography*, H. Booth, Ed. New York, NY: Plenum Press, 1975, pp. 71-90.

[Gre78] J. F. Greenleaf, S. K. Kenue, B. Rajagopalan, R. C. Bahn, and S. A. Johnson, "Breast imaging by ultrasonic computer-assisted tomography," in *Acoustical*

[Gre81] *Imaging,* A. Metherell, Ed. New York, NY: Plenum Press, 1978.
J. F. Greenleaf and R. C. Bahn, "Clinical imaging with transmissive ultrasonic computerized tomography," *IEEE Trans. Biomed. Eng.,* vol. BME-28, pp. 177-185, 1981.

[Gus78] D. E. Gustafson, M. J. Berggren, M. Singh, and M. K. Dewanjee, "Computed transaxial imaging using single gamma emitters," *Radiology,* vol. 129, pp. 187-194, Oct. 1978.

[Hal74] J. Hale, *The Fundamentals of Radiological Science.* Springfield, IL: Charles C. Thomas, Publisher, 1974.

[Haq78] P. Haque, D. Pisano, W. Cullen, and L. Meyer, "Initial performance evaluation of the CT 7000 scanner," presented at the 20th Meeting of A.A.P.M., Aug. 1978.

[Hef85] P. B. Heffernan and R. A. Robb, "Difference image reconstruction from a few projections for ND materials inspection," *Appl. Opt.,* vol. 24, pp. 4105-4110, Dec. 1, 1985.

[Her71] G. T. Herman and S. Rowland, "Resolution in ART: An experimental investigation of the resolving power of an algebraic picture reconstruction," *J. Theor. Biol.,* vol. 33, pp. 213-223, 1971.

[Her80] G. T. Herman, *Image Reconstructions from Projections.* New York, NY: Academic Press, 1980.

[Hin83] W. S. Hinshaw and A. H. Lent, "An introduction to NMR imaging: From the Bloch equation to the imaging equation," *Proc. IEEE,* vol. 71, pp. 338-350, Mar. 1983.

[Hof76] E. J. Hoffman, M. E. Phelps, N. A. Mullani, C. S. Higgins, and M. M. TerPogossian, "Design and performance characteristics of a whole body transaxial tomography," *J. Nucl. Med.,* vol. 17, pp. 493-502, 1976.

[Hsi76] R. C. Hsieh and W. G. Wee, "On methods of three-dimensional reconstruction from a set of radioisotope scintigrams," *IEEE Trans. Syst. Man Cybern.,* vol. SMC-6, pp. 854-862, Dec. 1976.

[ICR64] International Commission on Radiological Units and Measurements, "Physical aspects of irradiation," Rep. 10b. Bethesda, MD: ICRU Publications, 1964.

[Iwa75] K. Iwata and R. Nagata, "Calculation of refractive index distribution from interferograms using the Born and Rytov's approximations," *Japan. J. Appl. Phys.,* vol. 14, pp. 1921-1927, 1975.

[Jak76] C. V. Jakowatz, Jr. and A. C. Kak, "Computerized tomography using x-rays and ultrasound," Research Rep. TR-EE 76-26, School of Electrical Engineering, Purdue Univ., Lafayette, IN, 1976.

[Joh75] S. A. Johnson, J. F. Greenleaf, W. F. Samayoa, F. A. Duck, and J. D. Sjostrand, "Reconstruction of three-dimensional velocity fields and other parameters by acoustic ray tracing," in *Proc. 1975 Ultrasonic Symposium,* 1975, pp. 46-51.

[Jos78] P. M. Joseph and R. D. Spital, "A method for correcting bone induced artifacts in computed tomography scanners," *J. Comput. Assist. Tomog.,* vol. 2, pp. 100-108, Jan. 1978.

[Jos82] P. M. Joseph, "The effects of scatter in x-ray computed tomography," *Med. Phys.,* vol. 9, pp. 464-472, July/Aug. 1982.

[Kak78] A. C. Kak and K. A. Dines, "Signal processing of broadband pulsed ultrasound: Measurement of attenuation of soft biological tissues," *IEEE Trans. Biomed. Eng.,* vol. BME-25, pp. 321-344, July 1978.

[Kak79] A. C. Kak, "Computerized tomography with x-ray emission and ultrasound sources," *Proc. IEEE,* vol. 67, pp. 1245-1272, 1979.

[Kak81] ——, Guest Editor, Special Issue on Computerized Medical Imaging, *IEEE Transactions on Biomedical Engineering,* vol. BME-28, Feb. 1981.

[Kij78] D. K. Kijewski and B. E. Bjarngard, "Correction for beam hardening in computed tomography," *Med. Phys.,* vol. 5, pp. 209-214, 1978.

[Kno83] G. F. Knoll, "Single-emission computed tomography," *Proc. IEEE,* vol. 71, pp. 320-329, Mar. 1983.

[Kuc84] R. Kuc, "Estimating acoustic attenuation from reflected ultrasound signals: Comparison of spectral-shift and spectral-difference approaches," *IEEE Trans. Acoust. Speech Signal Processing,* vol. ASSP-32, pp. 1-7, Feb. 1984.

[Kuh63] D. E. Kuhl and R. Q. Edwards, "Image separation radio-isotope scanning," *Radiology*, vol. 80, pp. 653–661, 1963.

[Lip83] M. J. Lipton and C. B. Higgins, "Computed tomography: The technique and its use for the evaluation of cardiocirculatory anatomy and function," *Cardiology Clinics*, vol. 1, pp. 457–471, Aug. 1983.

[Lyt80] R. J. Lytle and K. A. Dines, "Iterative ray tracing between boreholes for underground image reconstruction," *IEEE Trans. Geosciences and Remote Sensing*, vol. GE-18, pp. 234–240, 1980.

[Mac83] A. Macovski, *Medical Imaging Systems*. Englewood Cliffs, NJ: Prentice-Hall, 1983.

[Man82] P. Mansfield and P. G. Morris, *NMR Imaging in Biomedicine*. New York, NY: Academic Press, 1982.

[Mar82] P. M. Margosian, "A redundant ray projection completion method for an inverse fan beam computed tomography system," *J. Comput. Assist. Tomog.*, vol. 6, pp. 608–613, June 1982.

[McC74] E. C. McCullough, Jr., H. L. Baker, O. W. Houser, and D. F. Reese, "An evaluation of the quantitative and radiation features of a scanning x-ray transverse axial tomograph: The EMI scanner," *Radiat. Phys.*, vol. 3, pp. 709–715, June 1974.

[McC75] E. C. McCullough, "Photon attenuation in computed tomography," *Med. Phys.*, vol. 2, pp. 307–320, 1975.

[McD75] W. D. McDavid, R. G. Waggener, W. H. Payne, and M. J. Dennis, "Spectral effects on three-dimensional reconstruction from x-rays," *Med. Phys.*, vol. 2, pp. 321–324, 1975.

[McD77] ———, "Correction for spectral artifacts in cross-sectional reconstruction from x-rays," *Med. Phys.*, vol. 4, pp. 54–57, 1977.

[McK81] G. C. McKinnon and R. H. T. Bates, "Towards imaging the beating heart usefully with a conventional CT scanner," *IEEE Trans. Biomed. Eng.*, vol. BME-28, pp. 123–127, Feb. 1981.

[Mil77] J. G. Miller, M. O'Donnell, J. W. Mimbs, and B. E. Sobel, "Ultrasonic attenuation in normal and ischemic myocardium," in *Proc. Second Int. Symp. on Ultrasonic Tissue Characterization, National Bureau of Standards*, 1977.

[Mil78] M. Millner, W. H. Payne, R. G. Waggener, W. D. McDavid, M. J. Dennis, and V. J. Sank, "Determination of effective energies in CT calibration," *Med. Phys.*, vol. 5, pp. 543–545, 1978.

[Mue80] R. K. Mueller, M. Kaveh, and R. D. Iversen, "A new approach to acoustic tomography using diffraction techniques," in *Acoustical Imaging*, vol. 8, A. Metherall, Ed. New York, NY: Plenum Press, 1980, pp. 615–628.

[Mul78] N. A. Mullani, C. S. Higgins, J. T. Hood, and C. M. Curie, "PETT IV: Design analysis and performance characteristics," *IEEE Trans. Nucl. Sci.*, vol. NS-25, pp. 180–183, Feb. 1978.

[Nap81] S. Napel, "Frequency estimation by coherent vector averaging for doppler blood flow analysis," Ph.D. thesis, Stanford Univ., Stanford, CA, 1981.

[Nor79a] S. J. Norton and M. Linzer, "Ultrasonic reflectivity tomography: Reconstruction with circular transducer arrays," *Ultrason. Imaging*, vol. 1, no. 2, pp. 154–184, Apr. 1979.

[Nor79b] ———, "Ultrasonic reflectivity tomography in three dimensions: Reconstruction with spherical transducer arrays," *Ultrason. Imaging*, vol. 1, no. 2, pp. 210–231, 1979.

[ODo85] M. O'Donnell and W. A. Edelstein, "NMR imaging in the presence of magnetic field inhomogeneities and gradient field nonlinearities," *Med. Phys.*, vol. 12, no. 1, pp. 20–26, Jan./Feb. 1985.

[Old61] W. H. Oldendorf, "Isolated flying spot detection of radiodensity discontinuities displaying the internal structural pattern of a complex object," *IRE Trans. Biomed. Eng.*, vol. BME-8, pp. 68–72, 1961.

[OSA85] Special Issue on Computerized Tomography, *Applied Optics*, vol. 24, Dec. 1, 1985.

[Per85] S. Persson and E. Ostman, "Use of computed tomography in NDT of polymeric

[Pes85]   materials,'' *Appl. Opt.*, vol. 24, pp. 4095–4104, Dec. 1, 1985.
[Pes85]   K. R. Peschmann, S. Napel, J. L. Couch, R. E. Rand, R. Alei, S. M. Ackelsberg, R. Gould, and D. P. Boyd, ''High-speed computed tomography: Systems and performance,'' *Appl. Phys.*, vol. 58, no. 1, pp. 4052–4060, Dec. 1, 1985.
[Phe75]   M. E. Phelps, E. J. Hoffman, and M. M. TerPogossian, ''Attenuation coefficients of various body tissues, fluids, and lesions at photon energies of 18 to 136 KeV,'' *Radiology*, vol. 117, pp. 573–583, 1975.
[Phe78]   M. E. Phelps, E. J. Hoffman, S. C. Huang, and D. E. Kuhl, ''ECAT: A new computerized tomographic imaging system for positron-emitting radiopharmaceuticals,'' *J. Nucl. Med.*, vol. 19, pp. 635–647, 1978.
[Pyk82]   I. L. Pykett, ''NMR imaging in medicine,'' *Sci. Amer.*, vol. 246, pp. 78–88, May 1982.
[Rad17]   J. Radon, ''Uber due bestimmung von funktionen durch ihre intergralwerte langs gewisser mannigfaltigkeiten'' (''On the determination of functions from their integrals along certain manifolds''), *Berichte Saechsische Akademie der Wissenschaften*, vol. 29, pp. 262–277, 1917. [See also: F. John, *Plane Wave and Spherical Means Applied to Partial Differential Equations*. New York, NY: Wiley-Interscience, 1955.]
[Ram71]   G. N. Ramachandran and A. V. Lakshminarayanan, ''Three dimensional reconstructions from radiographs and electron micrographs: Application of convolution instead of Fourier transforms,'' *Proc. Nat. Acad. Sci.*, vol. 68, pp. 2236–2240, 1971.
[Rob83]   R. A. Robb, E. A. Hoffman, L. J. Sinak, L. D. Harris, and E. L. Ritman, ''High-speed three-dimensional x-ray computed tomography: The dynamic spatial reconstructor,'' *Proc. IEEE*, vol. 71, pp. 308–319, Mar. 1983.
[Row69]   P. D. Rowley, ''Quantitative interpretation of three dimensional weakly refractive phase objects using holographic interferometry,'' *J. Opt. Soc. Amer.*, vol. 59, pp. 1496–1498, Nov. 1969.
[Sch84]   J. S. Schreiman, J. J. Gisvold, J. F. Greenleaf, and R. C. Bahn, ''Ultrasound computed tomography of the breast,'' *Radiology*, vol. 150, pp. 523–530, Feb. 1984.
[Sha76]   D. Shaw, *Fourier Transform N.M.R. Spectroscopy*. Amsterdam, the Netherlands: Elsevier Scientific Publishing, 1976.
[She77]   L. A. Shepp and J. A. Stein, ''Simulated reconstruction artifacts in computerized x-ray tomography,'' in *Reconstruction Tomography in Diagnostic Radiology and Nuclear Medicine*, M. M. TerPogossian *et al.*, Eds. Baltimore, MD: University Park Press, 1977.
[Shu77]   R. A. Schulz, E. C. Olson, and K. S. Han, ''A comparison of the number of rays vs. the number of views in reconstruction tomography,'' *Proc. S.P.I.E.*, vol. 127, pp. 313–320, 1977.
[Sny85]   R. Snyder and L. Hesselink, ''High-speed optical tomography for flow visualization,'' *Appl. Opt.*, vol. 24, pp. 4046–4051, Dec. 1, 1985.
[Swe73]   D. W. Sweeney and C. M. Vest, ''Reconstruction of three-dimensional refractive index fields from multi-directional interferometric data,'' *Appl. Opt.*, vol. 12, pp. 1649–1664, 1973.
[Tam78]   K. C. Tam, G. Chu, V. Perez-Mendez, and C. B. Lim, ''Three dimensional reconstruction in planar positron cameras using Fourier deconvolution of generalized tomograms,'' *IEEE Trans. Nucl. Sci.*, vol. NS-25, pp. 152–159, Feb. 1978.
[Ter67]   M. TerPogossian, *The Physical Aspects of Diagnostic Radiology*. New York, NY: Harper and Row, 1967.
[Ter78a]   M. M. TerPogossian, N. A. Mullani, J. Hood, C. S. Higgins, and C. M. Curie, ''A multislice positron emission computed tomography (PETT-IV) yielding transverse and longitudinal images,'' *Radiology*, vol. 128, pp. 477–484, Aug. 1978.
[Ter79b]   M. M. TerPogossian, N. A. Mullani, J. J. Hood, C. S. Higgins, and D. C. Ficke, ''Design consideration for a positron emission transverse tomography (PETT-V) for the imaging of the brain,'' *J. Comput. Assist. Tomog.*, vol. 2, pp. 439–444, Nov. 1978.
[Tre69]   O. Tretiak, M. Eden, and M. Simon, ''Internal structures for three dimensional images,'' in *Proc. 8th Int. Conf. on Med. Biol. Eng.*, Chicago, IL, 1969.

[Tre80] O. J. Tretiak and C. Metz, "The exponential radon transform," *SIAM J. Appl. Math.*, vol. 39, pp. 341–354, 1980.

[Uck85] H. Uckiyama, M. Nakajima, and S. Yuta, "Measurement of flame temperature distribution by IR emission computed tomography," *Appl. Opt.*, vol. 24, pp. 4111–4116, Dec. 1, 1985.

[Wan85] S. Y. Wang, Y. B. Huang, V. Pereira, and C. C. Gryte, "Applications of computed tomography to oil recovery from porous media," *Appl. Opt.*, vol. 24, pp. 4021–4027, Dec. 1, 1985.

[Wel77] P. N. T. Wells, "Ultrasonics in medicine and biology," *Phys. Med. Biol.*, vol. 22, pp. 629–669, 1977.

[Wil78] G. H. Williams, "The design of a rotational x-ray CT scanner," *Media (Proc. of MEDEX 78)*, vol. 6, no. 7, pp. 47–53, June 1978.

[Wre51] F. R. Wrenn, Jr., M. L. Good, and P. Handler, "The use of positron-emitting radioisotope for the localization of brain tumors," *Nature*, vol. 113, pp. 525–527, 1951.

[Yaf77] M. Yaffe, A. Fenster, and H. E. Johns, "Xenon ionization detectors for fan-beam computed tomography scanners," *J. Comput. Assist. Tomog.*, vol. 1, pp. 419–428, 1977.

[Yam77] Y. Yamamoto, C. J. Thompson, E. Meyer, J. S. Robertson, and W. Feindel, "Dynamic positron emission tomography for study of cerebral hemodynamics in a cross-section of the head using positron-emitting ^{68}Ga-EDTA and ^{77}Kr," *J. Comput. Assist. Tomog.*, vol. 1, pp. 43–56, Jan. 1977.

5 Aliasing Artifacts and Noise in CT Images

The errors discussed in the last chapter are fundamental to the projection process and depend upon the interaction of object inhomogeneities with the form of energy used. The effects of these errors can't be lessened by simply increasing the number of measurements in each projection or the total number of projections.

This chapter will focus on reconstruction errors of a different type: those caused either by insufficiency of data or by the presence of random noise in the measurements. An insufficiency of data may occur either through undersampling of projection data or because not enough projections are recorded. The distortions that arise on account of insufficiency of data are usually called the aliasing distortions. Aliasing distortions may also be caused by using an undersampled grid for displaying the reconstructed image.

5.1 Aliasing Artifacts

We will discuss aliasing from two points of view. First we will assume point sources and detectors and show the artifacts due to aliasing. With this assumption it is easy to show the effects of undersampling a projection, using too small a number of views, and choosing an incorrect reconstruction grid or filter. We will then introduce detectors and sources of nonzero width and discuss how they in effect help reduce the severity of aliasing distortions.

5.1.1 What Does Aliasing Look Like?

Fig. 5.1 shows 16 parallel beam reconstructions of an ellipse with various values of K, the number of projections, and N, the number of rays in each projection. The projections for the ellipse were generated as described in Chapter 3. The gray level inside the ellipse was 1 and the background 0 and the data were generated assuming a point source and point detector. To bring out all the artifacts, the reconstructed images were windowed between 0.1 and -0.1. (In other words, all the gray levels above 0.1 were set at white and all below -0.1 at black.) The images in Fig. 5.1 are displayed on a 128 × 128 matrix. Fig. 5.2 is a graphic depiction of the reconstructed numerical values on the middle horizontal lines for two of the images in Fig. 5.1. From

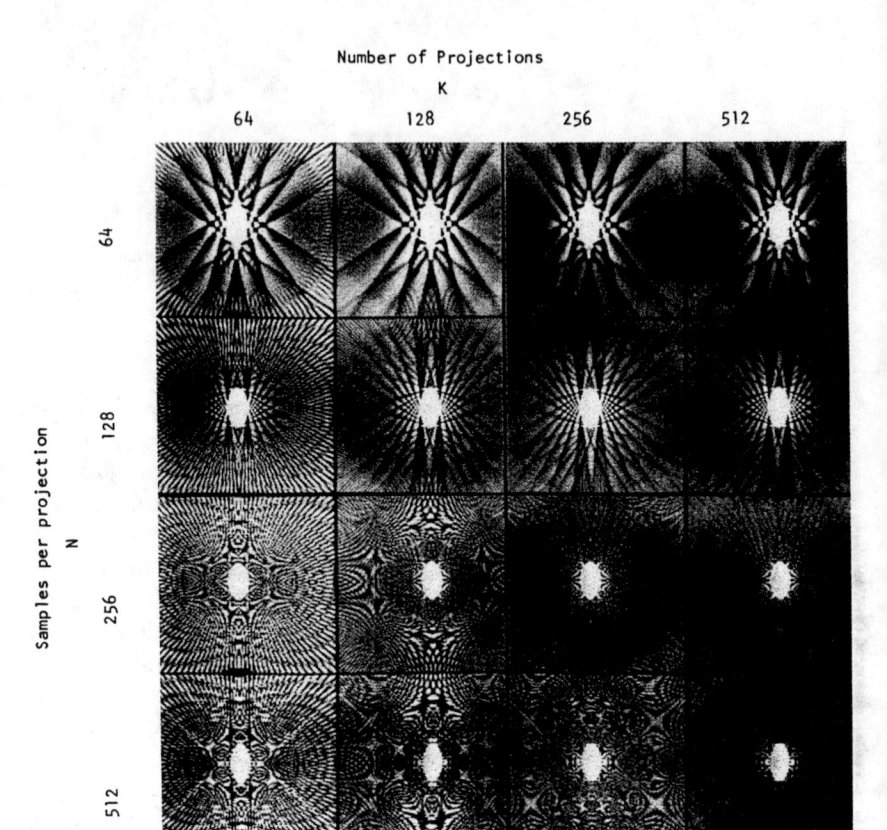

Fig. 5.1: *Sixteen reconstructions of an ellipse are shown for different values of K, the number of projections, and N, the number of rays in each projection. In each case the reconstructions were windowed to emphasize the distortions. (Courtesy of Carl Crawford of the General Electric Medical Systems Division in Milwaukee, WI.)*

Figs. 5.1 and 5.2 the following artifacts are evident: Gibbs phenomenon, streaks, and Moiré patterns.

We will now show that the streaks evident in Fig. 5.1 for the cases when N is small and K is large are caused by aliasing errors in the projection data. Note that a fundamental problem with tomographic images in general is that the objects (in this case an ellipse), and therefore their projections, are not bandlimited. In other words, the bandwidth of the projection data exceeds the highest frequency that can be recorded at a given sampling rate. To illustrate how aliasing errors enter the projection data assume that the Fourier transform $S_\theta(f)$ of a projection $P_\theta(t)$ looks as shown in Fig. 5.3(a). The bandwidth of this function is B as also shown there. Let's choose a sampling interval τ for sampling the projection. By the discussion in Chapter 2, with this sampling interval we can associate a measurement bandwidth W which is equal to $1/2\tau$. We will assume that $W < B$. It follows that the Fourier transform of the *samples* of the projection data is given by Fig. 5.3(b). We see that the information within the measurement band is contaminated by the tails (shaded areas) of the higher and lower replications of the original Fourier transform. This contaminating information constitutes the aliasing

178   COMPUTERIZED TOMOGRAPHIC IMAGING

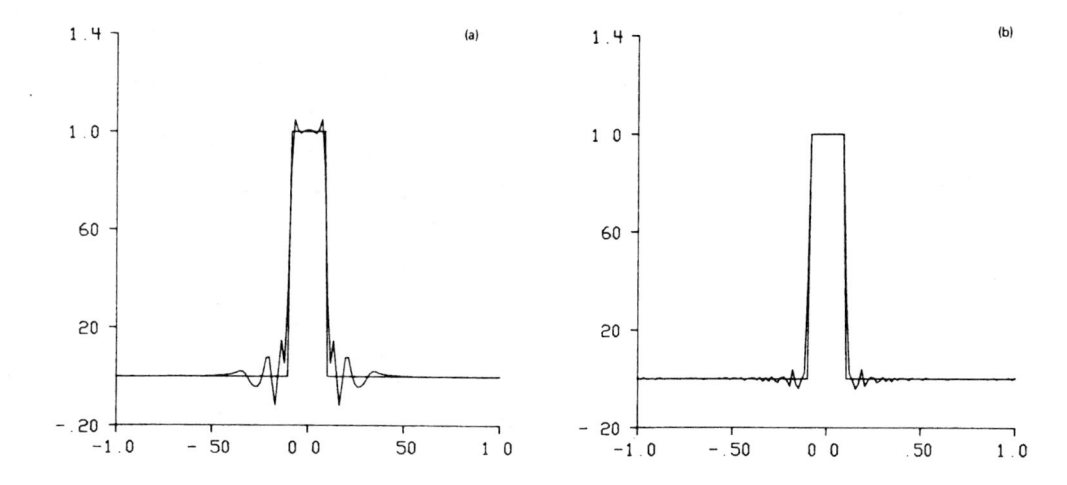

Fig. 5.2: *The center lines of the reconstructions shown in Fig. 5.1 for (a) $N = 64$, $K = 512$ and (b) $N = 512$, $K = 512$ are shown here. (From [Cra79].)*

errors in the sampled projection data. These contaminating frequencies constitute the aliased spectrum.

Backprojection is a linear process so the final image can be thought to be made up of two functions. One is the image made from the bandlimited projections degraded primarily by the finite number of projections. The second is the image made from the aliased portion of the spectrum in each projection.

The aliased portion of the reconstruction can be seen by itself by subtracting the transforms of the sampled projections from the corresponding theoretical transforms of the original projections. Then if this result is filtered as before, the final reconstructed image will be that of the aliased spectrum. We performed a computer simulation study along these lines for an elliptical object. In order to present the result of this study we first show in Fig. 5.4(a) the reconstruction of the ellipse for $N = 64$. (The number of projections was 512, which is large enough to preclude any artifacts due to insufficient number of views, and will remain the same for the discussion here.) We have subtracted the transform of each projection for the $N = 64$ case from the corresponding transform for the $N = 1024$ case. The latter was assumed to be the true transform because the projections are oversampled (at least in comparison to the $N = 64$ case). The reconstruction obtained from the difference data is shown in Fig. 5.4(b). Fig. 5.4(c) is the bandlimited image obtained by subtracting the aliased-spectrum image of Fig. 5.4(b) from the complete image shown in Fig. 5.4(a). Fig. 5.4(c) is the reconstruction that would be obtained provided the projection data for the $N = 64$ case were truly bandlimited (i.e., did not suffer from aliasing errors after sampling). The aliased-spectrum reconstruction in Fig. 5.4(b) and the absence of streaks in Fig. 5.4(c) prove our point that when the number of projections is large, the streaking artifacts are caused by aliasing errors in the projection data.

We will now present a plausible argument, first advanced by Brooks *et al.*

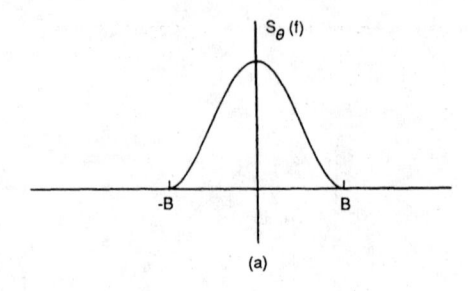

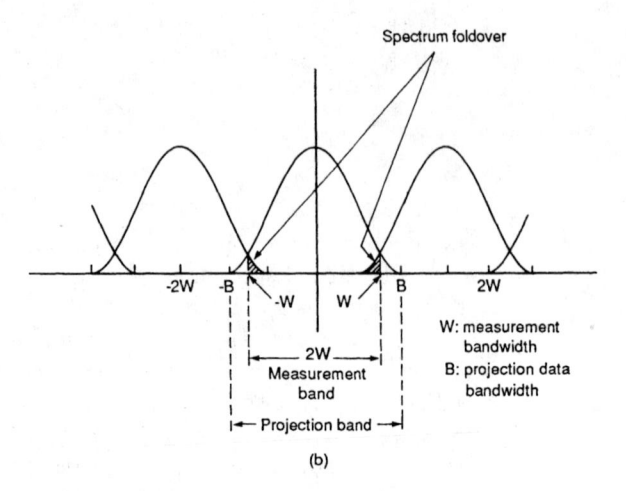

Fig. 5.3: *If a projection (a) is sampled at below the Nyquist rate (2B in this case), then aliasing will occur. As shown in (b) the result is aliasing or spectrum foldover. (Adapted from [Cra79].)*

[Bro79], for when a streak may be dark and when it may be light. Note that when an object is illuminated by a source, a projection of the object is formed at the detector array as shown in Fig. 5.5. If the object has a discontinuity at its edges, then the projection will also. We will now show how the position of this discontinuity with respect to the detector array has a bearing on the sign of the aliasing error. When the filtered projection is backprojected over the image array the sign of the error will determine the shade of the streak.

Consider sampling a projection described by

$$f(x) = \begin{cases} 1 & x > 0 \\ -1 & \text{elsewhere.} \end{cases} \quad (1)$$

The Fourier transform of this function is given by

$$F(\omega) = \frac{-2j}{\omega}. \quad (2)$$

For the purpose of sampling, we can imagine that the function f is multiplied by the function

$$h(x) = \sum_{k=-\infty}^{\infty} \delta(x - kT) \quad (3)$$

180   COMPUTERIZED TOMOGRAPHIC IMAGING

(a)

(b)

(c)

Fig. 5.4: *(a) Reconstruction of an ellipse with N = 64 and K = 512. (b) Reconstruction from only the aliased spectrum. Note that the streaks exactly match those in (a). (c) Image obtained by subtracting (b) from (a). This is the reconstruction that would be obtained provided the data for the N = 64 case were truly bandlimited. (From [Cra79].)*

where T represents the sampling interval of the projection. The Fourier transform of the sampling function is then given by

$$H(\omega) = \sum_{k=-\infty}^{\infty} \delta(\omega - k\omega_N) \qquad (4)$$

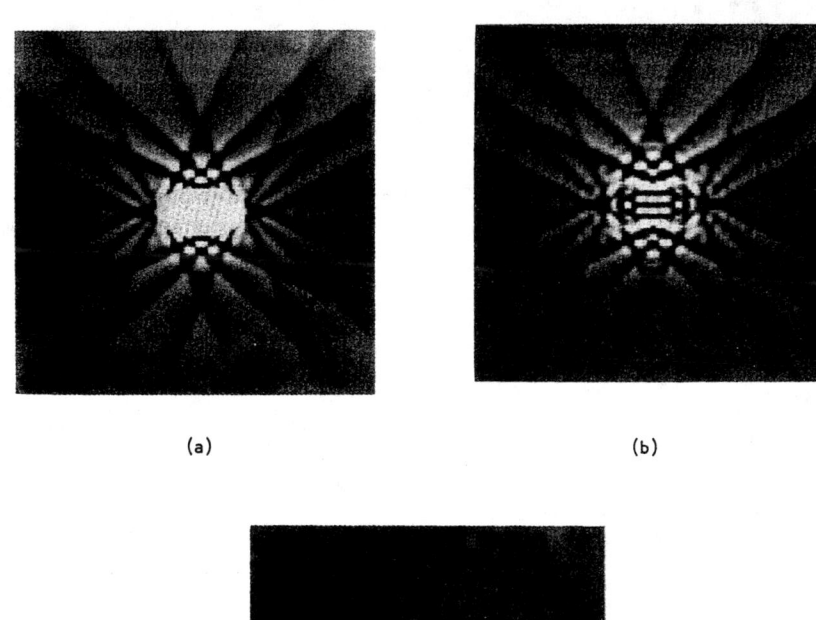

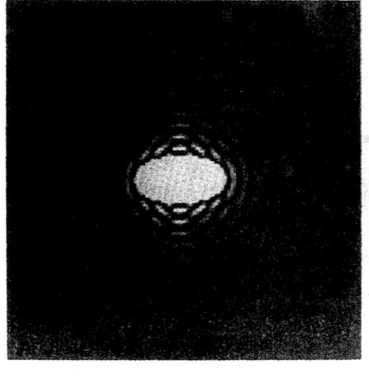

where $\omega_N = 2\pi/T$. Clearly, the Fourier transform of the sampled function is a convolution of the expressions in (2) and (4):

$$F_{\text{sampled}}(\omega) = \sum_{k=-\infty}^{\infty} \frac{-2j}{\omega + k\omega_N}. \qquad (5)$$

This function is shown in Fig. 5.6(a). Before these projection data can be backprojected they must be filtered by multiplying the Fourier transform of

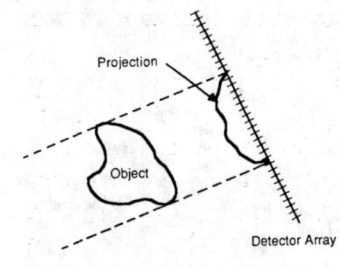

Fig. 5.5: *The projection of an object with sharp discontinuities will have significant high frequency energy.*

Fig. 5.6: *The aliasing due to undersampled projections is illustrated here. (a) shows the Fourier transform of an edge discontinuity. The aliased portions of the spectrum are shaded. (b) shows an approximation to the error when the sampling grid is aligned with the discontinuity and (c) shows the error when the discontinuity is shifted by 1/4 of the sampling interval. Note the magnitude of the error changes by more than a factor of 3 when the sampling grid shifts.*

the projection by $|\omega|/2\pi$. The filtered projection is then written

$$F'_{\text{sampled}}(\omega) = \sum_{k=-\infty}^{\infty} \frac{|\omega|}{2\pi} \frac{-2j}{\omega + k\omega_N}. \tag{6}$$

To study the errors due to aliasing, we will only consider the terms for $k = 1$ and $k = -1$, and assume that the higher order terms are negligible. Note that the zeroth order term is the edge information and is part of the desired reconstruction; the higher order terms are part of the error but will be small compared to the $k = \pm 1$ terms at low frequencies. The inverse Fourier transform of these two aliased terms is written as

$$f_{\text{error}}(x) \approx \frac{1}{2\pi} \int_{-\omega_N/2}^{\omega_N/2} \frac{|\omega|}{2\pi} \left[\frac{-2j}{\omega + \omega_N} + \frac{-2j}{\omega - \omega_N} \right] e^{-j\omega x} d\omega \tag{7}$$

and is shown in Fig. 5.6(b).

Now if the sampling grid is shifted by 1/4 of the sampling interval its Fourier transform is multiplied by $e^{+j\omega_N(T/4)}$ or

$$F_{\text{shifted}}(\omega) = \sum_{k=-\infty}^{\infty} \frac{|\omega|}{2\pi} \frac{-2j}{\omega + k\omega_N} e^{jk\omega_N(T/4)}. \tag{8}$$

This can be evaluated for the $k = 1$ and $k = -1$ terms to find the error integral is

$$f_{\text{shifted}}(x) \approx \frac{1}{2\pi} \int_{-\omega_N/2}^{\omega_N/2} \frac{|\omega|}{2\pi} \left[\frac{2}{\omega + \omega_N} - \frac{2}{\omega - \omega_N} \right] e^{-j\omega x} d\omega \tag{9}$$

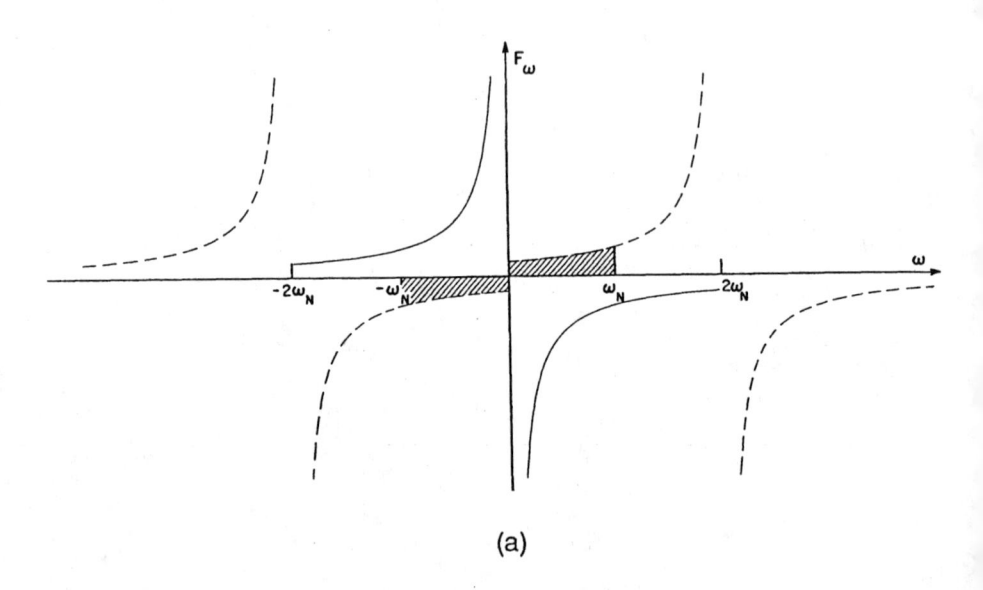

(a)

and is shown in Fig. 5.6(c). If the grid is shifted in the opposite direction, then the error will be similar but with the opposite sign.

As was done earlier in this section, consider the sampled projection to consist of two components: the true projection and the error term. The true projection data from each view will combine to form the desired image; the error in each projection will combine to form an image like that in Fig. 5.4(b). A positive error in a projection causes a light streak when the data are backprojected. Likewise, negative errors lead to dark streaks. As the view angle changes the size of the ellipse's "shadow" changes and the discontinuity moves with respect to the detector array. In addition, where the curvature of the object is large, the edge of the discontinuity will move rapidly which results in a large number of streaks.

The thin streaks that are evident in Fig. 5.1 for the cases of large N and small K (e.g., when $N = 512$ and $K = 64$) are caused by an insufficient number of projections. It is easily shown that when only a small number of filtered projections of a small object are backprojected, the result is a star-shaped pattern. This is illustrated in Fig. 5.7: in (a) are shown four projections of a point object, in (b) the filtered projections, and in (c) their backprojections.

The number of projections should be roughly equal to the number of rays in each projection. This can be shown analytically for the case of parallel projections by the following argument: By the Fourier Slice Theorem, the Fourier transform of each projection is a slice of the two-dimensional Fourier transform of the object. In the frequency domain shown in Fig. 5.8, each radial line, such as A_1A_2, is generated by one projection. If there are M_{proj}

Fig. 5.6: Continued.

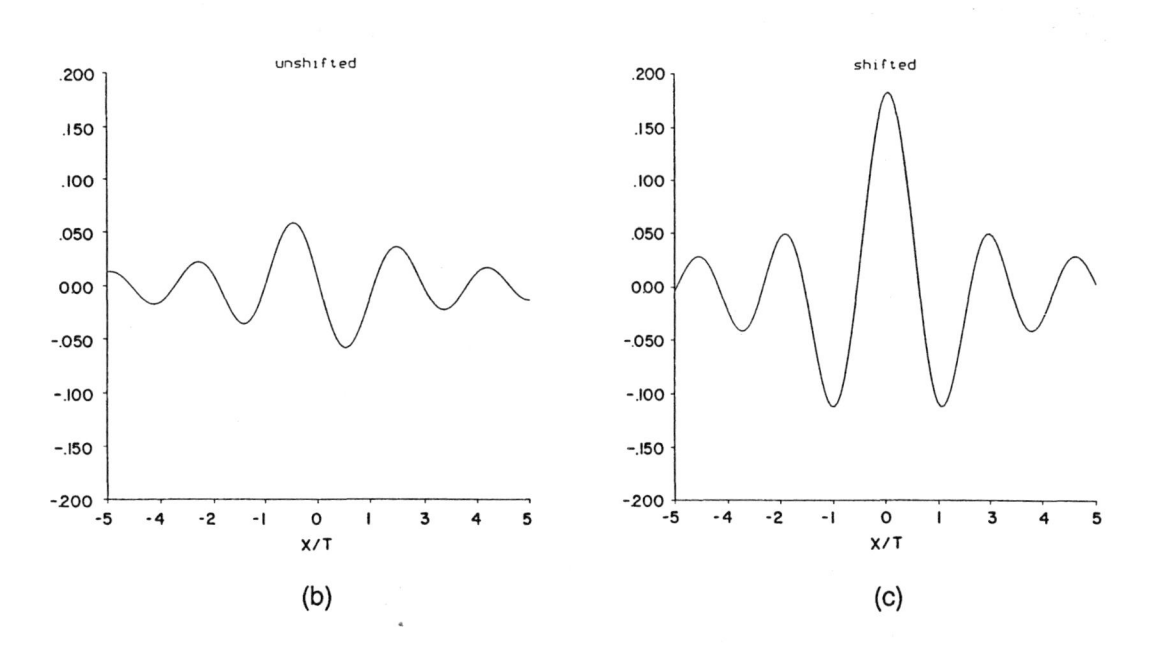

(b)

(c)

ALIASING ARTIFACTS AND NOISE IN CT IMAGES 183

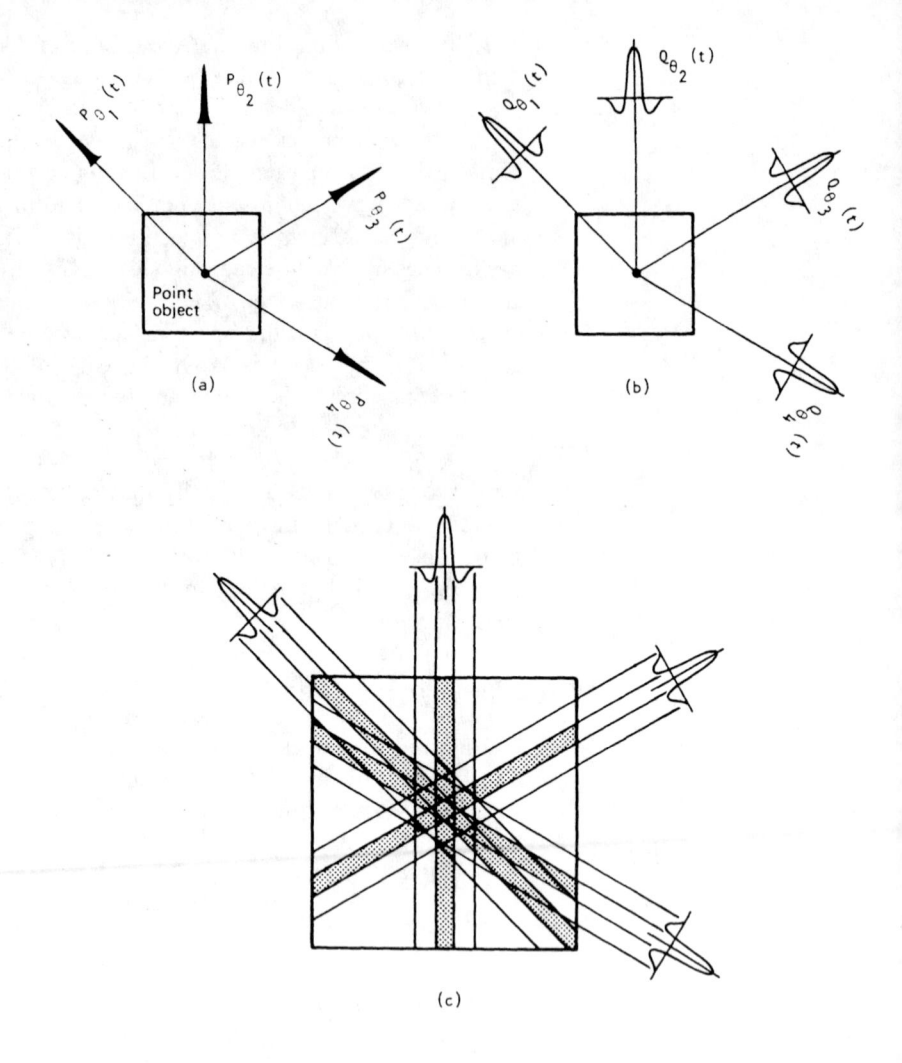

Fig. 5.7: *The backprojection operation introduces a star-shaped pattern to the reconstruction. (From [Ros82].)*

projections uniformly distributed over 180°, the angular interval δ between successive radial lines is given by

$$\delta = \frac{\pi}{M_{proj}}. \qquad (10)$$

If τ is the sampling interval used for each projection, the highest spatial frequency W measured for each projection will be

$$W = 1/2\tau. \qquad (11)$$

This is the radius of the disk shown in Fig. 5.8. The distance between consecutive sampling points on the periphery of this disk is equal to $\overline{A_2B_2}$ and

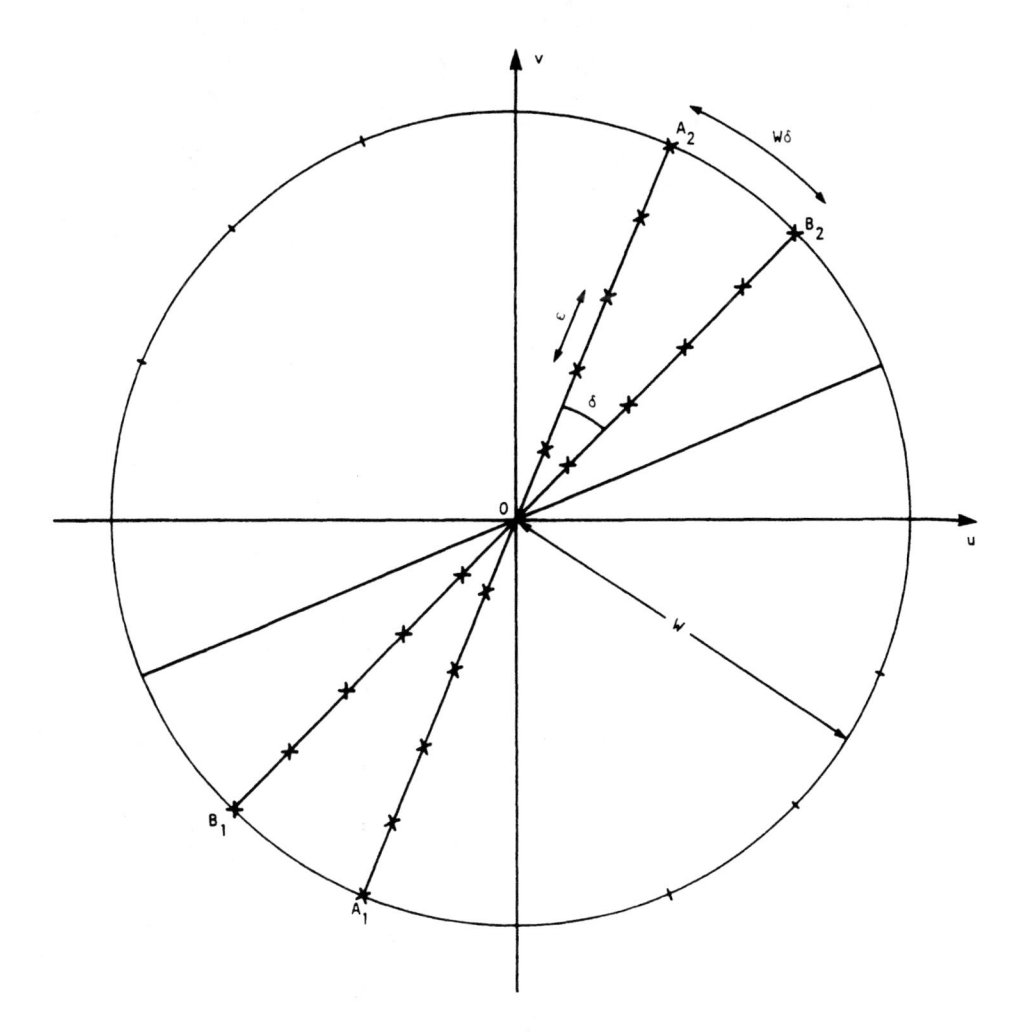

Fig. 5.8: *Frequency domain parameters pertinent to parallel projection data. (From [Kak84].)*

is given by

$$\overline{A_2B_2} = W\delta = \frac{1}{2\tau}\frac{\pi}{M_{\text{proj}}}. \qquad (12)$$

If there are N_{ray} sampling points in each projection, the total number of independent frequency domain sampling points on a line such as A_1A_2 will also be the same. Therefore, the distance ϵ between any two consecutive sampling points on each radial line in Fig. 5.8 will be

$$\epsilon = \frac{2W}{N_{\text{ray}}} = \frac{1}{\tau N_{\text{ray}}}. \qquad (13)$$

Because in the frequency domain the worst-case azimuthal resolution should

ALIASING ARTIFACTS AND NOISE IN CT IMAGES   185

be approximately the same as the radial resolution, we must have

$$\frac{1}{2\tau}\frac{\pi}{M_{\text{proj}}} \approx \frac{1}{\tau N_{\text{ray}}}, \qquad (14)$$

which is obtained by equating (12) and (13). Equation (14) reduces to

$$\frac{M_{\text{proj}}}{N_{\text{ray}}} \approx \frac{\pi}{2}, \qquad (15)$$

which implies that the number of projections should be roughly the same as the number of rays per projection.

The reader may have noticed that the thin streaks caused by an insufficient number of projections (see, e.g., the image for $N = 512$ and $K = 64$ in Fig. 5.1) appear broken. This is caused by two-dimensional aliasing due to the display grid being only 128×128. When, say, $N = 512$, the highest frequency in each projection can be 256 cycles per projection length, whereas the highest frequency that can be displayed on the image grid is 64 cycles per image width (or height). The effect of this two-dimensional aliasing is very pronounced in the left three images for the $N = 512$ row and the left two images for the $N = 256$ row in Fig. 5.1. As mentioned in Chapter 2, the artifacts generated by this two-dimensional aliasing are called Moiré patterns. These artifacts can be diminished by tailoring the bandwidth of the reconstruction kernel (filter) to match the display resolution.

From the computer simulation and analytical results presented in this section, one can conclude that for a well-balanced $N \times N$ reconstructed image, the number of rays in each projection should be roughly N and the total number of projections should also be roughly N.

5.1.2 Sampling in a Real System

In the previous section we described aliasing errors caused by undersampling the projections, number of views, and the reconstruction grid. In practice, these errors are somewhat mitigated by experimental considerations like the size of the detector aperture and the nonzero size of the x-ray source. Both these factors bring about a certain smoothing of the projections, and a consequent loss of information at the highest frequencies. In this section, we will demonstrate how these factors can be taken into account to determine the "optimum rate" at which a projection should be sampled.

In order to analyze the effect of a nonzero size for the detector aperture, note that this effect can be taken into account by convolving the ideal projection with the aperture function. Let the following function represent an aperture that is T_d units wide (we are only considering aperture widths along the projection, the width along the perpendicular direction being irrelevant to our discussion):

$$a(x) = \begin{cases} 1 & |x| \leq \dfrac{T_d}{2} \\ 0 & \text{elsewhere.} \end{cases} \quad (16)$$

The Fourier transform of this aperture function is given by

$$A(\omega) = T_d \text{ sinc } (\omega T_d/2). \quad (17)$$

In the frequency domain, the Fourier transform of the ideal projection is multiplied by this function, implying that we are in effect passing the projection through a low pass filter (LPF). Since the first zero of $A(\omega)$ is located at $2\pi/T_d$, it is not unreasonable to say that the effect of $A(\omega)$ is to filter out all frequencies higher than

$$\omega_{\text{LPF}} = \frac{2\pi}{T_d}. \quad (18)$$

In other words, we are approximating the aperture function in the frequency domain by

$$A'(\omega) = \begin{cases} T_d \text{ sinc } (\omega T_d/2) & |\omega| < \omega_{\text{LPF}} \\ 0 & \text{elsewhere.} \end{cases} \quad (19)$$

Let's say that we are using an array of detectors to measure a projection and that the array is characterized by T_s as the center-to-center spacing between the detectors. Measurement of the projection data is equivalent to multiplication of the low pass filtered projection with a train $d(x)$ of impulses, where $d(x)$ is given by

$$d(x) = \sum_{n=-\infty}^{\infty} \delta(x - nT_s) \quad (20)$$

whose Fourier transform is

$$D(\omega) = \frac{2\pi}{T_s} \sum_{n=-\infty}^{\infty} \delta\left(\omega - \frac{2\pi n}{T_s}\right). \quad (21)$$

In the frequency domain the effect of the detector aperture and sampling distance is shown in Fig. 5.9. We can now write the following expression for the recorded samples p_n of an ideal projection $p(x)$:

$$p_n = \delta(x - nT_s)[p(x) * a(x)] \quad (22)$$

or, equivalently,

$$p_n = \text{IFT}\{D(\omega) * [P(\omega) A'(\omega)]\} \quad (23)$$

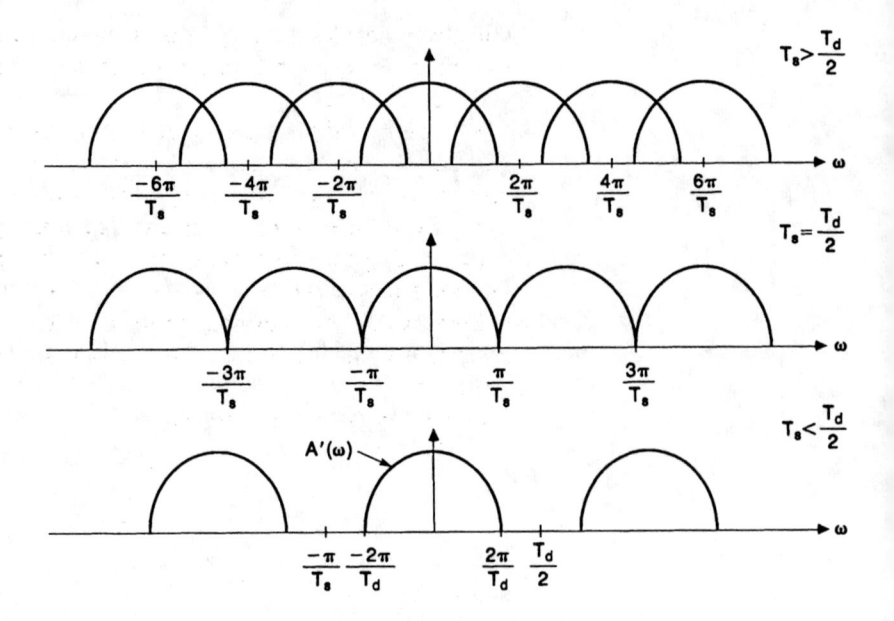

Fig. 5.9: *The Fourier transform of the detector array response is shown for three different detector spacings. For values of T_s such that $T_s > T_d/2$ there will be aliasing. If $T_s \leq T_d/2$, then aliasing is minimized.*

where $P(\omega)$ is the Fourier transform of the projection data and IFT is the inverse Fourier transform. Clearly, there will be aliasing in the sampled projections unless

$$T_s < \frac{T_d}{2}. \tag{24}$$

This relationship implies that we should have at least two samples per detector width [Jos80a].

There are several ways to measure multiple samples per detector width. With first-generation (parallel beam) scanners, it is simply a matter of sampling the detectors more often as the source–detector combination moves past the object. Increasing the sampling density can also be done in fourth-generation (fixed-detector) scanners by considering each detector as the apex of a fan. Now as the source rotates, each detector measures ray integrals and the ray density can be made arbitrarily dense by increasing the sampling rate for each detector.

For third-generation scanners a technique known as quarter detector offset is used. Recall that for a fan beam scanner only data for 180° plus the width of the fan need be collected; if a full 360° of data is collected then the rest of the data is effectively redundant. But if the detector array is offset by 1/4 of the detector spacing (ordinarily, the detector bank is symmetric with respect to the line joining the x-ray source and the center of rotation; by offset is meant translating the detector bank to the left or right, thereby causing rays in opposite views to be unique) and a full 360° of data is collected it is possible to use the extra views to obtain unique information about the object. This

188   COMPUTERIZED TOMOGRAPHIC IMAGING

effectively doubles the projection sampling frequency. Fig. 5.10 compares the effect of quarter detector offset on a first-generation and a third-generation scanner.

We will now discuss the second factor that causes projections to become blurred, namely, the size of the x-ray beam. As we will show, we can't account for the extent of blurring caused by this effect in as elegant a manner as we did for the detector aperture. The primary source of difficulty is that objects undergo different amounts of blurring depending upon how far away they are from the source of x-rays. Fig. 5.11 shows the effect of a source of nonzero width. As is evident from the figure, the effect on a projection is dependent upon where the object is located between the source and the detectors.

Simple geometrical arguments show that for a given point in the object, the size of its image at the detector array is given by

$$B_s = w_s \frac{D_d}{D_s} \tag{25}$$

where w_s is the width of the source and D_d and D_s are, respectively, the distances from the point in the object to the detectors and the source. This then would roughly be a measure of blurring introduced by a nonzero-width source in a parallel beam machine.

In a fan beam system, the above-mentioned blurring is exacerbated by the natural divergence of the fan. To illustrate our point, consider two detector lines for a fan beam system, as shown in Fig. 5.12. The projection data measured along the two lines would be identical except for stretching of the projection function along the detector arc as we go to the array farther away from the center. This stretch factor is given by (see Fig. 5.13)

$$\frac{D_s}{D_s + D_d} \tag{26}$$

where the distances D_s and D_d are for object points at the center of the scan. If we combine the preceding two equations, we obtain for a fan beam system the blurring caused by a nonzero-width source

$$B_s = w_s \frac{D_d}{D_s} \frac{D_s}{D_s + D_d} = w_s \frac{D_d}{D_s + D_d} \tag{27}$$

with the understanding that, rigorously speaking, this equation is only valid for object points close to the center of rotation.

Since the size of the image is dependent on the position along the ray integral this leads to a spatially varying blurring of the projection data. Near the detector the blurring will be small while near the source a point in the object could be magnified by a large amount. Since the system is linear each point in the object will be convolved with a scaled image of the source point and then projected onto the detector line.

5.2 Noise in Reconstructed Images

We will now consider the effect of noise in the projection data on a reconstructed image. There are two types of noise to be considered. The first, a continuously varying error due to electrical noise or roundoff errors, can be modeled as a simple additive noise. The reconstructed image can therefore be considered to be the sum of two images, the true image and that image resulting from the noise. The second type of noise is best exemplified by shot noise in x-ray tomography. In this case the magnitude of the possible error is a function of the number of x-ray photons that exit the object and the error analysis becomes more involved.

Fig. 5.10: *The ray paths for normal and quarter offset detectors are compared here. Each ray path is represented by plotting an asterisk at the point on the ray closest to the origin. In each case 6 projections of 10 rays each were gathered by rotating a full 360° around the object. (Note: normally only 180° of projection data is used for parallel projection reconstruction.) (a) shows parallel projections without quarter offset (note that the extra 180° of data is redundant). (b) is identical to (a) but the detector array has been shifted by a quarter of the sampling interval. (c) shows equiangular projections without quarter offset and (d) is identical to (c) but the detector array has been shifted by a quarter of the sampling interval.*

5.2.1 The Continuous Case

Consider the case where each projection, $P_\theta(t)$, is corrupted by additive noise $\nu_\theta(t)$. The measured projections, $P_\theta^m(t)$, are now given by

$$P_\theta^m(t) = P_\theta(t) + \nu_\theta(t). \tag{28}$$

We will assume that the noise is a stationary zero-mean random process and that its values are uncorrelated for any two rays in the system. Therefore,

$$E[\nu_{\theta_1}(t_1)\nu_{\theta_2}(t_2)] = S_0 \, \delta(\theta_1 - \theta_2)\delta(t_1 - t_2). \tag{29}$$

The reconstruction from the measured projection data is obtained by first

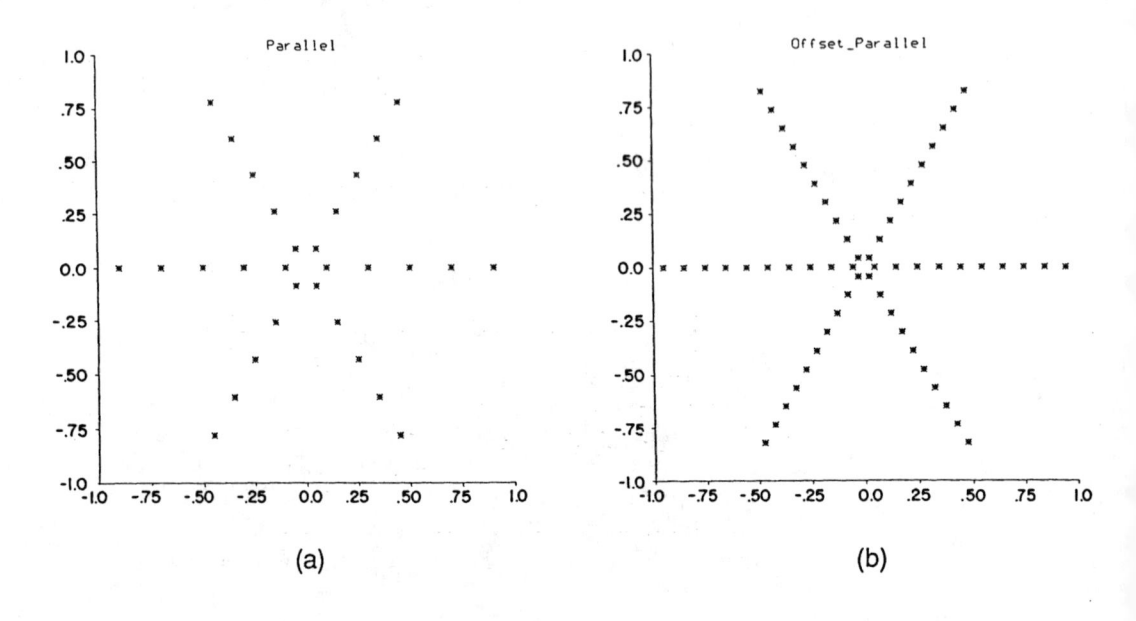

(a)   (b)

Fan_Beam

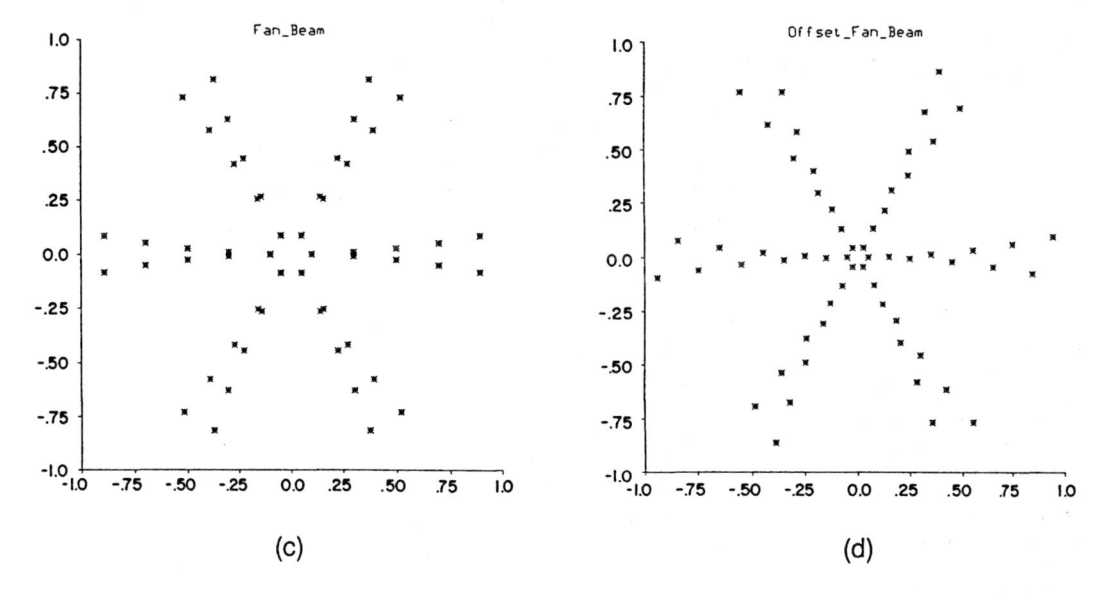

(c)

Offset_Fan_Beam

(d)

Fig. 5.10: *Continued.*

filtering each projection:

$$Q_\theta^m(t) = \int_{-\infty}^{\infty} S_\theta^m(w) |w| G(w) e^{j2\pi wt} \, dw \qquad (30)$$

where $S_\theta^m(w)$ is the Fourier transform of $P_\theta^m(t)$ and $G(w)$ is the smoothing filter used; and then backprojecting the filtered projections:

$$\hat{f}(x, y) = \int_0^\pi Q_\theta^m(x \cos \theta + y \sin \theta) \, d\theta \qquad (31)$$

where $\hat{f}(x, y)$ is the reconstructed approximation to the original image $f(x, y)$. For the purpose of noise calculations, we substitute (28) and (30) in (31) and write

$$\hat{f}(x, y) = \int_0^\pi \int_{-\infty}^{\infty} [S_\theta(w) + N_\theta(w)] |w| G(w) e^{j2\pi w(x \cos \theta + y \sin \theta)} \, dw \, d\theta$$

$$(32)$$

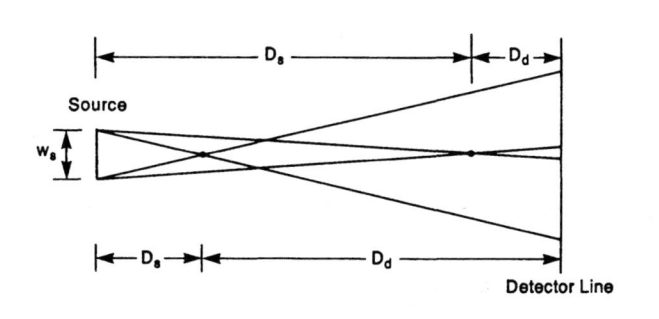

Fig. 5.11: *A finite source of width w_s will be imaged by each point in the object onto the detector line. The size of the image will depend on the ratio of D_s to D_d. The images of two points in the object are shown here.*

ALIASING ARTIFACTS AND NOISE IN CT IMAGES   191

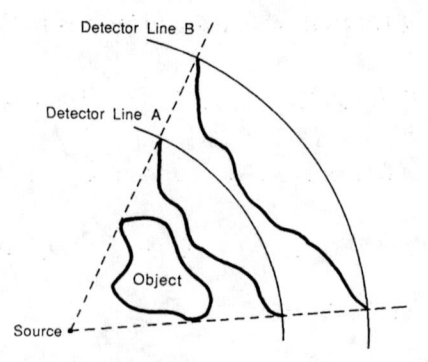

Fig. 5.12: *The magnification of a projection due to a fan beam system is shown here. To find the effect of the source or detector aperture on image resolution it is necessary to map the blurring of the projection into an equivalent object size.*

where, as before, $S_\theta(w)$ is the Fourier transform of the ideal projection $P_\theta(t)$, and $N_\theta(w)$ is the Fourier transform of the additive noise, $\nu_\theta(t)$. (Here we assume $N_\theta(w)$ exists in some sense. Note that in spite of our notation we are only dealing with projections with finite support.) Clearly,

$$N_\theta(w) = \int_{-\infty}^{\infty} \nu_\theta(t) e^{-j2\pi wt} \, dt \tag{33}$$

from which we can write

$$E[N_{\theta_1}(w_1) N^*_{\theta_2}(w_2)] = \int_{-\infty}^{\infty} \int_{-\infty}^{\infty} E[\nu_{\theta_1}(t_1) \nu_{\theta_2}(t_2)] e^{-j2\pi(w_1 t_2 - w_2 t_2)} \, dt_1 \, dt_2 \tag{34}$$

$$= S_0 \, \delta(w_1 - w_2) \delta(\theta_1 - \theta_2) \tag{35}$$

where we have used (29).

Since $N_\theta(w)$ is random, the reconstructed image given by (32) is also random. The mean value of $\hat{f}(x, y)$ is given by

$$E[\hat{f}(x, y)] = \int_0^\pi \int_{-\infty}^{\infty} [S_\theta(w) + E(N_\theta(w))] |w| G(w) e^{j2\pi w(x \cos\theta + y \sin\theta)} \, dw \, d\theta. \tag{36}$$

Since we are dealing with zero-mean noise, $E[\nu_\theta(t)] = 0$; hence, from (33)

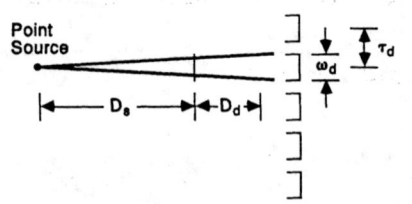

Fig. 5.13: *A finite detector aperture leads to a blurring of the object.*

we get $E[N_\theta(w)] = 0$. Substituting this in (36), we get

$$E[\hat{f}(x,y)] = \int_0^\pi \int_{-\infty}^\infty S_\theta(w)|w|G(w)e^{j2\pi w(x\cos\theta + y\sin\theta)} \, dw \, d\theta. \qquad (37)$$

Now the variance of noise at a point (x, y) in the reconstructed image is given by

$$\sigma_{\text{recon}}^2(x, y) = E[\hat{f}(x,y) - E(\hat{f}(x,y))]^2. \qquad (38)$$

Substituting (32) and (37), we get

$$\sigma_{\text{recon}}^2(x,y) = E\left|\int_0^\pi \int_{-\infty}^\infty N_\theta(w)|w|G(w)e^{j2\pi w(x\cos\theta + y\sin\theta)} \, dw \, d\theta\right|^2 \qquad (39)$$

$$= E\left[\int_0^\pi \int_{-\infty}^\infty N_\theta(w)|w|G(w)e^{j2\pi w(x\cos\theta + y\sin\theta)} \, dw \, d\theta\right]$$

$$\times \left[\int_0^\pi \int_{-\infty}^\infty N_\theta(w)|w|G(w)e^{j2\pi w(x\cos\theta + y\sin\theta)} \, dw \, d\theta\right]^* \qquad (40)$$

$$= \pi S_0 \int_{-\infty}^\infty |w|^2 |G(w)|^2 \, dw \qquad (41)$$

where we have used (35). Therefore, we may write

$$\frac{\sigma_{\text{recon}}^2}{S_0} = \pi \int_{-\infty}^\infty |w|^2 |G(w)|^2 \, dw \qquad (42)$$

where we have dropped the (x, y) dependence of σ_{recon}^2 since it has turned out to be independent of position in the picture plane.

Equation (42) says that in order to reduce the variance of noise in a reconstructed image, the filter function $G(w)$ must be chosen such that the area under the square of $|w|G(w)$ is as small as possible. But note that if there is to be no image distortion $|w|G(w)$ must be as close to $|w|$ as possible. Therefore, the choice of $G(w)$ depends upon the desired trade-off between image distortion and noise variance.

We will conclude this subsection by presenting a brief description of the spectral density of noise in a reconstructed image. To keep our presentation simple we will assume that the projections consist only of zero-mean white noise, $\nu_\theta(t)$. The reconstructed image from the noise projections is given by

$$\hat{f}(x,y) = \int_0^\pi \int_{-\infty}^\infty N_\theta(w)|w|G(w)e^{j2\pi w(x\cos\theta + y\sin\theta)} \, dw \, d\theta \qquad (43)$$

$$= \int_0^{2\pi} \int_0^\infty N_\theta(w) w G(w) e^{j2\pi w(x\cos\theta + y\sin\theta)} \, dw \, d\theta \qquad (44)$$

where, as before, $N_\theta(w)$ is the Fourier transform of $\nu_\theta(t)$. Now let $R(\alpha, \beta)$ be the autocorrelation function of the reconstructed image:

$$R(\alpha, \beta) \equiv E[\hat{f}(x+\alpha, y+\beta)\hat{f}(x, y)] = E[\hat{f}(x+\alpha, y+\beta)\hat{f}^*(x, y)] \quad (45)$$

$$= S_0 \int_0^{2\pi} d\theta \int_0^\infty dw\, w^2 |g(w)|^2 e^{j2\pi w(\alpha\cos\theta + \beta\sin\theta)}. \quad (46)$$

From this one can show that the spectral density of the reconstructed noise is dependent only on the distance from the origin in the frequency domain and is given by

$$S_\nu(w, \theta) = S_0 |G(w)|^2 w \quad \text{and} \quad \begin{matrix} w \geq 0 \\ 0 < \theta \leq 2\pi \end{matrix} \quad (47)$$

where, of course, w is always positive. This may be shown by first expressing the result for the autocorrelation function in polar coordinates

$$R(r, \phi) = S_0 \int_0^\pi d\theta \int_0^\infty dw\, w^2 |G(w)|^2 e^{j2\pi wr\cos(\theta - \phi)} \quad (48)$$

$$= S_0 \int_0^\infty w|G(w)|^2 w J_0(2\pi wr)\, dw \quad (49)$$

and recognizing the Hankel transform relationship between the autocorrelation function and the spectral density given above.

5.2.2 The Discrete Case

Although the continuous case does bring out the dependence of the noise variance in the reconstructed image on the filter used for the projection data, it is based on a somewhat unrealistic assumption. The assumption of stationarity which led to (29) implies that in any projection the variance of measurement noise for each ray is the same. This is almost never true in practice. The variance of noise is often signal dependent and this has an important bearing on the structure of noise in the reconstructed image.

As an illustration of the case of signal-dependent noise consider the case of x-ray computerized tomography. Let τ be the sampling interval and also the width of the x-ray beam, as illustrated in Fig. 5.14. If the width τ of the beam is small enough and the beam is monochromatic the integral of the attenuation function $\mu(x, y)$ along line AB in Fig. 5.14 is given by

$$P_\theta(t) \equiv \int_{\text{ray path } AB} \mu(x, y)\, ds \approx \ln N_{\text{in}} - \ln N_\theta(k\tau) \quad (50)$$

where $N_\theta(k\tau)$ denotes the value of N_d for the ray at location $(\theta, k\tau)$ as shown in the figure. Randomness in the measurement of $P_\theta(t)$ is introduced by statistical fluctuations in $N_\theta(k\tau)$. Note that in practice only $N_\theta(k\tau)$ is

$$P_\theta(k\tau) = \int_{\text{ray path AB}} \mu(x, y) \, ds = \ln \frac{N_{in}}{N_d}$$

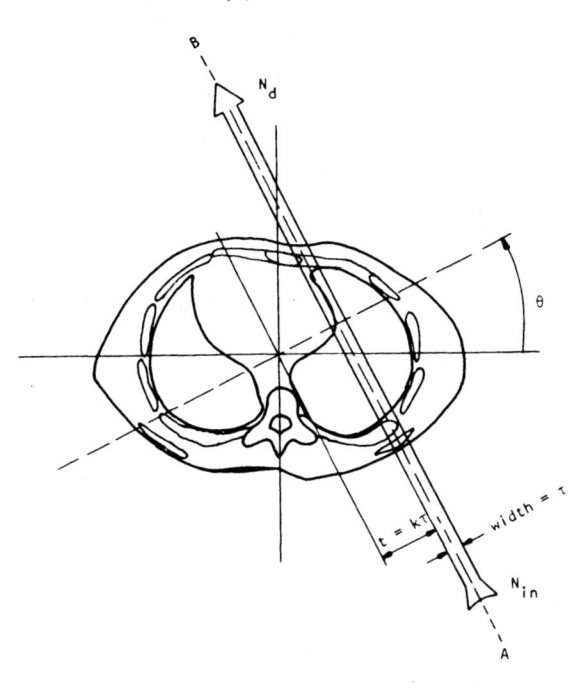

Fig. 5.14: *An x-ray beam with a width of τ is shown traveling through a cross section of the human body. (From [Kak79].)*

measured directly. The value of N_{in} for all rays is inferred by monitoring the x-ray source with a reference detector and from the knowledge of the spatial distribution of emitted x-rays. It is usually safe to assume that the reference x-ray flux is large enough so that N_{in} may be considered to be known with negligible error. In the rest of the discussion here we will assume that for each ray integral measurement N_{in} is a known deterministic constant, while on the other hand the directly measured quantity $N_\theta(k\tau)$ is a random variable. The randomness of $N_\theta(k\tau)$ is statistically described by the Poisson probability function [Ter67], [Pap65]:

$$p\{N_\theta(k\tau)\} = \frac{[\bar{N}_\theta(k\tau)]^{N_\theta(k\tau)}}{N_\theta(k\tau)!} e^{-\bar{N}_\theta(k\tau)} \qquad (51)$$

where $p\{\cdot\}$ denotes the probability and $\bar{N}_\theta(k\tau)$ the expected value of the measurement:

$$\bar{N}_\theta(k\tau) = E\{N_\theta(k\tau)\} \qquad (52)$$

where $E\{\ \}$ denotes statistical expectation. Note that the variance of each measurement is given by

$$\text{variance } \{N_\theta(k\tau)\} = \bar{N}_\theta(k\tau). \qquad (53)$$

ALIASING ARTIFACTS AND NOISE IN CT IMAGES 195

Because of the randomness in $N_\theta(k\tau)$ the true value of $P_\theta(k\tau)$ will differ from its measured value which will be denoted by $P_\theta^m(k\tau)$. To bring out this distinction we reexpress (50) as follows:

$$P_\theta^m(k\tau) = \ln N_{\text{in}} - \ln N_\theta(k\tau) \tag{54}$$

and

$$P_\theta(k\tau) = \int_{\text{ray}} \mu(x, y)\, ds. \tag{55}$$

By interpreting $e^{-P_\theta(k\tau)}$ as the probability that (along a ray such as the one shown in Chapter 4) a photon entering the object from side A will emerge (without scattering or absorption) at side B, one can show that

$$\bar{N}_\theta(k\tau) = N_{\text{in}} e^{-P_\theta(k\tau)}. \tag{56}$$

We will now assume that all fluctuations (departures from the mean) in $N_\theta(k\tau)$ that have a significant probability of occurrence are much less than the mean. With this assumption and using (50) and (51) it is easily shown that

$$E\{P_\theta^m(k\tau)\} = P_\theta(k\tau) \tag{57}$$

and

$$\text{variance } \{P_\theta^m(k\tau)\} = \frac{1}{\bar{N}_\theta(k\tau)}. \tag{58}$$

From the statistical properties of the measured projections, $P_\theta^m(k\tau)$, we will now derive those of the reconstructed image. Using the discrete filtered backprojection algorithms of Chapter 3, the relationship between the reconstruction at a point (x, y) and the *measured* projections is given by

$$\hat{f}(x, y) = \frac{\pi\tau}{M_{\text{proj}}} \sum_{i=1}^{M_{\text{proj}}} \sum_k P_{\theta_i}^m(k\tau) h(x \cos \theta_i + y \sin \theta_i - kT). \tag{59}$$

Using (57), (58), and (59), we get

$$E\{\hat{f}(x, y)\} = \frac{\pi\tau}{M_{\text{proj}}} \sum_{i=1}^{M_{\text{proj}}} \sum_k P_{\theta_i}(k\tau) h(x \cos \theta_i + y \sin \theta_i - k\tau) \tag{60}$$

and

$$\text{variance } \{\hat{f}(x, y)\} = \left(\frac{\pi\tau}{M_{\text{proj}}}\right)^2 \sum_i \sum_k$$

$$\frac{1}{\bar{N}_{\theta_i}(k\tau)} h^2(x \cos \theta_i + y \sin \theta_i - k\tau) \tag{61}$$

where we have used the assumption that fluctuations in $P_{\theta_i}^m(k\tau)$ are uncorrelated for different rays. Equation (60) shows that the expected value of the reconstructed image is equal to that made from the ideal projection data. Before we interpret (61) we will rewrite it as follows. In terms of the ideal projections, $P_\theta(k\tau)$, we define new projections as

$$V_\theta(k\tau) = e^{P_\theta(k\tau)} \tag{62}$$

and a new filter function, $h_v(t)$, as

$$h_v(t) = h^2(t). \tag{63}$$

Substituting (56), (62), and (63) in (61), we get

$$\text{variance } \{\hat{f}(x, y)\} = \left(\frac{\pi\tau}{M_{\text{proj}}}\right)^2 \frac{1}{N_{\text{in}}} \sum_i \sum_k V_\theta(k\tau)$$

$$\cdot h_v(x \cos \theta_i + y \sin \theta_i - k\tau). \tag{64}$$

We will now define a *relative-uncertainty image* as follows[1]:

$$\text{relative-uncertainty at } (x, y) = N_{\text{in}} \frac{\text{variance } \{\hat{f}(x, y)\}}{[\hat{f}(x, y)]^2}. \tag{65}$$

In computer simulation studies with this definition the relative-uncertainty image becomes independent of the number of incident photons used for measurements, and is completely determined by the choice of the phantom. Fig. 5.15(c) shows the relative-uncertainty image for the Shepp and Logan phantom (Fig. 5.15(b)) for $M_{\text{proj}} = 120$ and $\tau = 2/101$ and for $h(t)$ originally described in Chapter 3. Fig. 5.15(d) shows graphically the middle horizontal line through Fig. 5.15(c). The relative-uncertainty at (x, y) gives us a measure of how much confidence an observer might place in the reconstructed value at the point (x, y) vis-à-vis those elsewhere.

We will now derive some special cases of (64). Suppose we want to determine the variance of noise at the origin. From (64) we can write

$$\text{variance } \{\hat{f}(0, 0)\} = \left(\frac{\pi\tau}{M_{\text{proj}}}\right)^2 \sum_{i=1}^{M_{\text{proj}}} \sum_k \frac{1}{\bar{N}_{\theta_i}(k\tau)} h^2(k\tau) \tag{66}$$

where we have used the fact that $h(t)$ is an even function. Chesler *et al.* [Che77] have argued that since $h(k\tau)$ drops rapidly with k (see Chapter 3), it is safe to make the following approximation for objects that are approxi-

---

[1] This result only applies when compensators aren't used to reduce the dynamic range of the detector output signal. In noise analyses their effect can be approximately modeled by using different N_{in}'s for different rays.

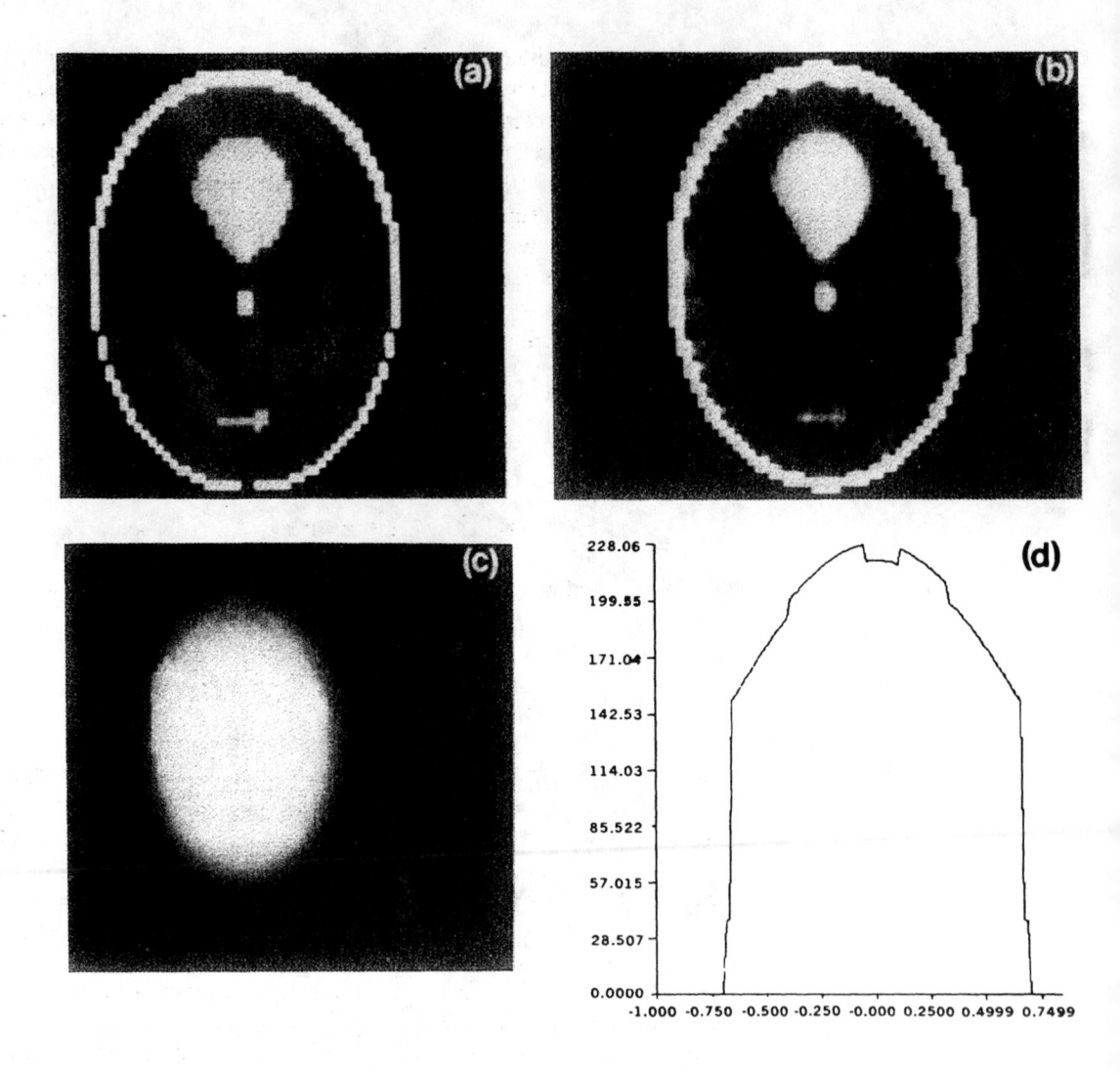

Fig. 5.15: *(a) A Shepp and Logan head phantom [She74] is shown here. (b) A reconstruction of the phantom from 120 projections and 101 rays in each parallel projection. The display matrix was 64 × 64. (c) The relative-uncertainty image for the reconstruction in (b). (d) A graphic depiction of the relative-uncertainty values through the middle horizontal line of (c). (From [Kak79].)*

mately homogeneous:

$$\text{variance } \{\hat{f}(0, 0)\} = \left(\frac{\pi\tau}{M_{\text{proj}}}\right)^2 \sum_k h^2(k\tau) \sum_{i=1}^{M_{\text{proj}}} \frac{1}{\bar{N}_{\theta_i}(0)} \quad (67)$$

which, when τ is small enough, may also be written as

$$\text{variance } \{\hat{f}(0, 0)\} = \left(\frac{\pi}{M_{\text{proj}}}\right)^2 \tau \int_{-\infty}^{\infty} h^2(t)\, dt \sum_{i=1}^{M_{\text{proj}}} \frac{1}{\bar{N}_{\theta_i}(0)} . \quad (68)$$

Note again that the $\bar{N}_{\theta_i}(0)$ are the mean number of exiting photons measured for the center ray in each projection. Using (68) Chesler *et al.* [Che77] have arrived at the very interesting result that (for the same uncertainty in measurement) the total number of photons per resolution element required for x-ray CT (using the filtered backprojection algorithm) is the same as that required for the measurement of attenuation of an isolated (excised) piece of the object with dimensions equal to those of the resolution element.

Now consider the case where the cross section for which the CT image is being reconstructed is circularly symmetric. The $\bar{N}_{\theta_i}(0)$'s for all i's will be equal; call their common value $\bar{N}_0$. That is, let

$$\bar{N}_0 = \bar{N}_{\theta_1}(0) = \bar{N}_{\theta_2}(0) = \cdots. \tag{69}$$

The expression (68) for the variance may now be written as

$$\text{variance } \{\hat{f}(0, 0)\} = \frac{\pi^2 \tau}{M_{\text{proj}} \bar{N}_0} \int_{-\infty}^{\infty} h^2(t)\, dt. \tag{70}$$

By Parseval's theorem this result may be expressed in the frequency domain as

$$\text{variance } \{\hat{f}(0, 0)\} = \frac{\pi^2 \tau}{M_{\text{proj}} \bar{N}_0} \int_{-1/2\tau}^{1/2\tau} |H(w)|^2\, dw \tag{71}$$

where τ is the sampling interval for the projection data. This result says that the variance of noise at the origin is proportional to the area under the square of the filter function used for reconstruction. This doesn't imply that this area could be made arbitrarily small since any major departure from the $|w|$ function will introduce spatial distortion in the image even though it may be less noisy. *None of the equations above should be construed to imply that the signal-to-noise ratio approaches zero as τ is made arbitrarily small.* Note from Chapter 4 that τ is also the width of the measurement beam. In any practical system, as τ is reduced $\bar{N}_0$ will decrease also.

The preceding discussion has resulted in expressions for the variance of noise in reconstructions made with a filtered backprojection algorithm for parallel projection data. As mentioned before, filtered backprojection algorithms have become very popular because of their accuracy. Still, given a set of projections, can there be an algorithm that might reconstruct an image with a smaller error? The answer to this question has been supplied by Tretiak [Tre78]. Tretiak has derived an algorithm-independent lower bound for the mean squared error in a reconstructed image and has argued that for the case of reconstructions from parallel projection data this lower bound is very close to the error estimates obtained by Brooks and DiChiro [Bro76] for the filtered backprojection algorithms, which leads to the conclusion that very little improvement can be obtained over the performance of such an algorithm.

5.3 Bibliographic Notes

Aliasing artifacts in tomographic imaging with nondiffracting sources have been studied by Brooks *et al.* [Bro78], [Bro79] and Crawford and Kak [Cra79]. A different analysis of the optimum number of rays and projections was presented in [Sch77] and reached nearly the same conclusion. A more detailed analysis is in [Jos80]. Excellent work describing the effects of sampling on CT images has been published in [Jos80], [Jos80b], [Bro79].

With regard to the properties of noise in images reconstructed with filtered backprojection, Shepp and Logan [She74] first showed that when filtered backprojection algorithms are used, the variance of the noise is directly proportional to the area under the square of the filter function. This derivation was based on the assumption that the variance of the measurement noise is the same for all the rays in the projection data, a condition which is usually not satisfied. The variance of the reconstruction was also studied by Gore and Tofts [Gor78]. This assumption was also used by Riederer *et al.* [Rie78] to derive the spectral density of the noise in a CT reconstruction.

A more general expression (not using this assumption) for the noise variance was derived by Kak [Kak79] who has also introduced the concept of "the relative-uncertainty image." For tomographic imaging with x-rays, Tretiak [Tre78] has derived an algorithm-independent lower bound on the noise variance in a reconstructed image. An explanation of the trade-offs between reconstruction noise in x-ray CT and image resolution is given in [Che77], [Alv79], [Kow77].

5.4 References

[Alv79] R. E. Alvarez and J. P. Stonestrom, "Optimal processing of computed tomography images using experimentally measured noise properties," *J. Comput. Tomog.*, vol. 3, no. 1, pp. 77-84, 1979.

[Bro76] R. A. Brooks and G. DiChiro, "Statistical limitations in x-ray reconstructive tomography," *Med. Phys.*, vol. 3, pp. 237-240, 1976.

[Bro78] R. A. Brooks, G. H. Weiss, and A. J. Talbert, "A new approach to interpolation in computed tomography," *J. Comput. Assist. Tomog.*, vol. 2, pp. 577-585, Nov. 1978.

[Bro79] R. A. Brooks, G. H. Glover, A. J. Talbert, R. L. Eisner, and F. A. DiBianca, "Aliasing: A source of streaks in computed tomograms," *J. Comput. Assist. Tomog.*, vol. 3, no. 4, pp. 511-518, Aug. 1979.

[Che77] D. A. Chesler, S. J. Riederer, and N. J. Pelc, "Noise due to photon counting statistics in computed x-ray tomography," *J. Comput. Assist. Tomog.*, vol. 1, pp. 64-74, Jan. 1977.

[Cra79] C. R. Crawford and A. C. Kak, "Aliasing artifacts in computerized tomography," *Appl. Opt.*, vol. 18, pp. 3704-3711, 1979.

[Gor78] J. C. Gore and P. S. Tofts, "Statistical limitations in computed tomography," *Phys. Med. Biol.*, vol. 23, pp. 1176-1182, 1978.

[Jos80a] P. M. Joseph, "The influence of gantry geometry on aliasing and other geometry dependent errors," *IEEE Trans. Nucl. Sci.*, vol. 27, pp. 1104-1111, 1980.

[Jos80b] P. M. Joseph, R. D. Spital, and C. D. Stockham, "The effects of sampling on CT images," *Comput. Tomog.*, vol. 4, pp. 189-206, 1980.

[Jos80] P. M. Joseph and R. A. Schulz, "View sampling requirements in fan beam computed tomography," *Med. Phys.*, vol. 7, no. 6, pp. 692-702, Nov./Dec. 1980.

[Kak79] A. C. Kak, "Computerized tomography with x-ray emission and ultrasound sources," *Proc. IEEE,* vol. 67, pp. 1245-1272, 1979.

[Kak84] ——, "Image reconstruction from projections," in *Digital Image Processing Techniques,* M. P. Ekstrom, Ed. New York, NY: Academic Press, 1984.

[Kow77] G. Kowalski, "Reconstruction of objects from their projections. The influence of measurement errors on the reconstruction," *IEEE Trans. Nucl. Sci.,* vol. NS-24, pp. 850-864, Feb. 1977.

[Pap65] A. Papoulis, *Probability, Random Variables, and Stochastic Processes.* New York, NY: McGraw-Hill, 1965 (2nd ed., 1984).

[Rie78] S. J. Riederer, N. J. Pelc, and D. A. Chesler, "The noise power spectrum in computer x-ray tomography," *Phys. Med. Biol.,* vol. 23, pp. 446-454, 1978.

[Ros82] A. Rosenfeld and A. C. Kak, *Digital Picture Processing,* 2nd ed. New York, NY: Academic Press, 1982.

[Sch77] R. A. Schulz, E. C. Olson, and K. S. Han, "A comparison of the number of rays vs the number of views in reconstruction tomography," *SPIE Conf. on Optical Instrumentation in Medicine VI,* vol. 127, pp. 313-320, 1977.

[She74] L. A. Shepp and B. F. Logan, "The Fourier reconstruction of a head section," *IEEE Trans. Nucl. Sci.,* vol. NS-21, pp. 21-43, 1974.

[Ter67] M. TerPogossian, *The Physical Aspects of Diagnostic Radiology.* New York, NY: Harper and Row, 1967.

[Tre78] O. J. Tretiak, "Noise limitations in x-ray computed tomography," *J. Comput. Assist. Tomog.,* vol. 2, pp. 477-480, Sept. 1978.

6 Tomographic Imaging with Diffracting Sources

Diffraction tomography is an important alternative to straight ray tomography. For some applications, the harm caused by the use of x-rays, an ionizing radiation, could outweigh any benefits that might be gained from the tomogram. This is one reason for the interest in imaging with acoustic or electromagnetic radiation, which are considered safe at low levels. In addition, these modalities measure the acoustic and electromagnetic refractive index and thus make available information that isn't obtainable from x-ray tomography.

As mentioned in Chapter 4, the accuracy of tomography using acoustic or electromagnetic energy and straight ray assumptions suffers from the effects of refraction and/or diffraction. These cause each projection to not represent integrals along straight lines but, in some cases where geometrical laws of propagation apply, paths determined by the refractive index of the object. When the geometrical laws of propagation don't apply, one can't even use the concept of line integrals—as will be clear from the discussions in this chapter.

There are two approaches to correcting these errors. One approach is to use an initial estimate of the refractive index to estimate the path each ray follows. This approach is known as algebraic reconstruction and, for weakly refracting objects, will converge to the correct refractive index distribution after a few iterations. We will discuss algebraic techniques in Chapter 7.

When the sizes of inhomogeneities in the object become comparable to or smaller than a wavelength, it is not possible to use ray theory (geometric propagation) based concepts; instead one must resort directly to wave propagation and diffraction based phenomena. In this chapter, we will show that if the interaction of an object and a field is modeled with the wave equation, then a tomographic reconstruction approach based on the Fourier Diffraction Theorem is possible for weakly diffracting objects. The Fourier Diffraction Theorem is very similar to the Fourier Slice Theorem of conventional tomography: In conventional (or straight ray) tomography, the Fourier Slice Theorem says that the Fourier transform of a projection gives the values of the Fourier transform of the object along a straight line. When diffraction effects are included, the Fourier Diffraction Theorem says that a "projection" yields the Fourier transform of the object over a semicircular arc. This result is fundamental to diffraction tomography.

In this chapter the basics of diffraction tomography are presented for application with acoustic, microwave, and optical energy. For each case we will start with the wave equation and use either the Born or the Rytov approximation to derive a simple expression that relates the scattered field to the object. This relationship will then be inverted for several measurement geometries to give an estimate of the object as a function of the scattered field. Finally, we will show simulations and experimental results that show the limitations of the method.

6.1 Diffracted Projections

Tomography with diffracting energy requires an entirely different approach to the manner in which projections are mathematically modeled. Acoustic and electromagnetic waves don't travel along straight rays and the projections aren't line integrals, so we will describe the flow of energy with a wave equation.

We will first consider the propagation of waves in homogeneous media, although our ultimate interest lies in imaging the inhomogeneities within an object. The propagation of waves in a homogeneous object is described by a wave equation, which is a second-order linear differential equation. Given such an equation and the "source" fields in an aperture, we can determine the fields everywhere else in the homogeneous medium.

There are no direct methods for solving the problem of wave propagation in an inhomogeneous medium; in practice, approximate formalisms are used that allow the theory of homogeneous medium wave propagation to be used for generating solutions in the presence of weak inhomogeneities. The better known among these approximate methods go under the names of Born and Rytov approximations.

Although in most cases we are interested in reconstructing three-dimensional objects, the diffraction tomography theory presented in this chapter will deal mostly with the two-dimensional case. Note that when a three-dimensional object can be assumed to vary only slowly along one of the dimensions, a two-dimensional theory can be readily applied to such an object. This assumption, for example, is often made in conventional computerized tomography where images are made of single slices of the object. In any case, we have two reasons for limiting our presentation to the two-dimensional case: First and most importantly, the ideas behind the theory are often easier to visualize (and certainly to draw) in two dimensions. Second, the technology has not yet made it practical to implement large three-dimensional transforms that are required for direct three-dimensional reconstructions of objects; furthermore, direct display of three-dimensional entities isn't easy.

6.1.1 Homogeneous Wave Equation

An acoustic pressure field or an electromagnetic field must satisfy the following differential equation [Goo68]:

$$\nabla^2 u(\vec{r}, t) - \frac{1}{c^2} \frac{\nabla^2}{dt^2} u(\vec{r}, t) = 0 \qquad (1)$$

where u represents the magnitude of the field as a function of position $\vec{r}$ and time t and c is the velocity of the field as a function of position.

This form of the wave equation is more complicated than needed; most derivations of diffraction tomography are done by considering only one temporal frequency at a time. This decomposition can be accomplished by finding the Fourier transform of the field with respect to time at each position $\vec{r}$. Note that the above differential equation is linear so that the solutions for different frequencies can be added to find additional solutions.

A field $u(\vec{r}, t)$ with a temporal frequency of ω radians per second (rps) satisfies the equation

$$[\nabla^2 + k^2(\vec{r})] u(\vec{r}, t) = 0 \qquad (2)$$

where $k(\vec{r})$ is the wavenumber of the field and is equal to

$$k(\vec{r}) = \frac{2\pi}{\lambda} = \frac{2\pi\omega}{c} \qquad (3)$$

where λ is the field's wavelength. At this point the field is at a single frequency and we will write it as

$$\text{Real Part } \{u(\vec{r}) e^{-j\omega t}\}. \qquad (4)$$

In this form it is easy to see that the time dependence of the field can be suppressed and the wave equation rewritten as

$$(\nabla^2 + k^2(\vec{r})) u(\vec{r}) = 0. \qquad (5)$$

For acoustic (or ultrasonic) tomography, $u(\vec{r})$ can be the pressure field at position $\vec{r}$. For the electromagnetic case, assuming the applicability of a scalar propagation equation, $u(\vec{r})$ may be set equal to the complex amplitude of the electric field along its polarization. In both cases, $u(\vec{r})$ represents the complex amplitude of the field.

For homogeneous media the wavenumber is constant and we can further simplify the wave equation. Setting the wavenumber equal to

$$k(\vec{r}) = k_0 \qquad (6)$$

the wave equation becomes

$$(\nabla^2 + k_0^2) u(\vec{r}) = 0. \qquad (7)$$

The vector gradient operator, ∇, can be expanded into its two-dimensional representation and the wave equation becomes

$$\frac{\partial^2 u(\vec{r})}{\partial x^2} + \frac{\partial^2 u(\vec{r})}{\partial y^2} + k_0^2 u(\vec{r}) = 0. \qquad (8)$$

As a trial solution we let

$$u(\vec{r}) = e^{j\vec{k}\cdot\vec{r}} \qquad (9)$$

where the vector $\vec{k} = (k_x, k_y)$ is the two-dimensional propagation vector and $u(\vec{r})$ represents a two-dimensional plane wave of spatial frequency $|\vec{k}|$. This form of $u(\vec{r})$ represents the basis function for the two-dimensional Fourier transform; using it, we can represent any two-dimensional function as a weighted sum of plane waves. Calculating the derivatives as indicated in (8), we find that only plane waves that satisfy the condition

$$|\vec{k}|^2 = k_x^2 + k_y^2 = k_0^2 \qquad (10)$$

satisfy the wave equation. This condition is consistent with our intuitive picture of a wave and our earlier description of the wave equation, since for any frequency wave only a single wavelength can exist no matter in which direction the wave propagates.

The homogeneous wave equation is a linear differential equation so we can write the general solution as a weighted sum of each possible plane wave solution. In two dimensions, at a temporal frequency of ω, the field $u(\vec{r})$ is given by

$$u(\vec{r}) = \frac{1}{2\pi}\int_{-\infty}^{\infty} \alpha(k_y)e^{j(k_x x + k_y y)}\,dk_y + \frac{1}{2\pi}\int_{-\infty}^{\infty} \beta(k_y)e^{j(-k_x x + k_y y)}\,dk_y \qquad (11)$$

where by (10)

$$k_x = \sqrt{k_0^2 - k_y^2}. \qquad (12)$$

The form of this equation might be surprising to the reader for two reasons. First we have split the integral into two parts. We have chosen to represent the coefficients of waves traveling to the right by $\alpha(k_y)$ and those of waves traveling to the left by $\beta(k_y)$. In addition, we have set the limits of the integrals to go from $-\infty$ to ∞. For k_y^2 greater than k_0^2, the radical in (12) becomes imaginary and the plane wave becomes an evanescent wave. These are valid solutions to the wave equation, but because k_y is imaginary, the exponential has a real or attenuating component. This real component causes the amplitude of the wave to either grow or decay exponentially. In practice, these evanescent waves only occur to satisfy boundary conditions, always decaying rapidly far from the boundary, and can often be ignored at a distance greater than 10λ from an inhomogeneity.

We will now show by using the plane wave representation that it is possible to express the field anywhere in terms of the fields along a line. The three-dimensional version of this idea gives us the field in three-space if we know the field at all points on a plane.

Consider a source of plane waves to the left of a vertical line as shown in Fig. 6.1. If we take the one-dimensional Fourier transform of the field along

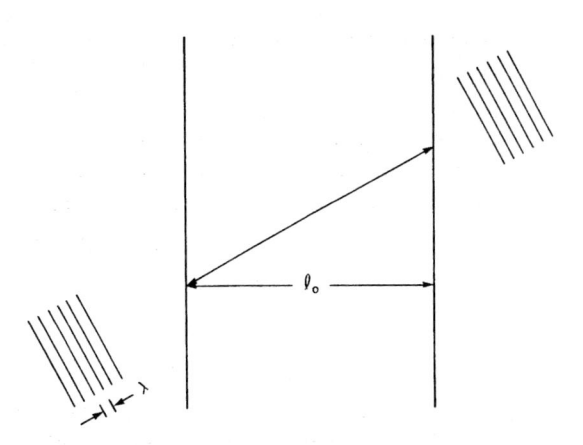

Fig. 6.1: *A plane wave propagating between two planes undergoes a phase shift dependent on the distance between the planes and the direction of the plane wave.*

the vertical line, we can decompose the field into a number of one-dimensional components. Each of these one-dimensional components can then be attributed to one of the valid plane wave solutions to the homogeneous wave equation, because for any one spatial frequency component, k_y, there can exist only two plane waves that satisfy the wave equation. Since we have already constrained the incident field to propagate to the right (all sources are to the left of the measurement line), a one-dimensional Fourier component at a frequency of k_y can be attributed to a two-dimensional wave with a propagation vector of $(\sqrt{k_0^2 - k_y^2}, k_y)$.

We can put this on a more mathematical basis if we compare the one-dimensional Fourier transform of the field to the general form of the wave equation. If we ignore waves that are traveling to the left, then the general solution to the wave equation becomes

$$u(\vec{r}) = \frac{1}{2\pi} \int_{-\infty}^{\infty} \alpha(k_y) e^{j(k_x x + k_y y)} \, dk_y. \tag{13}$$

If we also move the coordinate system so that the measurement line is at $x = 0$, the expression for the field becomes equal to the one-dimensional Fourier transform of the amplitude distribution function $\alpha(k_y)$.

$$u(0, y) = \frac{1}{2\pi} \int_{-\infty}^{\infty} \alpha(k_y) e^{j k_y y} \, dk_y. \tag{14}$$

If we invert the transform relationship, this equation tells us that the amplitude distribution function can be obtained from the fields on the line $x = 0$ by

$$\alpha(k_y) = \text{Fourier transform of } \{u(0, y)\}. \tag{15}$$

This amplitude distribution function can then be substituted into the equation for $u(\vec{r})$ to obtain the fields everywhere right of the line $x = 0$.

We will now show how it is possible to relate fields on two parallel lines. Again consider the situation diagrammed in Fig. 6.1. If we know a priori that all the sources for the field are positioned, for example, to the left of the line at $x = l_0$, then we can decompose the field $u(x = l_0, y)$ into its plane wave components. Given a plane wave $u_{\text{plane wave}}(x = l_0, y) = \alpha e^{j(k_x l_0 + k_y y)}$ the field undergoes a phase shift as it propagates to the line $x = l_1$, and we can write

$$u_{\text{plane wave}}(x = l_1, y) = \alpha e^{j(k_x l_0 + k_y y)} e^{jk_x(l_1 - l_0)} = u_{\text{plane wave}}(x = l_0, y) e^{jk_x(l_1 - l_0)}. \tag{16}$$

Thus the complex amplitude of the plane wave at $x = l_1$ is related to its complex amplitude at $x = l_0$ by a factor of $e^{jk_x(l_1 - l_0)}$.

The complete process of finding the field at a line $x = l_1$ follows in three steps:

1) Take the Fourier transform of $u(x = l_0, y)$ to find the Fourier decomposition of u as a function of k_y.
2) Propagate each plane wave to the line $x = l_1$ by multiplying its complex amplitude by the phase factor $e^{jk_x(l_1 - l_0)}$ where, as before, $k_x = \sqrt{k_0^2 - k_y^2}$.
3) Find the inverse Fourier transform of the plane wave decomposition to find the field at $u(x = l_1, y)$.

These steps can be reversed if, for some reason, one wished to implement on a computer the notion of backward propagation; more on that subject later.

6.1.2 Inhomogeneous Wave Equation

For imaging purposes, our main interest lies in inhomogeneous media. We, therefore, write a more general form of the wave equation as

$$[\nabla^2 + k(\vec{r})^2] u(\vec{r}) = 0. \tag{17}$$

For the electromagnetic case, if we ignore the effects of polarization we can consider $k(\vec{r})$ to be a scalar function representing the refractive index of the medium. We now write

$$k(\vec{r}) = k_0 n(\vec{r}) = k_0[1 + n_\delta(\vec{r})] \tag{18}$$

where k_0 represents the average wavenumber of the medium and $n_\delta(\vec{r})$ represents the refractive index deviations. In general, we will assume that the object has a finite size and therefore $n_\delta(\vec{r})$ is zero outside the object. Rewriting the wave equation we find

$$(\nabla^2 + k_0^2) u(\vec{r}) = -k_0^2 [n(\vec{r})^2 - 1](\vec{r}) u(\vec{r}) \tag{19}$$

where $n(\vec{r})$ is the electromagnetic refractive index of the media and is given by

$$n(\vec{r}) = \sqrt{\frac{\mu(\vec{r})\epsilon(\vec{r})}{\mu_0 \epsilon_0}}. \tag{20}$$

Here we have used μ and ϵ to represent the magnetic permeability and dielectric constant and the subscript zero to indicate their average values. This new term, on the right-hand side of (19), is known as a forcing function for the differential equation $(\nabla^2 + k_0^2)u(\vec{r})$.

Note that (19) is a *scalar* wave propagation equation. Its use implies that there is no depolarization as the electromagnetic wave propagates through the medium. It is known [Ish78] that the depolarization effects can be ignored only if the wavelength is much smaller than the correlation size of the inhomogeneities in the object. If this condition isn't satisfied, then strictly speaking we must use the following vector wave propagation equation:

$$\nabla^2 \vec{E}(rv) + k_0^2 n^2 \vec{E}(\vec{r}) - 2\nabla \left[\frac{\nabla n}{n} \cdot \vec{E} \right] = 0 \tag{21}$$

where $\vec{E}$ is the electric field vector. A vector theory for diffraction tomography based on this equation has yet to be developed.

For the acoustic case, first-order approximations give us the following wave equation [Kak85], [Mor68]:

$$(\nabla^2 + k_0^2)u(\vec{r}) = -k_0^2[n^2(\vec{r}) - 1]u(\vec{r}) \tag{22}$$

where n is the *complex refractive index* at position $\vec{r}$, and is equal to

$$n(\vec{r}) = \frac{c_0}{c(\vec{r})} \tag{23}$$

where c_0 is the propagation velocity in the medium in which the object is immersed and $c(\vec{r})$ is the propagation velocity at location $\vec{r}$ in the object. For the acoustic case where only compressional waves in a viscous compressible fluid are involved, we have

$$c(\vec{r}) = \frac{1}{\sqrt{\rho(\vec{r})\kappa(\vec{r})}} \tag{24}$$

where ρ and κ are the *local density* and the *complex compressibility* at location $\vec{r}$.

The forcing function in (22) is only valid provided we can ignore the first and higher order derivatives of the medium parameters. If these higher order derivatives can't be ignored, the exact form for the wave equation must be used:

$$(\nabla^2 + k_0^2)u(\vec{r}) = k_0^2 \gamma_\kappa u - \nabla \cdot (\gamma_\rho \nabla u) \tag{25}$$

where

$$\gamma_\kappa = \frac{\kappa - \kappa_0}{\kappa_0} \qquad (26)$$

$$\gamma_\rho = \frac{\rho - \rho_0}{\rho}. \qquad (27)$$

κ_0 and ρ_0 are either the compressibility and the density of the medium in which the object is immersed, or the average compressibility and the density of the object, depending upon how the process of imaging is modeled. On the other hand, if the object is a solid and can be modeled as a linear isotropic viscoelastic medium, the forcing function possesses another more complicated form. Since this form involves tensor notation, it will not be presented here and the interested reader is referred to [Iwa75].

Due to the similarities of the electromagnetic and acoustic wave equations, a general form of the wave equation for the small perturbation case can be written as

$$(\nabla^2 + k_0^2)u(\vec{r}) = -o(\vec{r})u(\vec{r}) \qquad (28)$$

where

$$o(\vec{r}) = k_0^2[n^2(\vec{r}) - 1]. \qquad (29)$$

This allows us to describe the math involved in diffraction tomography independent of the form of energy used to illuminate the object.

We will consider the field, $u(\vec{r})$, to be the sum of two components, $u_0(\vec{r})$ and $u_s(\vec{r})$. The component $u_0(\vec{r})$, known as the incident field, is the field present without any inhomogeneities, or, equivalently, a solution to the equation

$$(\nabla^2 + k_0^2)u_0(\vec{r}) = 0. \qquad (30)$$

The component $u_s(\vec{r})$, known as the scattered field, will be that part of the total field that can be attributed solely to the inhomogeneities. What we are saying is that with $u_0(\vec{r})$ as the solution to the above equation, we want the field $u(\vec{r})$ to be given by $u(\vec{r}) = u_0(\vec{r}) + u_s(\vec{r})$. Substituting the wave equation for u_0 and the sum representation for u into (28), we get the following wave equation for just the scattered component:

$$(\nabla^2 + k_0^2)u_s(\vec{r}) = -u(\vec{r})o(\vec{r}). \qquad (31)$$

The scalar Helmholtz equation (31) can't be solved for $u_s(\vec{r})$ directly, but a solution can be written in terms of the Green's function [Mor53]. The Green's function, which is a solution of the differential equation

$$(\nabla^2 + k_0^2)g(\vec{r}|\vec{r}\,') = -\delta(\vec{r} - \vec{r}\,'), \qquad (32)$$

is written in three-space as

$$g(\vec{r}|\vec{r}\,') = \frac{e^{jk_0 R}}{4\pi R} \qquad (33)$$

with

$$R = |\vec{r} - \vec{r}\,'|. \qquad (34)$$

In two dimensions the solution of (32) is written in terms of a zero-order Hankel function of the first kind, and can be expressed as

$$g(\vec{r}\,'|\vec{r}\,') = \frac{j}{4} H_0^{(1)}(k_0 R). \qquad (35)$$

In both cases, the Green's function, $g(\vec{r}|\vec{r}\,')$, is only a function of the difference $\vec{r} - \vec{r}\,'$ so we will often represent the function as simply $g(\vec{r} - \vec{r}\,')$. Because the object function in (32) represents a point inhomogeneity, the Green's function can be considered to represent the field resulting from a single point scatterer.

It is possible to represent the forcing function of the wave equation as an array of impulses or

$$o(\vec{r})u(\vec{r}) = \int o(\vec{r}\,')u(\vec{r}\,')\delta(\vec{r}-\vec{r}\,')\,d\vec{r}\,'. \qquad (36)$$

In this equation we have represented the forcing function of the inhomogeneous wave equation as a summation of impulses weighted by $o(\vec{r})u(\vec{r})$ and shifted by $\vec{r}$. The Green's function represents the solution of the wave equation for a single delta function; because the left-hand side of the wave equation is linear, we can write a solution by summing up the scattered field due to each individual point scatterer.

Using this idea, the total field due to the impulse $o(\vec{r}\,')u(\vec{r}\,')\delta(\vec{r} - \vec{r}\,')$ is written as a summation of scaled and shifted versions of the impulse response, $g(\vec{r})$. This is a simple convolution and the total radiation from all sources on the right-hand side of (31) must be given by the following superposition:

$$u_s(\vec{r}) = \int g(\vec{r}-\vec{r}\,')o(\vec{r}\,')u(\vec{r}\,')\,d\vec{r}\,'. \qquad (37)$$

At first glance it might appear that this is the solution we need for the scattered field, but it is not that simple. We have written an integral equation for the scattered field, u_s, in terms of the total field, $u = u_0 + u_s$. We still need to solve this equation for the scattered field and we will now discuss two approximations that allow this to be done.

6.2 Approximations to the Wave Equation

In the last section we derived an inhomogeneous integral equation to represent the scattered field, $u_s(\vec{r})$, as a function of the object, $o(\vec{r})$. This equation can't be solved directly, but a solution can be written using either of the two approximations to be described here. These approximations, the Born and the Rytov, are valid under different conditions but the form of the resulting solutions is quite similar. These approximations are the basis of the Fourier Diffraction Theorem.

Mathematically speaking, (37) is a Fredholm equation of the second kind. A number of mathematicians have presented works describing the solution of scattering integrals [Hoc73], [Col83] which should be consulted for the theory behind the approximations we will present.

6.2.1 The First Born Approximation

The first Born approximation is the simpler of the two approaches. Recall that the total field, $u(\vec{r})$, is expressed as the sum of the incident field, $u_0(\vec{r})$, and a small perturbation, $u_s(\vec{r})$, or

$$u(\vec{r}) = u_0(\vec{r}) + u_s(\vec{r}). \tag{38}$$

The integral of (37) is now written as

$$u_s(\vec{r}) = \int g(\vec{r}-\vec{r}\,')o(\vec{r}\,')u_0(\vec{r}\,')\,d\vec{r}\,' + \int g(\vec{r}-\vec{r}\,')o(\vec{r}\,')u_s(\vec{r}\,')\,d\vec{r}\,' \tag{39}$$

but if the scattered field, $u_s(\vec{r})$, is small compared to $u_0(\vec{r})$ the effects of the second integral can be ignored to arrive at the approximation

$$u_s(\vec{r}) \simeq u_B(\vec{r}) = \int g(\vec{r}-\vec{r}\,')o(\vec{r}\,')u_0(\vec{r}\,')\,d\vec{r}\,'. \tag{40}$$

An even better estimate can be found by substituting $u_0(\vec{r}) + u_B(\vec{r})$ for $u_0(\vec{r})$ in (40) to find

$$u_B^{(2)}(\vec{r}) = \int g(\vec{r}-\vec{r}\,')o(\vec{r}\,')[u_0(\vec{r}\,') + u_B(\vec{r}\,')]\,d\vec{r}\,'. \tag{41}$$

In general, the ith-order Born field can be written

$$u_B^{(i+1)}(\vec{r}) = \int g(\vec{r}-\vec{r}\,')o(\vec{r}\,')[u_0(\vec{r}\,') + u_B^{(i)}(\vec{r}\,')]\,d\vec{r}\,'. \tag{42}$$

An alternate representation is possible if we write

$$u(\vec{r}) = u_0(\vec{r}) + u_1(\vec{r}) + u_2(\vec{r}) + \cdots \tag{43}$$

where

$$u_{(i+1)}(\vec{r}) = \int u_i(\vec{r}\,')o(\vec{r}\,')g(\vec{r}-\vec{r}\,')\,d\vec{r}\,'. \tag{44}$$

By expanding (42) it is possible to see that an approximate expression for the scattered field, $u_B^{(i)}$, is

$$u_B^{(i)}(\vec{r}) = \sum_{j=0}^{i} u_j(\vec{r}) \qquad (45)$$

and in the limit

$$u(\vec{r}) \simeq u_0(\vec{r}) + u_1(\vec{r}) + u_2(\vec{r}) + u_3(\vec{r}) + \cdots . \qquad (46)$$

This representation (46) has a more intuitive interpretation. The Green's function gives the scattered field due to a point scatterer and thus the integral of (42) can be interpreted as calculating the first-order scattered field due to the field u_i. For this reason the first-order Born approximation represents the first-order scattered field and u_i represents the ith-order scattered field.

The result can also be interpreted in terms of the Huygens principle; each point in the object produces a scattered field proportional to the scattering potential at the site of the scatterer. Each of these partial scattered fields interacts with the other scattering centers in the object and if the Born series converges the total field is the sum of the partial scattered fields.

While the higher order Born series does provide a good model of the scattering process, reconstruction algorithms based on this series have yet to be developed. These algorithms are currently being researched; in the meantime, we will study reconstruction algorithms based on first-order approximations [Bar78], [Sla85].

The first Born approximation is valid only when the scattered field,

$$u_s(\vec{r}) = u(\vec{r}) - u_0(\vec{r}), \qquad (47)$$

is smaller than the incident field, u_0. If the object is a homogeneous cylinder it is possible to express this condition as a function of the size of the object and the refractive index. Let the incident wave, $u_0(\vec{r})$, be an electromagnetic plane wave propagating in the direction of the unit vector, $\vec{s}$. For a large object, the field inside the object will not be well approximated by the incident field

$$u(\vec{r}) = u_{\text{object}}(\vec{r}) \neq A e^{jk_0 \vec{s} \cdot \vec{r}} \qquad (48)$$

but instead will be a function of the change in refractive index, n_δ. Along a line through the center of the cylinder and parallel to the direction of propagation of the incident plane wave, the field inside the object becomes a slow (or fast) version of the incident wave, that is,

$$u_{\text{object}}(\vec{r}) = A e^{jk_0(1+n_\delta)\vec{s} \cdot \vec{r}}. \qquad (49)$$

Since the wave is propagating through the object, the phase difference between the incident field and the field inside the object is approximately equal to the integral through the object of the change in refractive index. For a homogeneous cylinder of radius a, the total phase shift through the object becomes

$$\text{Phase Change} = 4\pi n_\delta \frac{a}{\lambda} \tag{50}$$

where λ is the wavelength of the incident wave. For the Born approximation to be valid, a necessary condition is that the change in phase between the incident field and the wave propagating through the object be less than π. This condition can be expressed mathematically as

$$an_\delta < \frac{\lambda}{4}. \tag{51}$$

6.2.2 The First Rytov Approximation

Another approximation to the scattered field is the Rytov approximation which is valid under slightly different restrictions. It is derived by considering the total field to be represented as a complex phase or [Ish78]

$$u(\vec{r}) = e^{\phi(\vec{r})} \tag{52}$$

and rewriting the wave equation (17)

$$(\nabla^2 + k^2)u = 0 \tag{17}$$

as

$$\nabla^2 e^\phi + k^2 e^\phi = 0 \tag{53}$$

$$\nabla[\nabla\phi e^\phi] + k^2 e^\phi = 0 \tag{54}$$

$$\nabla^2 \phi e^\phi + (\nabla\phi)^2 e^\phi + k^2 e^\phi = 0 \tag{55}$$

and finally

$$(\nabla\phi)^2 + \nabla^2\phi + k_0^2 = -o(\vec{r}). \tag{56}$$

(Although all the fields, ϕ, are a function of $\vec{r}$, to simplify the notation the argument of these functions will be dropped.) Expressing the total complex phase, ϕ, as the sum of the incident phase function ϕ_0 and the scattered complex phase ϕ_s or

$$\phi(\vec{r}) = \phi_0(\vec{r}) + \phi_s(\vec{r}) \tag{57}$$

where

$$u_0(\vec{r}) = e^{\phi_0(\vec{r})}, \tag{58}$$

we find that

$$(\nabla\phi_0)^2 + 2\nabla\phi_0 \cdot \nabla\phi_s + (\nabla\phi_s)^2 + \nabla^2\phi_0 + \nabla^2\phi_s + k_0^2 + o(\vec{r}) = 0. \quad (59)$$

As in the Born approximation, it is possible to set the zero perturbation equation equal to zero. Doing this, we find that

$$k_0^2 + (\nabla\phi_0)^2 + \nabla^2\phi_0 = 0. \quad (60)$$

Substituting this into (59) we get

$$2\nabla\phi_0 \cdot \nabla\phi_s + \nabla^2\phi_s = -(\nabla\phi_s)^2 - o(\vec{r}). \quad (61)$$

This equation is still inhomogeneous but can be linearized by considering the relation

$$\nabla^2(u_0\phi_s) = \nabla(\nabla u_0 \cdot \phi_s + u_0\nabla\phi_s) \quad (62)$$

or by expanding the first derivative on the right-hand side of this equation

$$\nabla^2(u_0\phi_s) = \nabla^2 u_0 \cdot \phi_s + 2\nabla u_0 \cdot \nabla\phi_s + u_0\nabla^2\phi_s. \quad (63)$$

Using a plane wave for the incident field,

$$u_0 = Ae^{jk_0\vec{s}\cdot\vec{r}}, \quad (64)$$

we find

$$\nabla^2 u_0 = -k_0^2 u_0 \quad (65)$$

so that (63) may be rewritten as

$$2u_0\nabla\phi_0 \cdot \nabla\phi_s + u_0\nabla^2\phi_s = \nabla^2(u_0\phi_s) + k_0^2 u_0\phi_s. \quad (66)$$

This result can be substituted into (61) to find

$$(\nabla^2 + k_0^2)u_0\phi_s = -u_0[(\nabla\phi_s)^2 + o(\vec{r})]. \quad (67)$$

The solution to this differential equation can again be expressed as an integral equation. This becomes

$$u_0\phi_s = \int_{V'} g(\vec{r}-\vec{r}\,')\, u_0[(\nabla\phi_s)^2 + o(\vec{r}\,')]\, d\vec{r}\,'. \quad (68)$$

Using the Rytov approximation we assume that the term in brackets in the above equation can be approximated by

$$(\nabla\phi_s)^2 + o(\vec{r}) \simeq o(\vec{r}). \quad (69)$$

When this is done, the first-order Rytov approximation to the function $u_0\phi_s$ becomes

$$u_0\phi_s = \int_{V'} g(\vec{r}-\vec{r}\,')u_0(\vec{r}\,')o(\vec{r}\,')\, d\vec{r}\,'. \quad (70)$$

Thus ϕ_s, the complex phase of the scattered field, is given by

$$\phi_s(\vec{r}) = \frac{1}{u_0(\vec{r})} \int_{V'} g(\vec{r}-\vec{r}')u_0(\vec{r}')o(\vec{r}') \, d\vec{r}'. \tag{71}$$

Substituting the expression for u_B given in (40), we find that

$$\phi_s(\vec{r}) = \frac{u_B(\vec{r})}{u_0(\vec{r})}. \tag{72}$$

The Rytov approximation is valid under a less restrictive set of conditions than the Born approximation [Che60], [Kel69]. In deriving the Rytov approximation we made the assumption that

$$(\nabla \phi_s)^2 + o(\vec{r}) \simeq o(\vec{r}). \tag{73}$$

Clearly this is true only when

$$o(\vec{r}) \gg (\nabla \phi_s)^2. \tag{74}$$

If $o(\vec{r})$ is written in terms of the change in refractive index

$$o(\vec{r}) = k_0^2[n^2(\vec{r}) - 1] = k_0^2[(1 + n_\delta(\vec{r}))^2 - 1] \tag{29}$$

and the square of the refractive index is expanded to find

$$o(\vec{r}) = k_0^2[(1 + 2n_\delta(\vec{r}) + n_\delta^2(\vec{r})) - 1] \tag{75}$$

$$o(\vec{r}) = k_0^2[2n_\delta(\vec{r}) + n_\delta^2(\vec{r})]. \tag{76}$$

To a first approximation, the object function is linearly related to the refractive index or

$$o(\vec{r}) \simeq 2k_0^2 n_\delta(\vec{r}). \tag{77}$$

The condition needed for the Rytov approximation (see (74)) can be rewritten as

$$n_\delta \gg \frac{(\nabla \phi_s)^2}{k_0^2}. \tag{78}$$

This can be justified by observing that to a first approximation the scattered phase, ϕ_s, is linearly dependent on the refractive index change, n_δ, and therefore the first term in (73) can be safely ignored for small n_δ.

Unlike the Born approximation, the size of the object is not a factor in the Rytov approximation. The term $\nabla \phi_s$ is the change in the complex scattered phase per unit distance and by dividing by the wavenumber

$$k_0 = \frac{2\pi}{\lambda} \tag{79}$$

we find a necessary condition for the validity of the Rytov approximation is

$$n_\delta \gg \left[\frac{\nabla \phi_s \lambda}{2\pi}\right]^2. \tag{80}$$

Unlike the Born approximation, it is the change in scattered phase, ϕ_s, over one wavelength that is important and not the total phase. Thus, because of the ∇ operator, the Rytov approximation is valid when the phase change over a single wavelength is small.

Since the imaging process is carried out in terms of the field, u_B, defined in the previous subsection, we need to show a Rytov approximation expression for u_B. Estimating $u_B(\vec{r})$ for the Rytov case is slightly more difficult. In an experiment the total field, $u(\vec{r})$, is measured. An expression for $u_B(\vec{r})$ is found by recalling the expression for the Rytov solution to the total wave

$$u(\vec{r}) = u_0 + u_s(\vec{r}) = e^{\phi_0 + \phi_s} \tag{81}$$

and then rearranging the exponentials to find

$$u_s = e^{\phi_0 + \phi_s} - e^{\phi_0} \tag{82}$$

$$u_s = e^{\phi_0}(e^{\phi_s} - 1) \tag{83}$$

$$u_s = u_0(e^{\phi_s} - 1). \tag{84}$$

Inverting this to find an estimate for the scattered phase, ϕ_s, we obtain

$$\phi_s(\vec{r}) = \ln\left[\frac{u_s}{u_0} + 1\right]. \tag{85}$$

Expanding ϕ_s in terms of (72) we obtain the following estimate for the Rytov estimate of $u_B(\vec{r})$:

$$u_B(\vec{r}) = u_0(\vec{r}) \ln\left[\frac{u_s}{u_0} + 1\right]. \tag{86}$$

Since the natural logarithm is a multiple-valued function, one must be careful at each position to choose the correct value. For continuous functions this isn't difficult because only one value will satisfy the continuity requirement. On the other hand, for discrete (or sampled) signals the choice isn't nearly as simple and one must resort to a phase unwrapping algorithm to choose the proper phase. (Phase unwrapping has been described in a number of works [Tri77], [OCo78], [Kav84], [McG82].) Due to the "+1" factor inside the logarithmic term, this is only a problem if u_s is on the order of or larger than u_0. Thus both the Born and the Rytov techniques can be used to estimate $u_B(\vec{r})$.

While the Rytov approximation is valid over a larger class of objects, it is possible to show that the Born and the Rytov approximations produce the same result for objects that are small and deviate only slightly from the average refractive index of the medium. Consider first the Rytov approximation to the scattered wave. This is given by

$$u(\vec{r}) = e^{\phi_0 + \phi_s}. \tag{87}$$

Substituting an expression for the scattered phase, (72), and the incident field, (64), we find

$$u(\vec{r}) = e^{jk_0\vec{s}\cdot\vec{r} + \exp(-jk_0\vec{s}\cdot\vec{r})u_B(\vec{r})} \tag{88}$$

or

$$u(\vec{r}) = u_0(\vec{r})e^{\exp(-jk_0\vec{s}\cdot\vec{r})u_B(\vec{r})}. \tag{89}$$

For small u_B, the first exponential can be expanded in terms of its power series. Throwing out all but the first two terms we find that

$$u(\vec{r}) = u_0(\vec{r})[1 + e^{-jk_0\vec{s}\cdot\vec{r}}u_B(\vec{r})] \tag{90}$$

or

$$u(\vec{r}) = u_0(\vec{r}) + u_B(\vec{r}). \tag{91}$$

Thus for very small objects and perturbations the Rytov solution is approximately equal to the Born solution given in (40).

The similarity between the expressions for the first-order Born and Rytov solutions will form the basis of our reconstructions. In the Born approximation we measure the complex amplitude of the scattered field and use this as an estimate of the function u_B, while in the Rytov case we estimate u_B from the phase of the scattered field. Since the Rytov approximation is considered more accurate than the Born approximation it should provide a better estimate of u_B. In Section 6.5, after we have derived reconstruction algorithms based on the Fourier Diffraction Theorem, we will discuss simulations comparing the Born and the Rytov approximations.

6.3 The Fourier Diffraction Theorem

Fundamental to diffraction tomography is the *Fourier Diffraction Theorem,* which relates the Fourier transform of the measured forward scattered data with the Fourier transform of the object. *The theorem is valid when the inhomogeneities in the object are only weakly scattering.* The statement of the theorem is as follows:

> When an object, $o(x, y)$, is illuminated with a plane wave as shown in Fig. 6.2, the Fourier transform of the forward scattered field measured on line TT' gives the values of the 2-D transform, $O(\omega_1, \omega_2)$, of the object along a semicircular arc in the frequency domain, as shown in the right half of the figure.

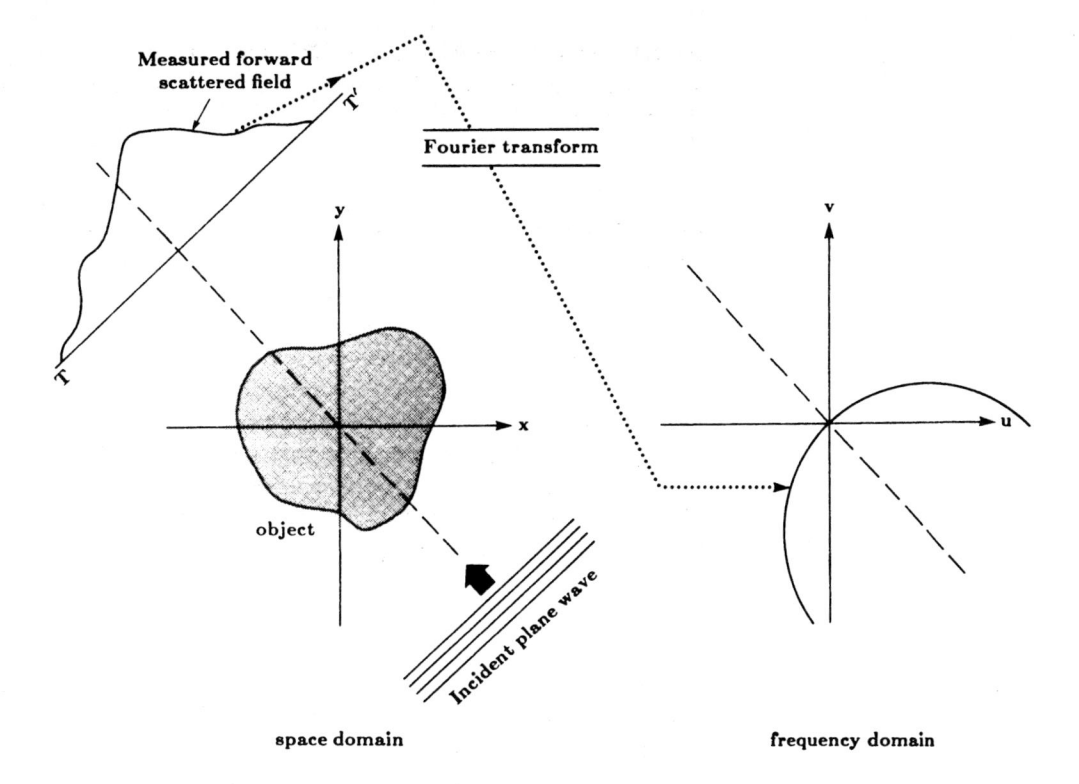

Fig. 6.2: *The Fourier Diffraction Theorem relates the Fourier transform of a diffracted projection to the Fourier transform of the object along a semicircular arc. (From [Sla83].)*

The importance of the theorem is made obvious by noting that if an object is illuminated by plane waves from many directions over 360°, the resulting circular arcs in the (ω_1, ω_2)-plane will fill up the frequency domain. The function $o(x, y)$ may then be recovered by Fourier inversion.

Before giving a short proof of the theorem, we would like to say a few words about the dimensionality of the object vis-à-vis that of the wave fields. Although the theorem talks about a two-dimensional object, what is actually meant is an object that doesn't vary in the z direction. In other words, the theorem is about any cylindrical object whose cross-sectional distribution is given by the function $o(x, y)$. The forward scattered fields are measured on a line of detectors along TT' in Fig. 6.2. If a truly three-dimensional object were illuminated by the plane wave, the forward scattered fields would now have to be measured by a planar array of detectors. The Fourier transform of the fields measured by such an array would give the values of the 3-D transform of the object over a spherical surface. This was first shown by Wolf [Wol69]. More recent expositions are given in [Nah82] and [Dev84], where the authors have also presented a new synthetic aperture procedure for a full three-dimensional reconstruction using only two rotational positions of the object. In this chapter, however, we will continue to work with two-dimensional objects in the sense described here. A recent work describing some of the errors in this approach is [LuZ84].

Earlier in this chapter, we expressed the scattered field due to a weakly scattering object as the convolution

$$u_B(\vec{r}) = \int o(\vec{r}\,')u_0(\vec{r}\,')g(\vec{r}-\vec{r}\,')\,d\vec{r}\,' \tag{92}$$

where $u_B(\vec{r})$ represents the complex amplitude of the field as in the Born approximation, or the incident field, $u_0(\vec{r})$, times the complex scattered phase, $\phi_s(\vec{r})$, as in the Rytov approximation. Starting from this integral there are two approaches to the derivation of the Fourier Diffraction Theorem. Many researchers [Mue79], [Gre78], [Dev82] have expanded the Green's function into its plane wave decomposition and then noted the similarity of the resulting expression and the Fourier transform of the object. The alternative approach consists of taking the Fourier transform of both sides of (92). In this work we will present both approaches to the derivation of the Fourier Diffraction Theorem; the first because the math is more straightforward, the second because it provides a greater insight into the difference between transmission and reflection tomography.

6.3.1 Decomposing the Green's Function

We will first consider the decomposition of the Green's function into its plane wave components.

The integral equation for the scattered field (92) can be considered as a convolution of the Green's function, $g(\vec{r} - \vec{r}\,')$, and the product of the object function, $o(\vec{r}\,')$, and the incident field, $u_0(\vec{r}\,')$. Consider the effect of a single plane wave illuminating an object. The forward scattered field will be measured at the receiver line as is shown in Fig. 6.3.

A single plane wave in two dimensions can be represented as

$$u_0(\vec{r}) = e^{j\vec{K}\cdot\vec{r}} \tag{93}$$

where $\vec{K} = (k_x, k_y)$ satisfies the relationship

$$k_0^2 = k_x^2 + k_y^2. \tag{94}$$

From earlier in this chapter, the two-dimensional Green's function is given by

$$g(\vec{r}|\vec{r}\,') = \frac{j}{4} H_0(k_0|\vec{r}-\vec{r}\,'|) \tag{95}$$

and H_0 is the zero-order Hankel function of the first kind. The function H_0 has the plane wave decomposition [Mor53]

$$H_0(k|\vec{r}-\vec{r}\,'|) = \frac{1}{\pi}\int_{-\infty}^{\infty} \frac{1}{\beta} e^{j[\alpha(x-x')+\beta|y-y'|]}\,d\alpha \tag{96}$$

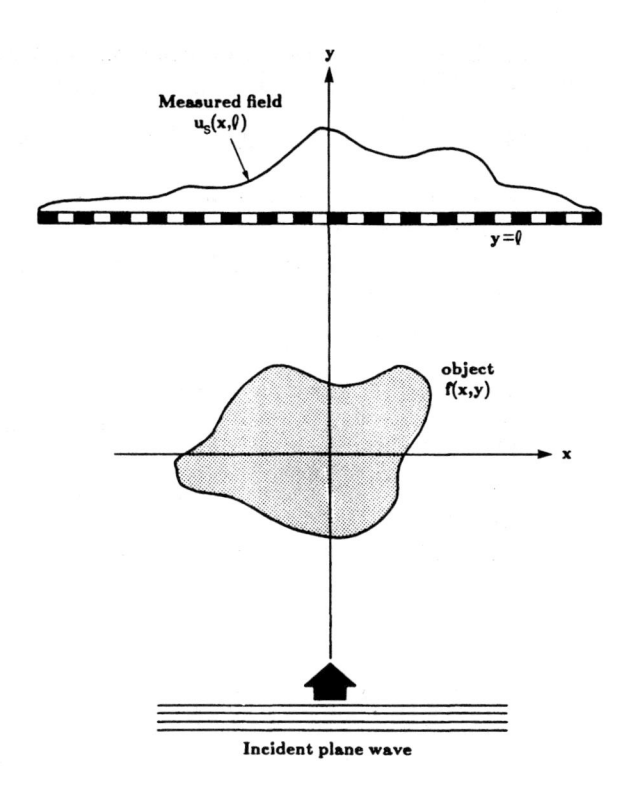

Fig. 6.3: *A typical diffraction tomography experiment is shown. Here a single plane wave is used to illuminate the object and the scattered field is measured on the far side of the object. This is transmission tomography. (From [Pan83].)*

where $\vec{r} = (x, y)$, $\vec{r}' = (x', y')$ and

$$\beta = \sqrt{k_0^2 - \alpha^2} \ . \tag{97}$$

Basically, (96) expresses a cylindrical wave, H_0, as a superposition of plane waves. At all points, the wave centered at $\vec{r}'$ is traveling outward; for points such that $y > y'$ the plane waves propagate upward while for $y < y'$ the plane waves propagate downward. In addition, for $|\alpha| \leq k_0$, the plane waves are of the ordinary type, propagating along the direction given by $\tan^{-1}(\beta/\alpha)$. However, for $|\alpha| > k_0$, β becomes imaginary, the waves decay exponentially and they are called *evanescent waves*. Evanescent waves are usually of no significance beyond about 10 wavelengths from the source.

Substituting this expression, (96), into the expression for the scattered field, (92), the scattered field can now be written

$$u_B(\vec{r}) = \frac{j}{4\pi} \int o(\vec{r}') u_0(\vec{r}') \int_{-\infty}^{\infty} \frac{1}{\beta} e^{j[\alpha(x-x')+\beta|y-y'|]} \, d\alpha \, d\vec{r}' . \tag{98}$$

In order to show the first steps in the proof of this theorem, we will now assume for notational convenience that the direction of the incident plane wave is along the positive y-axis. Thus the incident field will be given by

$$u_0(\vec{r}) = e^{j\vec{s}_0 \cdot \vec{r}} \tag{99}$$

where $\vec{s}_0 = (0, k_0)$. Since in transmission imaging the scattered fields are measured by a linear array located at $y = l_0$, where l_0 is greater than any y-coordinate within the object (see Fig. 6.3), the term $|y - y'|$ in the above expression may simply be replaced by $l_0 - y'$ and the resulting form may be rewritten

$$u_B(x, y = l_0) = \frac{j}{4\pi} \int_{-\infty}^{\infty} d\alpha \int \frac{o(\vec{r}')}{\beta} e^{j[\alpha(x-x') + \beta(l_0 - y')]} e^{jk_0 y'} \, d\vec{r}'. \tag{100}$$

Recognizing part of the inner integral as the two-dimensional Fourier transform of the object function evaluated at a frequency of $(\alpha, \beta - k_0)$ we find

$$u_B(x, y = l_0) = \frac{j}{4\pi} \int_{-\infty}^{\infty} \frac{1}{\beta} e^{j(\alpha x + \beta l_0)} O(\alpha, \beta - k_0) \, d\alpha \tag{101}$$

where O has been used to designate the two-dimensional Fourier transform of the object function.

Let $U_B(\omega, l_0)$ denote the Fourier transform of the one-dimensional scattered field, $u_B(x, l_0)$, with respect to x, that is,

$$U_B(\omega, l_0) = \int_{-\infty}^{\infty} u_B(x, l_0) e^{-j\omega x} \, dx. \tag{102}$$

As mentioned before, the physics of wave propagation dictate that the highest angular spatial frequency in the measured scattered field on the line $y = l_0$ is unlikely to exceed k_0. Therefore, in almost all practical situations, $U_s(\omega, l_0) = 0$ for $|\omega| > k_0$. This is consistent with neglecting the evanescent modes as described earlier.

If we take the Fourier transform of the scattered field by substituting (101) into (102) and using the following property of Fourier integrals

$$\int_{-\infty}^{\infty} e^{j(\omega - \alpha)x} \, dx = 2\pi \delta(\omega - \alpha) \tag{103}$$

where $\delta(\cdot)$ is the Dirac delta function we discussed in Chapter 2, we find

$$U_B(\alpha, l_0) = \frac{j}{2\sqrt{k_0^2 - \alpha^2}} e^{j\sqrt{k_0^2 - \alpha^2}\, l_0} O(\alpha, \sqrt{k_0^2 - \alpha^2} - k_0) \quad \text{for } |\alpha| < k_0. \tag{104}$$

This expression relates the two-dimensional Fourier transform of the object to the one-dimensional Fourier transform of the field at the receiver line. The factor

$$\frac{j}{2\sqrt{k_0^2-\alpha^2}} e^{j\sqrt{k_0^2-\alpha^2}l_0} \tag{105}$$

is a simple constant for a fixed receiver line. As α varies from $-k_0$ to k_0, the coordinates $(\alpha, \sqrt{k_0^2 - \alpha^2} - k_0)$ in the Fourier transform of the object function trace out a semicircular arc in the (u, v)-plane as shown in Fig. 6.2. This proves the theorem.

To summarize, if we take the Fourier transform of the forward scattered data when the incident illumination is propagating along the positive y-axis, the resulting transform will be zero for angular spatial frequencies $|\alpha| > k_0$. For $|\alpha| < k_0$, the transform of the data gives values of the Fourier transform of the object on the semicircular arc shown in Fig. 6.2 in the (u, v)-plane. The endpoints of the semicircular arc are at a distance of $\sqrt{2}k_0$ from the origin in the frequency domain.

6.3.2 Fourier Transform Approach

Another approach to the derivation of the Fourier Diffraction Theorem is possible if the scattered field

$$u_B(\vec{r}) = \int o(\vec{r}\,')u_0(\vec{r}\,')g(\vec{r}-\vec{r}\,')\,d\vec{r}\,' \tag{106}$$

is considered entirely in the Fourier domain. The plots of Fig. 6.4 will be used to illustrate the various transformations that take place. Again, consider the effect of a single plane wave illuminating an object. The forward scattered field will be measured at the receiver line as is shown in Fig. 6.3.

The integral equation for the scattered field, (106), can be considered as a convolution of the Green's function, $g(\vec{r} - \vec{r}\,')$, and the product of the object function, $o(\vec{r}\,')$, and the incident field, $u_0(\vec{r}\,')$. First define the following Fourier transform pairs:

$$o(\vec{r}) \leftrightarrow O(\vec{K})$$

$$g(\vec{r}-\vec{r}\,') \leftrightarrow G(\vec{K}) \tag{107}$$

$$u(\vec{r}) \leftrightarrow U(\vec{K}).$$

The integral solution to the wave equation, (40), can now be written in terms of these Fourier transforms, that is,

$$U_s(\vec{\Lambda}) = G(\vec{\Lambda})\{O(\vec{\Lambda}) * U_0(\vec{\Lambda})\} \tag{108}$$

where $*$ has been used to represent convolution and $\vec{\Lambda} = (\alpha, \gamma)$. In (93) an expression for u_0 was presented. Its Fourier transform is given by

$$U_0(\vec{\Lambda}) = 2\pi\delta(\vec{\Lambda} - \vec{K}) \tag{109}$$

(a)

(b)

(c)

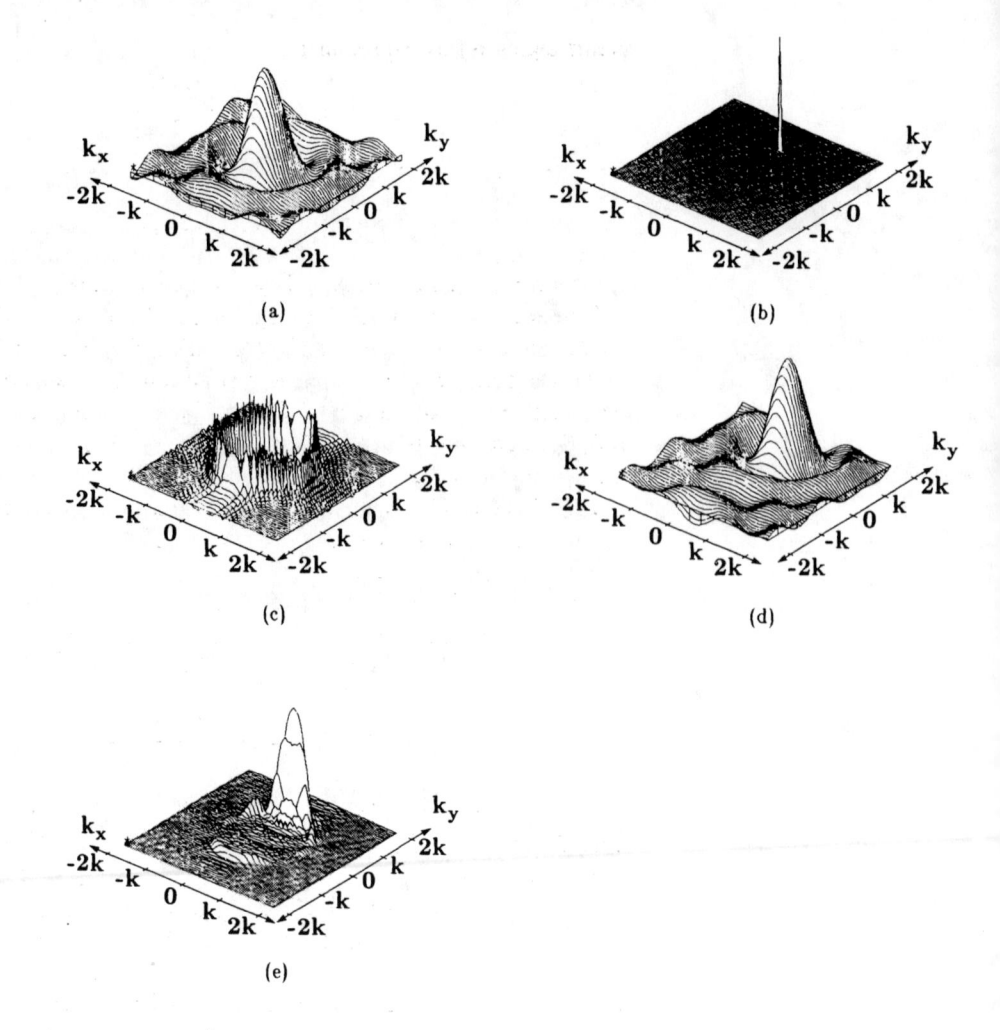

(d)

(e)

Fig. 6.4: *Two-dimensional Fourier representation of the Helmholtz equation. (a) is the Fourier transform of the object, in this case a cylinder, (b) is the Fourier transform of the incident field, (c) is the Fourier transform of the Green's function in (95), (d) shows the frequency domain convolution of (a) and (b), and finally (e) is the product in the frequency domain of (c) and (d). (From [Sla83].)*

and thus the convolution of (108) becomes a shift in the frequency domain or

$$O(\vec{\Lambda}) * U_0(\vec{\Lambda}) = 2\pi O(\vec{\Lambda} - \vec{K}). \tag{110}$$

This convolution is illustrated in Figs. 6.4(a)–(c) for a plane wave propagating with direction vector, $\vec{K} = (0, k_0)$. Fig. 6.4(a) shows the Fourier transform of a single cylinder of radius 1λ and Fig. 6.4(b) shows the Fourier transform of the incident field. The resulting multiplication in the space domain or convolution in the frequency domain is shown in Fig. 6.4(c).

To find the Fourier transform of the Green's function the Fourier transform of (32) is calculated to find

$$(-\Lambda^2 + k_0^2) G(\vec{\Lambda} | \vec{r}\,') = -e^{-j\vec{\Lambda} \cdot \vec{r}\,'}. \tag{111}$$

Rearranging terms we see that

$$G(\vec{\Lambda}\,|\vec{r}\,') = \frac{e^{-j\vec{\Lambda}\cdot\vec{r}}}{\Lambda^2 - k_0^2} \quad (112)$$

which has a singularity for all $\vec{\Lambda}$ such that

$$|\Lambda|^2 = \alpha^2 + \gamma^2 = k_0^2. \quad (113)$$

An approximation to $G(\vec{\Lambda})$ is shown in Fig. 6.4(d).

The Fourier transform representation in (112) can be misleading because it represents a point scatterer as both a sink and a source of waves. A single plane wave propagating from left to right can be considered in two different ways depending on your point of view. From the left side of the scatterer, the point scatterer represents a sink to the wave, while to the right of the scatterer the wave is spreading from a source point. Clearly, it's not possible for a scatterer to be both a point source and a sink. Later, when our expression for the scattered field is inverted, it will be necessary to choose a solution that leads to outgoing waves only.

The effect of the convolution shown in (106) is a multiplication in the frequency domain of the shifted object function, (110), and the Green's function, (112), evaluated at $\vec{r}\,' = 0$. The scattered field is written as

$$U_s(\vec{\Lambda}) = 2\pi \frac{O(\vec{\Lambda} - \vec{K})}{\Lambda^2 - k^2}. \quad (114)$$

This result is shown in Fig. 6.4(e) for a plane wave propagating along the y-axis. Since the largest frequency domain components of the Green's function satisfy (113), the Fourier transform of the scattered field is dominated by a shifted and sampled version of the object's Fourier transform.

We will now derive an expression for the field at the receiver line. For simplicity we will continue to assume that the incident field is propagating along the positive y-axis or $\vec{K} = (0, k_0)$. The scattered field along the receiver line $(x, y = l_0)$ is simply the inverse Fourier transform of the field in (114). This is written as

$$u(x, y = l_0) = \frac{1}{4\pi^2} \int_{-\infty}^{\infty}\int_{-\infty}^{\infty} U_s(\vec{\Lambda}) e^{j\vec{\Lambda}\cdot\vec{r}}\, d\alpha\, d\gamma \quad (115)$$

which, using (114), can be expressed as

$$u_s(x, y = l_0) = \frac{1}{4\pi^2} \int_{-\infty}^{\infty}\int_{-\infty}^{\infty} \frac{O(\alpha, \gamma - k_0)}{\alpha^2 + \gamma^2 - k_0^2} e^{j(\alpha x + \gamma l_0)}\, d\alpha\, d\gamma. \quad (116)$$

We will first find the integral with respect to γ. For a given α, the integral has a singularity for

$$\gamma_{1,2} = \pm\sqrt{k_0^2 - \alpha^2}. \quad (117)$$

Using contour integration we can evaluate the integral with respect to γ along the path shown in Fig. 6.5. By adding $1/2\pi$ of the residue at each pole we find

$$u_s(x, y) = \frac{1}{2\pi} \int \Gamma_1(\alpha; y) e^{j\alpha x} \, d\alpha + \frac{1}{2\pi} \int \Gamma_2(\alpha; y) e^{j\alpha x} \, d\alpha \quad (118)$$

where

$$\Gamma_1 = \frac{jO(\alpha, \sqrt{k_0^2 - \alpha^2} - k_0)}{2\sqrt{k_0^2 - \alpha^2}} e^{j\sqrt{k_0^2 - \alpha^2} l_0} \quad (119)$$

$$\Gamma_2 = \frac{-jO(\alpha, \sqrt{k_0^2 - \alpha^2} - k_0)}{2\sqrt{k_0^2 - \alpha^2}} e^{-j\sqrt{k_0^2 - \alpha^2} l_0}. \quad (120)$$

Examining the above pair of equations we see that Γ_1 represents the solution in terms of plane waves traveling along the positive y-axis, while Γ_2 represents plane waves traveling in the $-y$ direction.

As was discussed earlier, the Fourier transform of the Green's function (112) represents the field due to both a point source and a point sink, but the two solutions are distinct for receiver lines that are outside the extent of the object. First consider the scattered field along the line $y = l_0$ where l_0 is greater than the y-coordinate of all points in the object. Since all scattered fields originate in the object, plane waves propagating along the positive y-axis represent outgoing waves while waves propagating along the negative y-axis represent waves due to a point sink. Thus for $y >$ object (i.e., the receiver line is above the object) the outgoing scattered waves are represented by Γ_1 or

$$u_s(x, y) = \frac{1}{2\pi} \int \Gamma_1(\alpha; y) e^{j\alpha x} \, d\alpha, \quad y > \text{object}. \quad (121)$$

Conversely, for a receiver along a line $y = l_0$ where l_0 is less than the y-coordinate of any point in the object, the scattered field is represented by Γ_2 or

$$u_s(x, y) = \frac{1}{2\pi} \int \Gamma_2(\alpha; y) e^{j\alpha x} \, d\alpha, \quad y < \text{object}. \quad (122)$$

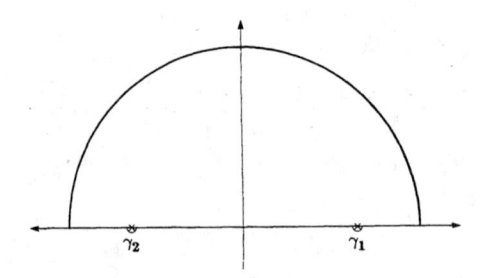

Fig. 6.5: *Integration path in the complex plane for inverting the two-dimensional Fourier transform of the scattered field. The correct pole must be chosen to lead to outgoing fields. (From [Sla84].)*

In general, the scattered field will be written as

$$u_s(x, y) = \frac{1}{2\pi} \int \Gamma(\alpha; y) e^{j\alpha x} \, d\alpha \tag{123}$$

and it will be understood that values that lead only to outgoing waves should be chosen for the square root in the expression for Γ.

Taking the Fourier transform of both sides of (123) we find that

$$\int u(x, y = l_0) e^{-j\alpha x} \, dx = \Gamma(\alpha, l_0). \tag{124}$$

But since by (119) and (120), $\Gamma(\alpha, l_0)$ is equal to a phase shifted version of the object function, the Fourier transform of the scattered field along the line $y = l_0$ is related to the Fourier transform of the object along a circular arc. The use of the contour integration is further justified by noting that only those waves that satisfy the relationship

$$\alpha^2 + \gamma^2 = k_0^2 \tag{125}$$

will be propagated and thus it is safe to ignore all waves not on the k_0-circle.

This result is diagrammed in Fig. 6.6. The circular arc represents the locus of all points (α, γ) such that $\gamma = \sqrt{k_0^2 - \alpha^2}$. The solid line shows the outgoing waves for a receiver line at $y = l_0$ above the object. This can be considered transmission tomography. Conversely, the broken line indicates the locus of solutions for the reflection tomography case, or $y = l_0$ is below the object.

6.3.3 Short Wavelength Limit of the Fourier Diffraction Theorem

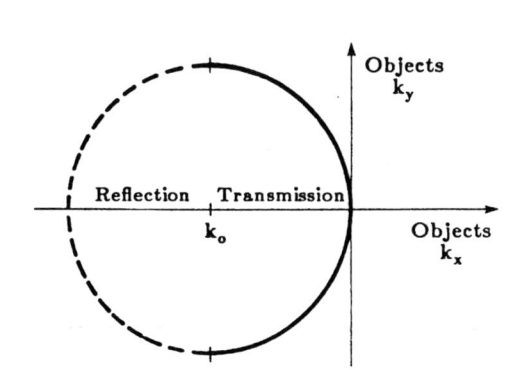

Fig. 6.6: *Estimates of the two-dimensional Fourier transform of the object are available along the solid arc for transmission tomography and the broken arc for reflection tomography. (Adapted from [Sla84].)*

While at first the derivations of the Fourier Slice Theorem and the Fourier Diffraction Theorem seem quite different, it is interesting to note that in the limit of very high energy waves or, equivalently, very short wavelengths the Fourier Diffraction Theorem approaches the Fourier Slice Theorem. Recall that the Fourier transform of a diffracted projection corresponds to samples of the two-dimensional Fourier transform of an object along a semicircular arc.

The radius of the arc shown in Fig. 6.2 is equal to k_0 which is given by

$$k_0 = \frac{2\pi}{\lambda} \qquad (126)$$

and λ is the wavelength of the energy. As the wavelength is decreased, the wavenumber, k_0, and the radius of the arc in the object's Fourier domain grow. This process is illustrated in Fig. 6.7 where we have shown the semicircular arcs resulting from diffraction experiments at seven different frequencies.

An example might make this idea clearer. An ultrasonic tomography experiment might be carried out at a frequency of 5 MHz which corresponds to a wavelength in water of 0.3 mm. This corresponds to a k_0 of 333 radians/meter. On the other hand, a hypothetical coherent x-ray source with a 100-keV beam has a wavelength of 0.012 μM. The result is that a diffraction experiment with x-rays can give samples along an arc of radius 5×10^8 radians/meter. Certainly for all physiological features (i.e., resolutions of < 1000 radians/meter) the arc could be considered to be a straight line and the Fourier Slice Theorem an excellent model for relating the transforms of the projections with the transform of the object.

6.3.4 The Data Collection Process

The best that can be hoped for in any tomographic experiment is to estimate the Fourier transform of the object for all frequencies within a disk centered at the origin. For objects whose spectra have no frequency content outside the disk, the reconstruction procedure is perfect.

There are several different procedures that can be used to estimate the object function from the scattered field. A single plane wave provides exact information (up to a frequency of $\sqrt{2}k_0$) about the Fourier transform of the object along a semicircular arc. Two of the simplest procedures involve

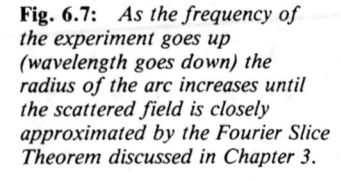

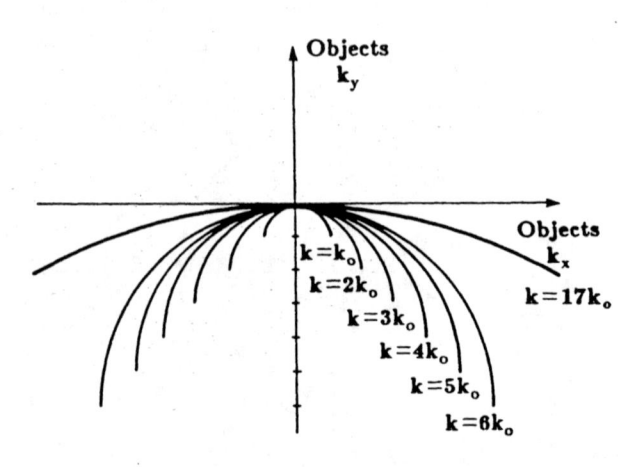

Fig. 6.7: *As the frequency of the experiment goes up (wavelength goes down) the radius of the arc increases until the scattered field is closely approximated by the Fourier Slice Theorem discussed in Chapter 3.*

changing the orientation and frequency of the incident plane waves to move the frequency domain arcs to a new position. By appropriately choosing an orientation and a frequency it is possible to estimate the Fourier transform of the object at any given frequency. In addition, it is possible to change the radius of the semicircular arc by varying the frequency of the incident field and thus generating an estimate of the entire Fourier transform of the object.

The most straightforward data collection procedure was discussed by Mueller *et al.* [Mue80] and consists of rotating the object and measuring the scattered field for different orientations. Each orientation will produce an estimate of the object's Fourier transform along a circular arc and these arcs will rotate as the object is rotated. When the object has rotated through a full 360° an estimate of the object will be available for the entire Fourier disk.

The coverage for this method is shown in Fig. 6.8 for a simple experiment with eight projections of nine samples each. Notice that there are two arcs that pass through each point of Fourier space. Generally, it will be necessary to choose one estimate as better.

On the other hand, if the reflected data are collected by measuring the field on the same side of the object as the source, then estimates of the object are available for frequencies greater than $\sqrt{2}k_0$. This follows from Fig. 6.6.

Nahamoo and Kak [Nah82], [Nah84] and Devaney [Dev84] have proposed a method that requires only two rotational views of an object. Consider an arbitrary source of waves in the transmitter plane as shown in Fig. 6.9. The

Fig. 6.8: *With plane wave illumination, estimates of the object's two-dimensional Fourier transform are available along the circular arcs.*

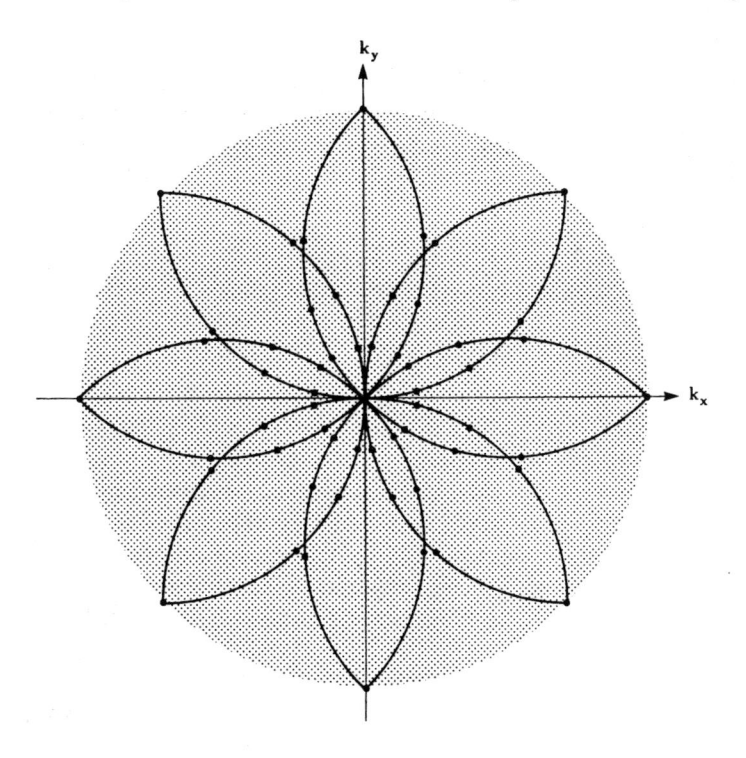

TOMOGRAPHIC IMAGING WITH DIFFRACTING SOURCES

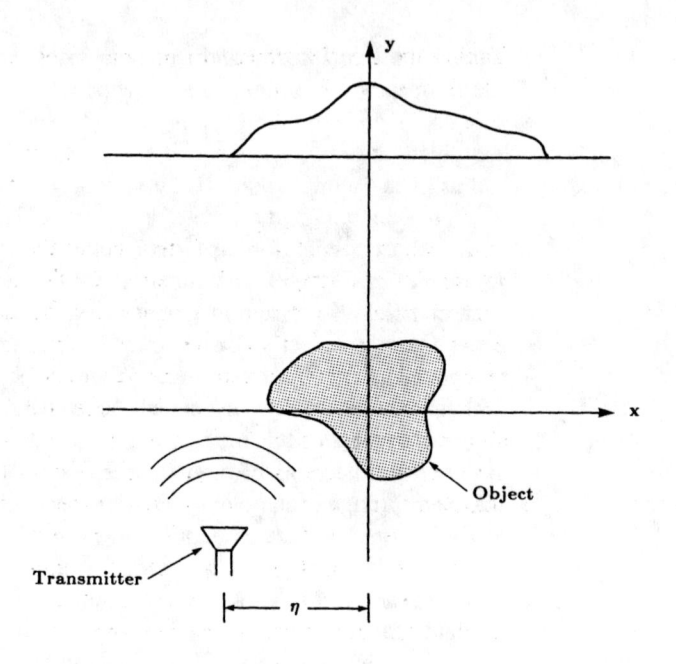

Fig. 6.9: *A typical synthetic aperture tomography experiment is shown. A transmitter is scanned past the object. For each transmitter position the scattered field is measured. Later, appropriate phases are added to the projections to synthesize any incident plane wave. (From [Sla83].)*

transmitted field, u_t, can be represented as a weighted set of plane waves by taking the Fourier transform of the transmitter aperture function [Goo68]. Doing this we find

$$u_t(x) = \frac{1}{4\pi^2} \int_{-\infty}^{\infty} A_t(k_x) e^{jk_x x} \, dk_x. \tag{127}$$

Moving the source to a new position, η, the plane wave decomposition of the transmitted field becomes

$$u_t(x; \eta) = \frac{1}{4\pi^2} \int_{-\infty}^{\infty} (A_t(k_x) e^{jk_x \eta}) e^{jk_x x} \, dk_x. \tag{128}$$

Given the plane wave decomposition, the incident field in the plane follows simply as

$$u_i(\eta; x, y) = \int_{-\infty}^{\infty} \left(\frac{1}{4\pi^2} A_t(k_x) e^{jk_x \eta} \right) e^{j(k_x x + k_y y)} \, dk_x. \tag{129}$$

In (124) we presented an equation for the scattered field from a single plane wave. Because of the linearity of the Fourier transform the effect of each plane wave, $e^{j(k_x x + k_y y)}$, can be weighted by the expression in brackets above and superimposed to find the Fourier transform of the total scattered field due to the incident field $u_t(x; \eta)$ as [Nah82]

$$U_s(\eta; \alpha) = \int_{-\infty}^{\infty} (A_t(k_x) e^{jk_x \eta}) \frac{O(\alpha - k_x, \gamma - k_y)}{j2\gamma} \, dk_x. \tag{130}$$

Taking the Fourier transform of both sides with respect to the transmitter position, η, we find that

$$U_s(k_x; \alpha) = A_t(k_x) \frac{O(\alpha - k_x, \gamma - k_y)}{j2\gamma}. \tag{131}$$

By collecting the scattered field along the receiver line as a function of transmitter position, η, we have an expression for the scattered field. Like the simpler case with plane wave incidence, the scattered field is related to the Fourier transform of the object along an arc. Unlike the previous case, though, the coverage due to a single view of the object is a pair of circular disks as shown in Fig. 6.10. Here a single view consists of transmitting from all positions in a line and measuring the scattered field at all positions along the receiver line. By rotating the object by 90° it is possible to generate the complementary disk and to fill the Fourier domain.

The coverage shown in Fig. 6.10 is constructed by calculating $(\vec{K} - \vec{\Lambda})$ for all vectors $(\vec{K})$ and $(\vec{\Lambda})$ that satisfy the experimental constraints. Not only must each vector satisfy the wave equation but it is also necessary that only forward traveling plane waves be used. The broken line in Fig. 6.10 shows the valid propagation vectors $(-\vec{\Lambda})$ for the transmitted waves. To each possible vector $(-\vec{\Lambda})$ a semicircular set of vectors representing each possible received wave can be added. The locus of received plane waves is shown as a solid semicircle centered at each of the transmitted waves indicated by an ×.

Fig. 6.10: *Estimates of the Fourier transform of an object in the synthetic aperture experiment are available in the shaded region.*

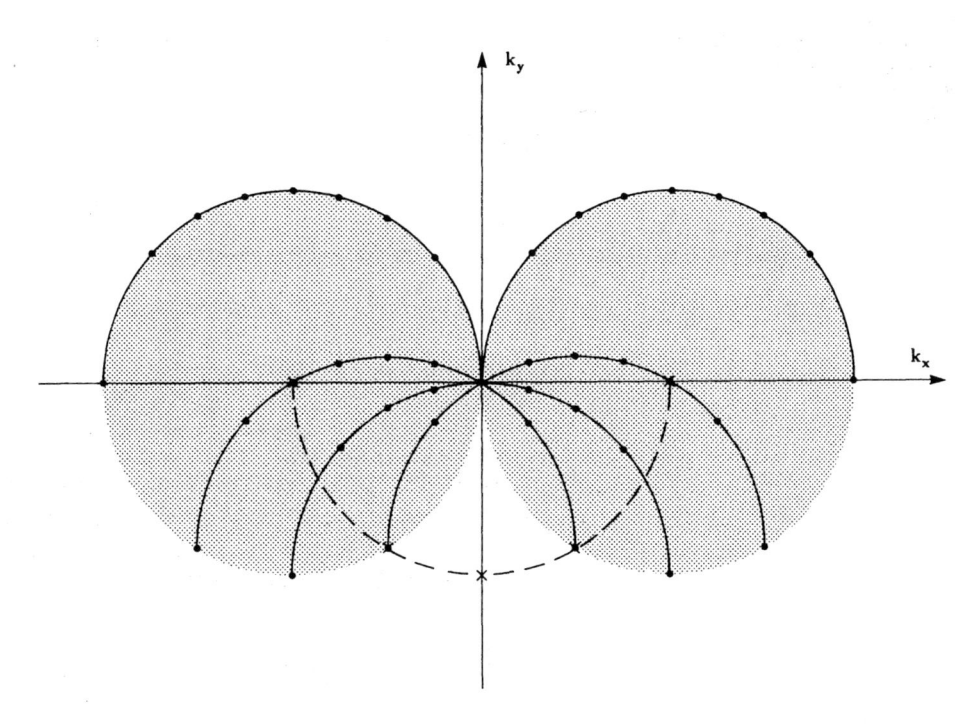

The entire coverage for the synthetic aperture approach is shown as the shaded areas.

In geophysical imaging it is not possible to generate or receive waves from all positions around the object. If it is possible to drill a borehole, then it is possible to perform vertical seismic profiling (VSP) [Dev83] and obtain information about most of the object. A typical experiment is shown in Fig. 6.11. So as to not damage the borehole, acoustic waves are generated at the surface using acoustic detonators or other methods and the scattered field is measured in the borehole.

The coverage in the frequency domain is similar to the synthetic aperture approach in [Nah84]. Plane waves at an arbitrary downward direction are synthesized by appropriately phasing the transmitting transducers. The receivers will receive any waves traveling to the right. The resulting coverage for this method is shown in Fig. 6.12(a). If we further assume that the object function is real valued, we can use the symmetry of the Fourier transform for real-valued functions to obtain the coverage in Fig. 6.12(b).

It is also possible to perform such experiments with broadband illumination [Ken82]. So far we have only considered narrow band illumination wherein the field at each point can be completely described by its complex amplitude.

Now consider a transducer that illuminates an object with a plane wave of the form $A_t(t)$. It can still be called a plane wave because the amplitude of the

Fig. 6.11: *A typical vertical seismic profiling (VSP) experiment.*

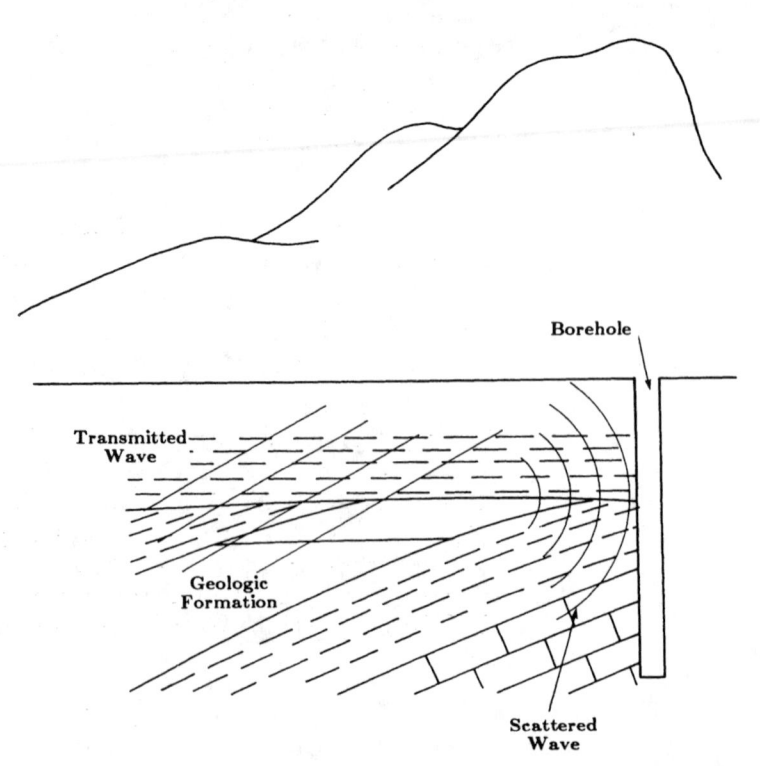

232   COMPUTERIZED TOMOGRAPHIC IMAGING

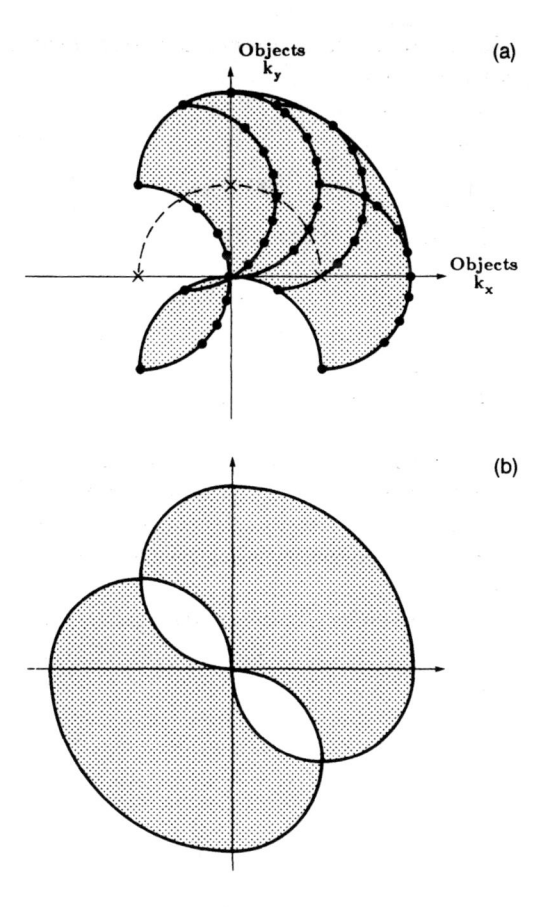

Fig. 6.12: *Available estimate of the Fourier transform of an object for a VSP experiment (a). If the object function is real valued, then the symmetry of the Fourier transform can be used to estimate the object in the region shown in (b).*

field along planes perpendicular to the direction of travel is constant. Taking the Fourier transform in the time domain we can decompose this field into a number of experiments, each at a different temporal frequency, ω. We let

$$A_t(x, y, \omega) = \int_{-\infty}^{\infty} A_t(x, y, t) e^{+j\omega t} \, dt \qquad (132)$$

where the sign on the exponential is positive because of the convention defined in Section 6.1.1.

Given the amplitude of the field at each temporal frequency, it is straightforward to decompose the field into plane wave components by finding its Fourier transform along the transmitter plane. Each plane wave component is then described as a function of spatial frequency, $k_\omega = \sqrt{k_x^2 + k_y^2}$, and temporal frequency, ω. The temporal frequency ω is related to k_ω by

$$k_\omega = \frac{c}{\omega} \qquad (133)$$

TOMOGRAPHIC IMAGING WITH DIFFRACTING SOURCES

where c is the speed of propagation in the media and the wave vector (k_x, k_y) satisfies the wave equation

$$k_x^2 + k_y^2 = k_\omega^2. \tag{134}$$

If a unit amplitude plane wave illumination of spatial frequency k_x and a temporal frequency ω leads to a scattered plane wave with amplitude $u_s(k_x, \omega)$, then the total scattered field is given by a weighted superposition of the scattered fields or

$$u_s(x, y; t) = \frac{1}{2\pi} \int_{-\infty}^{\infty} d\omega \int_{-k_\omega}^{k_\omega} dk_x A_t(k_x, \omega) e^{-j\omega t} u_s(k_x, \omega; y) e^{j(k_x x + k_y y)}. \tag{135}$$

For plane wave incidence the coverage for this method is shown in Fig. 6.13(a). Fig. 6.13(b) shows that by doing four experiments at 0, 90, 180, and 270° it is possible to gather information about the entire object.

6.4 Interpolation and a Filtered Backpropagation Algorithm for Diffracting Sources

In our proof of the Fourier Diffraction Theorem, we showed that when an object is illuminated with a plane wave traveling in the positive y direction, the Fourier transform of the forward scattered fields gives values of the arc shown in Fig. 6.2. Therefore, if an object is illuminated from many different directions, we can, in principle, fill up a disk of diameter $\sqrt{2}k$ in the frequency domain with samples of $O(\omega_1, \omega_2)$, which is the Fourier transform of the object, and then reconstruct the object by direct Fourier inversion. Therefore, we can say that diffraction tomography determines the object up to a maximum angular spatial frequency of $\sqrt{2}k$. To this extent, the reconstructed object is a low pass version of the original. In practice, the loss of resolution caused by this bandlimiting is negligible, being more influenced by considerations such as the aperture sizes of the transmitting and receiving elements, etc.

The fact that the frequency domain samples are available over circular arcs, whereas for convenient display it is desirable to have samples over a rectangular lattice, is a source of computational difficulty in reconstruction algorithms for diffracting tomography. To help the reader visualize the distribution of the available frequency domain information, we have shown in Fig. 6.8 the sampling points on a circular arc grid, each arc in this grid corresponding to the transform of one projection. It should also be clear from this figure that by illuminating the object over 360° a *double* coverage of the frequency domain is generated; note, however, that this double coverage is uniform. We may get a complete coverage of the frequency domain with illumination restricted to a portion of 360°; however, in that case there would

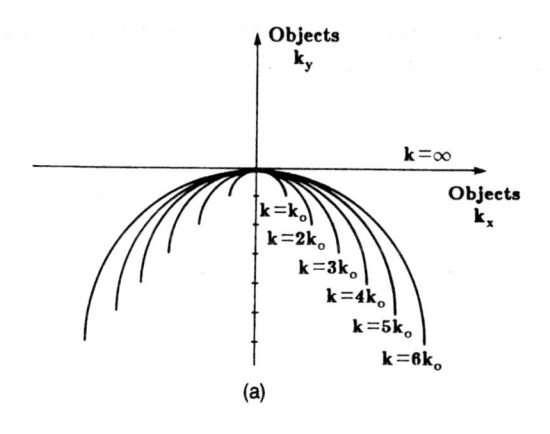

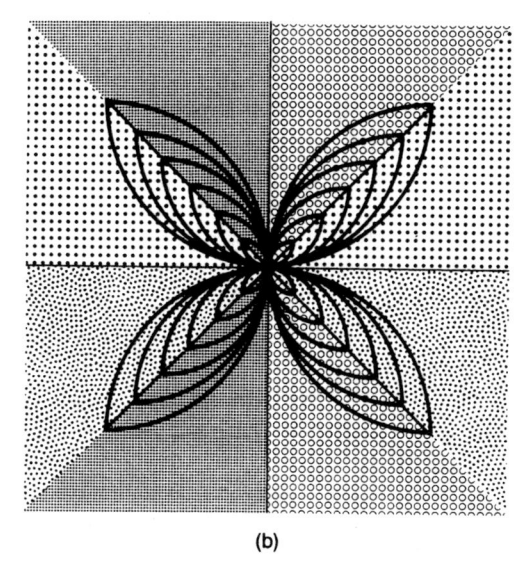

Fig. 6.13: *(a) Estimates of the Fourier transform of an object for broadband illumination. With four views the coverage shown in (b) is possible.*

be patches in the (ω_1, ω_2)-plane where we would have a double coverage. In reconstructing from circular arc grids to rectangular grids, it is often easier to contend with a uniform double coverage, as opposed to a coverage that is single in most areas and double in patches.

However, for some applications that do not lend themselves to data collection from all possible directions, it is useful to bear in mind that it is not necessary to go completely around an object to get complete coverage of the frequency domain. In principle, it should be possible to get an equal quality reconstruction when illumination angles are restricted to a 180° plus an interval, the angles in excess of 180° being required to complete the coverage of the frequency domain.

There are two computational strategies for reconstructing the object from the measurements of the scattered field. As pointed out in [Sou84a], the two algorithms can be considered as interpolation in the frequency domain and interpolation in the space domain; and are analogous to the direct Fourier inversion and backprojection algorithms of conventional tomography. Unlike conventional tomography, where backprojection is the preferred approach, the computational expense of space domain interpolation of diffracted projections makes frequency domain interpolation the preferred approach for diffraction tomography reconstructions.

The remainder of this section will consist of derivations of the frequency domain and space domain interpolation algorithms. In both cases we will assume plane wave illumination; the reader is referred to [Dev82], [Pan83] for reconstruction algorithms for the synthetic aperture approach and to [Sou84b] for the general case.

6.4.1 Frequency Domain Interpolation

There are two schemes for frequency domain interpolation. The more conventional approach is polynomial based and assumes that the data near each grid point can be approximated by polynomials. This is the classical numerical analysis approach to the problem. A second approach is known as the unified frequency domain reconstruction (UFR) and interpolates data in the frequency domain by assuming that the space domain reconstruction should be spatially limited. We will first describe polynomial interpolation.

In order to discuss the frequency domain interpolation between a circular arc grid on which the data are generated by diffraction tomography and a rectangular grid suitable for image reconstruction, we must first select parameters for representing each grid and then write down the relationship between the two sets of parameters.

In (104), $U_B(\omega, l_0)$ was used to denote the Fourier transform of the transmitted data when an object is illuminated with a plane wave traveling along the positive y direction. We now use $U_{B,\phi}(\omega)$ to denote this Fourier transform, where the subscript ϕ indicates the angle of illumination. This angle is measured as shown in Fig. 6.14. Similarly, $Q(\omega, \phi)$ will be used to indicate the values of $O(\omega_1, \omega_2)$ along a semicircular arc oriented at an angle ϕ as shown in Fig. 6.15 or

$$Q(\omega, \sqrt{k_0^2-\omega^2}-k_0), \qquad |\omega|<k_0. \qquad (136)$$

Therefore, when an illuminating plane wave is incident at angle ϕ, the equality in (104) can be rewritten as

$$U_{B,\phi}(\omega)=\frac{j}{2}\frac{1}{\sqrt{k^2-\omega^2}} \exp[j\ell\sqrt{k^2-\omega^2}]Q(\omega, \phi) \qquad \text{for } |\omega|<k. \quad (137)$$

In most cases the transmitted data will be uniformly sampled in space, and a *discrete* Fourier transform of these data will generate uniformly spaced

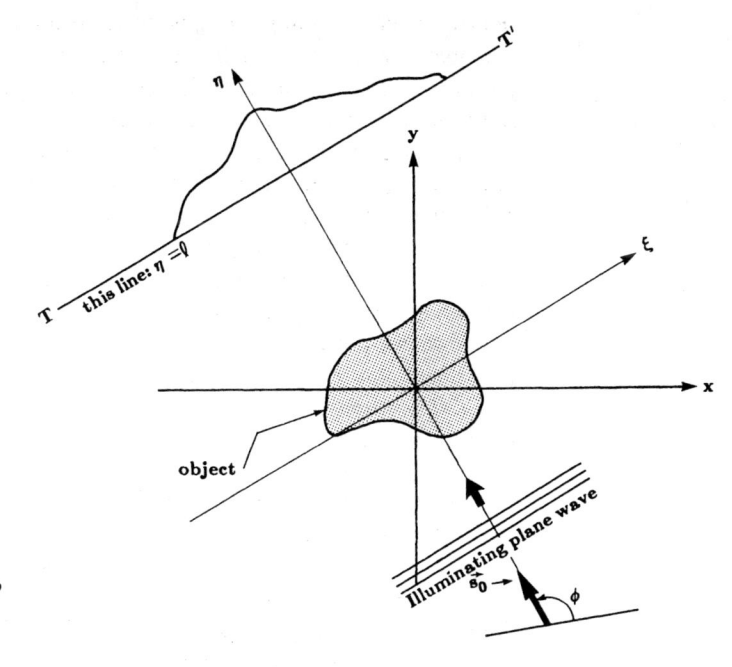

Fig. 6.14: The angle ϕ is used to identify each diffraction projection. (From [Pan83].)

Fig. 6.15: Each projection is measured using the $\phi - \omega$ coordinate system shown here. (From [Kak85].)

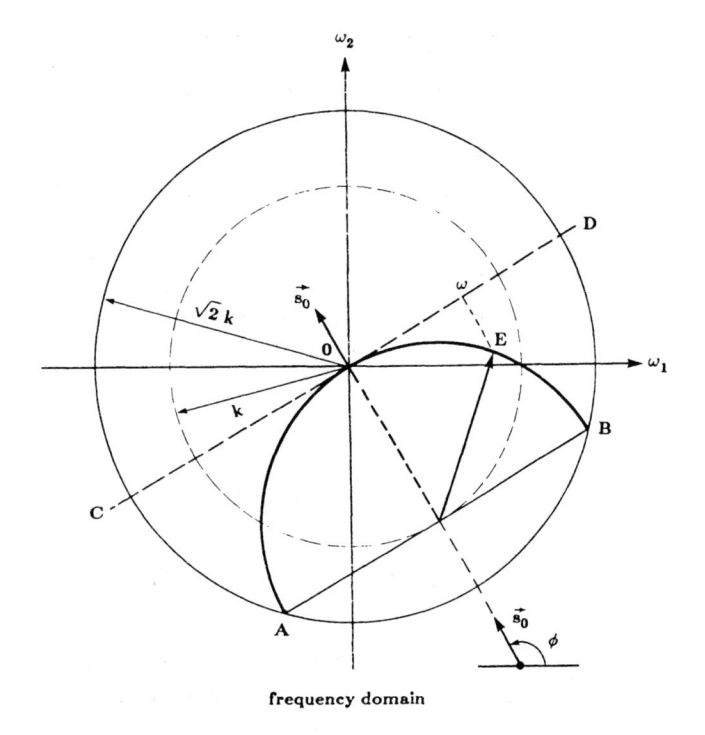

TOMOGRAPHIC IMAGING WITH DIFFRACTING SOURCES 237

samples of $U_{B,\phi}(\omega)$ in the ω domain. Since $Q(\omega)$ is the Fourier transform of the object along the circular arc AOB in Fig. 6.15 and since κ is the projection of a point on the circular arc on the tangent line CD, the uniform samples of Q in κ translate into nonuniform samples along the arc AOB as shown in Fig. 6.16. We will therefore designate each point on the arc AOB by its (ω, ϕ) parameters. [Note that (ω, ϕ) are *not* the polar coordinates of a point on arc AOB in Fig. 6.15. Therefore, ω is *not* the radial distance in the (ω_1, ω_2)-plane. For point E shown, the parameter ω is obtained by projecting E onto line CD.] We continue to denote the rectangular coordinates in the frequency domain by (ω_1, ω_2).

Before we present relationships between (ω, ϕ) and (ω_1, ω_2), it must be mentioned that we must consider separately the points generated by the AO and OB portions of the arc AOB as ϕ is varied from 0 to 2π. We do this because, as mentioned before, the arc AOB generates a double coverage of the frequency domain, as ϕ is varied from 0 to 2π, which is undesirable for discussing a one-to-one transformation between the (ω, ϕ) parameters and the (ω_1, ω_2) coordinates.

We now reserve (ω, ϕ) parameters to denote the arc grid generated by the portion OB as shown in Fig. 6.15. It is important to note that for this arc grid, ω varies from 0 to k and ϕ from 0 to 2π.

We now present the transformation equations between (ω, ϕ) and (ω_1, ω_2). We accomplish this in a slightly roundabout manner by first defining polar

Fig. 6.16: *Uniformly sampling the projection in the space domain leads to uneven spacing of the samples of the Fourier transform of the object along the semicircular arc. (Adapted from [Pan83].)*

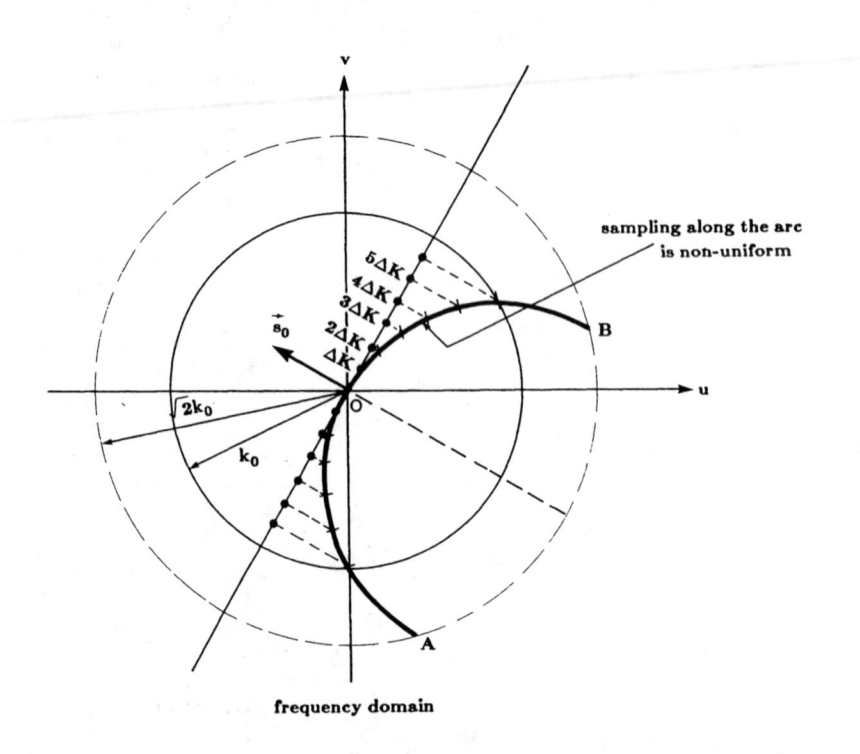

coordinates (Ω, θ) in the (ω_1, ω_2)-plane as shown in Fig. 6.17. In order to go from (ω_1, ω_2) to (ω, ϕ), we will first transform from the former coordinates to (Ω, θ) and then from (Ω, θ) to (ω, ϕ). The rectangular coordinates (ω_1, ω_2) are related to the polar coordinates (Ω, θ) by (Fig. 6.17)

$$\Omega = \sqrt{\omega_1^2 + \omega_2^2} \tag{138}$$

$$\theta = \tan^{-1}\left(\frac{\omega_2}{\omega_1}\right). \tag{139}$$

In order to relate (Ω, θ) to (ω, ϕ), we now introduce a new angle β, which is the angular position of a point (ω_1, ω_2) on arc OB in Fig. 6.17. Note from the figure that the point characterized by angle β is also characterized by parameter ω. The relationship between ω and β is given by

$$\omega = k \sin \beta. \tag{140}$$

The following relationship exists between the polar coordinates (Ω, θ) on the one hand and the parameters β and ϕ on the other:

$$\beta = 2 \sin^{-1} \frac{\Omega}{2k} \tag{141}$$

$$\phi = \theta + \frac{\pi}{2} + \frac{\beta}{2}. \tag{142}$$

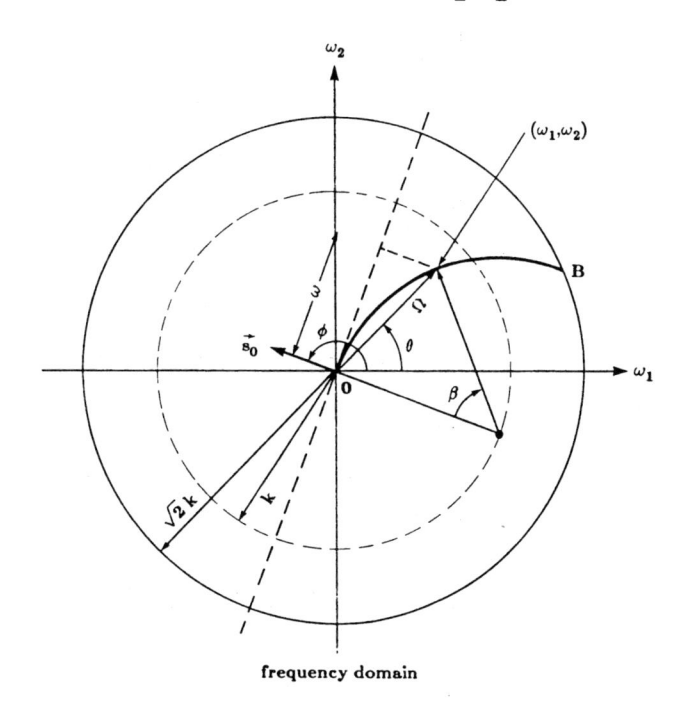

Fig. 6.17: *A second change of variables is used to relate the projection data to the object's Fourier transform. (From [Kak85] as modified from [Pan83].)*

By substituting (141) in (140) and then using (138), we can express ω in terms of ω_1 and ω_2. The result is shown below.

$$\omega = k \sin\left\{ 2 \sin^{-1}\left(\frac{\sqrt{\omega_1^2 + \omega_2^2}}{2k}\right)\right\}. \tag{143}$$

Similarly, by substituting (139) and (141) in (142), we obtain

$$\phi = \tan^{-1}\left(\frac{\omega_2}{\omega_1}\right) + \sin^{-1}\left(\frac{\sqrt{\omega_1^2 + \omega_2^2}}{2k}\right) + \frac{\pi}{2}. \tag{144}$$

These are our transformation equations for interpolating from the (ω, ϕ) parameters used for data representation to the (ω_1, ω_2) parameters needed for inverse transformation. To convert a particular rectangular point into (ω, ϕ) domain, we substitute its ω_1 and ω_2 values in (143) and (144). The resulting values for ω and ϕ may not correspond to any for which $Q(\omega, \phi)$ is known. By virtue of (137), $Q(\omega, \phi)$ will only be known over a uniformly sampled set of values for ω and ϕ. In order to determine Q at the calculated ω and ϕ, we use the following procedure. Given $N_\omega \times N_\phi$ uniformly located samples, $Q(\omega_i, \phi_j)$, we calculate a bilinearly interpolated value of this function at the desired ω and ϕ by using

$$Q(\omega, \phi) = \sum_{i=1}^{N_\omega} \sum_{j=1}^{N_\phi} Q(\omega_i, \phi_j) h_1(\omega - \omega_i) h_2(\phi - \phi_j), \tag{145}$$

where

$$h_1(\omega) = \begin{cases} 1 - \dfrac{|\omega|}{\Delta\omega} & |\omega| \leq \Delta\omega \\ 0 & \text{otherwise} \end{cases} \tag{146}$$

$$h_2(\phi) = \begin{cases} 1 - \dfrac{|\phi|}{\Delta\phi} & |\phi| \leq \Delta\phi \\ 0 & \text{otherwise}; \end{cases} \tag{147}$$

$\Delta\phi$ and $\Delta\omega$ are the sampling intervals for ϕ and ω, respectively. When expressed in the manner shown above, bilinear interpolation may be interpreted as the output of a filter whose impulse response is $h_1 h_2$.

The results obtained with bilinear interpolation can be considerably improved if we first increase the sampling density in the (ω, ϕ)-plane by using the computationally efficient method of zero-extending the two-dimensional inverse *fast Fourier transform* (FFT) of the $Q(\omega_i, \phi_j)$ matrix. The technique consists of first taking a two-dimensional inverse FFT of the $N_\omega \times N_\phi$ matrix consisting of the $Q(\omega_i, \phi_j)$ values, zero-extending the resulting $N_\omega \times N_\phi$

array of numbers to, let's say, $mN_\omega \times nM_\phi$, and then taking the FFT of this new array. The result is an mn-fold increase in the density of samples in the (ω, ϕ)-plane. After computing $Q(\omega, \phi)$ at each point of a rectangular grid by the procedure outlined above, the object $f(x, y)$ is obtained by a simple 2-D inverse FFT.

A different approach to frequency domain interpolation, called the unified frequency domain (UFR) interpolation, was proposed by Kaveh et al. [Kav84]. In this approach an interpolating function is derived by taking into account the object's spatial support. Consider an object's Fourier transform as might be measured in a diffraction tomography experiment. If the Fourier domain data are denoted by $F(u, v)$, then a reconstruction can be written

$$f(x, y) = i(x, y) \text{ IFT } \{F(u, v)\} \tag{148}$$

where the indicator function is given by

$$i(x, y) = \begin{cases} 1 & \text{where the object is known to have support} \\ 0 & \text{elsewhere.} \end{cases} \tag{149}$$

If the Fourier transform of $i(x, y)$ is $I(u, v)$, then the spatially limited reconstruction can be rewritten

$$f(x, y) = \text{IFT } \{I(u, v) * F(u, v)\} \tag{150}$$

by noting that multiplication in the space domain is equivalent to convolution in the frequency domain. To perform the inverse Fourier transform fast it is necessary to have the Fourier domain data on a rectangular grid. First consider the frequency domain convolution; once the data are available on a rectangular grid the inverse Fourier transform can easily be calculated as it is for polynomial interpolation.

The frequency domain data for the UFR reconstruction can be written as

$$F(u, v) = \iint I(u - u', v - v') F(u', v') \, du' \, dv'. \tag{151}$$

Now recall that the experimental data, $F(u', v')$, are only available on the circular arcs in the $\phi - \omega$ space shown in Fig. 6.15. By using the change of variables

$$\begin{bmatrix} u' \\ v' \end{bmatrix} = \begin{bmatrix} T_1(\phi, \omega) \\ T_2(\phi, \omega) \end{bmatrix} = \begin{bmatrix} \cos \phi & -\sin \phi \\ \sin \phi & \cos \phi \end{bmatrix} \begin{bmatrix} \sqrt{k_0^2 - \omega^2} - k_0 \\ \omega \end{bmatrix} \tag{152}$$

and the Jacobian of the transformation given by

$$J(\phi, \omega) = \left| \frac{\partial(u', v')}{\partial(\phi, \omega)} \right| \tag{153}$$

the convolution can be rewritten

$$F(u, v) = \iint J(\phi, \omega) I(u - T_1(\phi, \omega),$$
$$v - T_2(\phi, \omega)) F(T_1(\phi, \omega), T_2(\phi, \omega))\, d\phi\, d\omega. \quad (154)$$

This convolution integral gives us a means to get the frequency domain data on a rectangular grid and forms the heart of the UFR interpolation algorithm.

This integral can be easily discretized by replacing each integral with a summation over the projection angle, ϕ, and the spatial frequency of the received field, ω. The frequency domain data can now be written as

$$F(u, v) = \Delta_\phi \Delta_\omega \Sigma\Sigma J(\phi, \omega)$$
$$I(u - T_1(\phi, \omega), v - T_2(\phi, \omega))$$
$$F(T_1(\phi, \omega), T_2(\phi, \omega)) \quad (155)$$

where Δ_ϕ and Δ_ω represent the sampling intervals in the $\phi - \omega$ space.

If the indicator function, $i(x, y)$, is taken to be 1 only within a circle of radius R, then its Fourier transform is written

$$I(u, v) = \frac{J_1(R\sqrt{u^2+v^2})}{R\sqrt{u^2+v^2}}. \quad (156)$$

A further simplification of this algorithm can be realized by noting that only the main lobe of the Bessel function will contribute much to the summation in (155). Thus a practical implementation can ignore all but the main lobe. This drastically reduces the computational complexity of the algorithm and leads to a reconstruction scheme that is only slightly more complicated than bilinear interpolation.

6.4.2 Backpropagation Algorithms

It has recently been shown by Devaney [Dev82] and Kaveh et al. [Kav82] that there is an alternative method for reconstructing images from the diffracted projection data. This procedure, called the *filtered backpropagation method,* is similar in spirit to the filtered backprojection technique of x-ray tomography. Unfortunately, whereas the filtered backprojection algorithms possess efficient implementations, the same can't be said for the filtered backpropagation algorithms. The latter class of algorithms is computationally intensive, much more so than the interpolation procedure discussed above. With regard to accuracy, they don't seem to possess any particular advantage especially if the interpolation is carried out after increasing the sampling density by the use of appropriate zero-padding as discussed above.

We will follow the derivation of the backpropagation algorithm as first presented by Devaney [Dev82]. First consider the inverse Fourier transform of the object function,

$$o(\vec{r}) = \frac{1}{(2\pi)^2} \int_{-\infty}^{\infty} \int_{-\infty}^{\infty} O(\vec{K}) e^{j\vec{K}\cdot\vec{r}} d\vec{K}. \quad (157)$$

This integral most commonly represents the object function in terms of its Fourier transform in a rectangular coordinate system representing the frequency domain. As we have already discussed, a diffraction tomography experiment measures the Fourier transform of the object along circular arcs; thus it will be easier to perform the integration if we modify it slightly to use the projection data more naturally. We will use two coordinate transformations to do this: the first one will exchange the rectangular grid for a set of semicircular arcs and the second will map the arcs into their plane wave decomposition.

We first exchange the rectangular grid for semicircular arcs. To do this we represent $\vec{K} = (k_x, k_y)$ in (157) by the vector sum

$$\vec{K} = k_0(\vec{s} - \vec{s}_0) \quad (158)$$

where $\vec{s}_0 = (\cos \phi_0, \sin \phi_0)$ and $\vec{s} = (\cos \chi, \sin \chi)$ are unit vectors representing the direction of the wave vector for the transmitted and the received plane waves, respectively. This coordinate transformation is illustrated in Fig. 6.18.

Fig. 6.18: *The $k_0\vec{r}_0$ and $k_0\vec{s}$ used in the backpropagation algorithm are shown here. (From [Pan83].)*

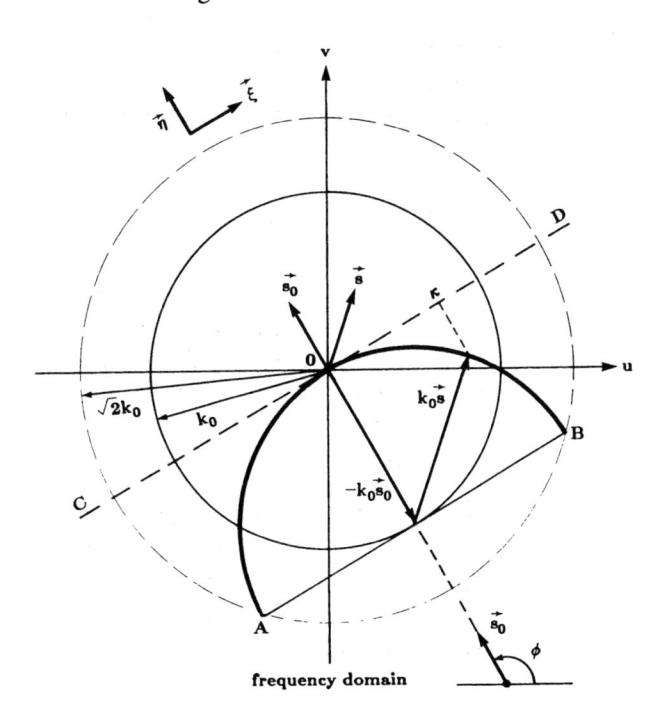

To find the Jacobian of this transformation write

$$k_x = k_0 (\cos \chi - \cos \phi_0) \tag{159}$$

$$k_y = k_0 (\sin \chi - \sin \phi_0) \tag{160}$$

and

$$dk_x dk_y = |k_0^2 \sin (\chi - \phi_0)| \, d\chi \, d\phi_0 \tag{161}$$

$$= k_0 \sqrt{1 - \cos^2 (\chi - \phi_0)} \, d\chi \, d\phi_0 \tag{162}$$

$$= k_0 \sqrt{1 - (\vec{s} \cdot \vec{s}_0)^2} \, d\chi \, d\phi_0 \tag{163}$$

and then (157) becomes

$$o(\vec{r}) = \frac{1}{(2\pi)^2} \left(\frac{1}{2}\right) k_0^2$$

$$\cdot \int_0^{2\pi} \int_0^{2\pi} \sqrt{1 - (\vec{s} \cdot \vec{s}_0)^2} \, O[k_o(\vec{s} - \vec{s}_0)] \, e^{jk_0(\vec{s} - \vec{s}_0) \cdot \vec{r}} \, d\chi \, d\phi_0. \tag{164}$$

The factor of 1/2 is necessary because as discussed in Section 6.4.1 the (χ, ϕ_0) coordinate system gives a double coverage of the (k_x, k_y) space.

This integral gives an expression for the scattered field as a function of the (χ, ϕ_0) coordinate system. The data that are collected will actually be a function of ϕ_0, the projection angle, and κ, the one-dimensional frequency of the scattered field along the receiver line. To make the final coordinate transformation we take the angle χ to be relative to the (κ, γ) coordinate system. This is a more natural representation since the data available in a diffraction tomography experiment lie on a semicircle and therefore the data are available only for $0 \leq \chi \leq \pi$. We can rewrite the χ integral in (164) by noting

$$\cos \chi = \kappa/k_0 \tag{165}$$

$$\sin \chi = \gamma/k_0 \tag{166}$$

and therefore

$$d\chi = \frac{-1}{k_0 \gamma} \, d\kappa. \tag{167}$$

The χ integral becomes

$$\frac{1}{k_0} \int_{-k_0}^{k_0} \frac{d\kappa}{\gamma} |\kappa| O[k_0(\vec{s} - \vec{s}_0)] e^{jk(\vec{s} - \vec{s}_0) \cdot \vec{r}} \, d\kappa. \tag{168}$$

Using the Fourier Diffraction Theorem as represented by (104) we can approximate the Fourier transform of the object function, O, by a simple function of the first-order Born field, u_B, at the receiver line. Thus the object function in (168) can be written

$$O[k_0(\vec{s}-\vec{s}_0)] = -2\gamma j U_B(\kappa, \gamma - k_0)e^{-j\gamma l_0}. \tag{169}$$

In addition, if a rotated coordinate system is used for $\vec{r} = (\xi, \eta)$ where

$$\xi = x \sin \phi - y \cos \phi \tag{170}$$

and

$$\eta = x \cos \phi + \sin \phi, \tag{171}$$

then the dot product $k_0(\vec{s} - \vec{s}_0)$ can be written

$$\kappa\xi + (\gamma - k_0)\eta. \tag{172}$$

Fig. 6.19: *In backpropagation the projection is backprojected with a depth-dependent filter function. At each depth, η, the filter corresponds to propagating the field a distance of $\Delta\eta$. (From [Sla83].)*

The coordinates (ξ, η) are illustrated in Fig. 6.19. Using the results above we can now write the χ integral of (164) as

$$\frac{2j}{k_0} \int_{-k_0}^{k_0} d\kappa |\kappa| U_B(\kappa, \gamma - k_0) e^{-j\gamma l_0} e^{\kappa\xi + (\gamma - k_0)\eta} \tag{173}$$

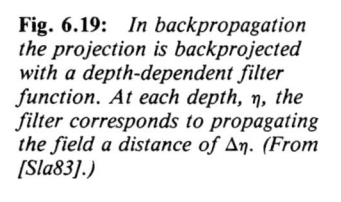

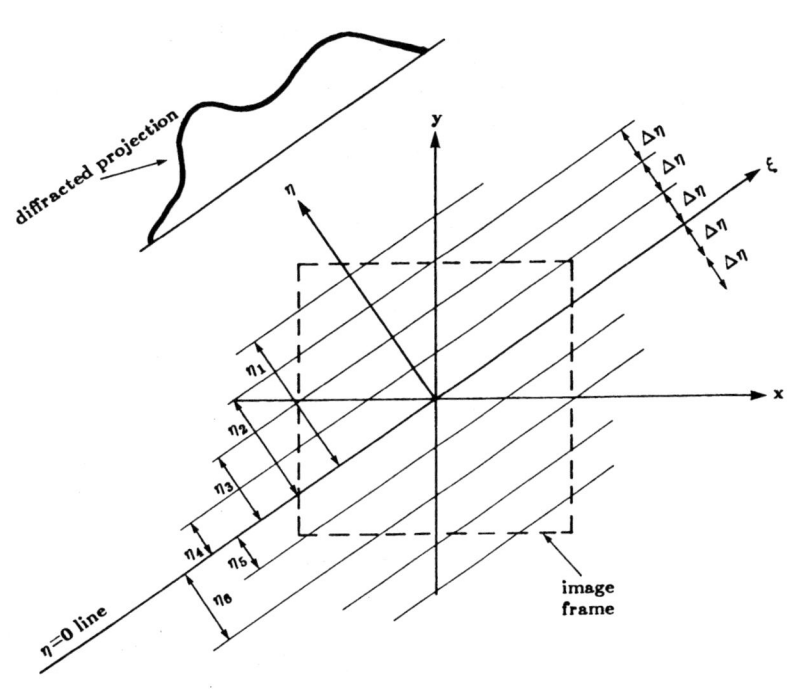

TOMOGRAPHIC IMAGING WITH DIFFRACTING SOURCES

and the equation for the object function in (164) becomes

$$o(\vec{r}) = \frac{jk_0}{(2\pi)^2} \int_0^{2\pi} d\phi_0 \int_{-k_0}^{k_0} d\kappa |\kappa| U_B(\kappa, \gamma - k_0) e^{-j\gamma l_0} e^{j\kappa\xi + j(\gamma - k_0)\eta}. \quad (174)$$

To bring out the filtered backpropagation implementation, we write here separately the inner integration:

$$\Pi_\phi(\xi, \eta) = \frac{1}{2\pi} \int_{-\infty}^{\infty} \Gamma_\phi(\omega) H(\omega) G_\eta(\omega) \exp(j\omega\xi) \, d\omega \quad (175)$$

where

$$H(\omega) = |\omega|, \qquad |\omega| \leq k_0, \quad (176)$$

$$= 0, \qquad |\omega| > k_0 \quad (177)$$

$$G_\eta(\omega) = \exp[j(\sqrt{k_0^2 - \omega^2} - k_0)\eta], \qquad |\omega| \leq k_0, \quad (178)$$

$$= 0, \qquad |\omega| > k \quad (179)$$

and

$$\Gamma_\phi(\omega) = U_B(\kappa, \gamma - k_0) e^{-j\gamma l_0}. \quad (180)$$

Without the extra filter function $G_\eta(\omega)$, the rest of (175) would correspond to the filtering operation of the projection data in x-ray tomography. The filtering as called for by the transfer function $G_\eta(\omega)$ is depth dependent due to the parameter η, which is equal to $x \cos \phi + y \sin \phi$.

In terms of the filtered projections $\Pi_\phi(\xi, \eta)$ in (175), the reconstruction integral of (174) may be expressed as

$$f(x, y) = \frac{1}{2\pi} \int_0^{2\pi} d\phi \, \Pi_\phi(x \sin \phi - y \cos \phi, x \cos \phi + y \sin \phi). \quad (181)$$

The computational procedure for reconstructing an image on the basis of (175) and (181) may be presented in the form of the following steps:

Step 1: In accordance with (175), filter each projection with a separate filter for each depth in the image frame. For example, if we chose only nine depths as shown in Fig. 6.19, we would need to apply nine different filters to the diffracted projection shown there. (In most cases for a 128 × 128 reconstruction grid, the number of discrete depths chosen for filtering the projection will also be around 128. If there are much less than 128, spatial resolution will suffer.)

Step 2: To each pixel (x, y) in the image frame, in accordance with (181), allocate a value of the filtered projection that corresponds to the nearest depth line. Since it is unlikely that a discrete implementation of (175) will lead to data at the precise location of each pixel, some form of polynomial interpolation (i.e., bilinear) will lead to better reconstructions.

Step 3: Repeat the preceding two steps for all projections. As a new projection is taken up, add its contribution to the current sum at pixel (x, y).

The depth-dependent filtering in Step 1 makes this algorithm computationally very demanding. For example, if we choose N_η depth values, the processing of each projection will take $(N_\eta + 1)$ fast Fourier transforms (FFTs). If the total number of projections is N_ϕ, this translates into $(N_\eta + 1)N_\phi$ FFTs. For most $N \times N$ reconstructions, both N_η and N_ϕ will be approximately equal to N. Therefore, Devaney's filtered backpropagation algorithm will require approximately N^2 FFTs compared to $4N$ FFTs for frequency domain interpolation. (For precise comparisons, we must mention that the FFTs for the case of frequency domain interpolation are longer due to zero-padding.)

Devaney [Dev82] has also proposed a modified filtered backpropagation algorithm, in which $G_\eta(\omega)$ is simply replaced by a single $G_{\eta_0}(\omega)$ where $\eta_0 = x_0 \cos \phi + y_0 \sin \phi$, (x_0, y_0) being the coordinates of the point where local accuracy in reconstruction is desired. (Elimination of depth-dependent filtering reduces the number of FFTs to $2N_\phi$.)

6.5 Limitations

There are several factors that limit the accuracy of diffraction tomography reconstructions. These limitations are caused both by the approximations that must be made in the derivation of the reconstruction process and the experimental factors.

The mathematical and experimental effects limit the reconstruction in different ways. The most severe mathematical limitations are imposed by the Born and the Rytov approximations. These approximations are fundamental to the reconstruction process and limit the range of objects that can be examined. On the other hand, it is only possible to collect a finite amount of data and this gives rise to errors in the reconstruction which can be attributed to experimental limitations. Up to the limit in resolution caused by evanescent waves, and given a perfect reconstruction algorithm, it is possible to improve a reconstruction by collecting more data. It is important to understand the experimental limitations so that the experimental data can be used efficiently.

6.5.1 Mathematical Limitations

Computer simulations were performed to study several questions posed by diffraction tomography. In diffraction tomography there are different approximations involved in the forward and inverse directions. In the forward process it is necessary to assume that the object is weakly scattering so that either the Born or the Rytov approximation can be used. Once an expression for the scattered field is derived it is necessary not only to measure the scattered fields but then numerically implement the inversion process.

By carefully designing the simulations it is possible to separate the effects of the approximations. To study the effects of the Born and the Rytov approximations it is necessary to calculate (or even measure) the exact fields and then use the best possible (most exact) reconstruction formulas available. The difference between the reconstruction and the actual object is a measure of the quality of the approximations.

6.5.2 Evaluation of the Born Approximation

The exact field for the scattered field from a cylinder, as shown by Weeks [Wee64] and by Morse and Ingard [Mor68], was calculated for cylinders of various sizes and refractive indexes. In the simulations that follow a single plane wave of unit wavelength was incident on the cylinder and the scattered field was measured along a line at a distance of 100 wavelengths from the origin. In addition, all refractive index changes were modeled as monopole scatterers. By doing this the directional dependence of dipole scatterers didn't have to be taken into account.

At the receiver line the received wave was measured at 512 points spaced at 1/2 wavelength intervals. In all cases the rotational symmetry of a single cylinder at the origin was used to reduce the computation time of the simulations.

The results shown in Fig. 6.20 are for cylinders of four different refractive indexes. In addition, Fig. 6.21 shows plots of the reconstructions along a line through the center of each cylinder. Notice that the y-coordinate of the center line is plotted in terms of change from unity.

The simulations were performed for refractive indexes that ranged from a 0.1% change (refractive index of 1.001) to a 20% change (refractive index of 1.2). For each refractive index, cylinders of size 1, 2, 4, and 10 wavelengths were reconstructed. This gives a range of phase changes across the cylinder (see (50)) from 0.004π to 16π.

Clearly, all the cylinders of refractive index 1.001 in Fig. 6.20 were perfectly reconstructed. As (50) predicts, the results get worse as the product of refractive index and radius gets larger. The largest refractive index that was successfully reconstructed was for the cylinder in Fig. 6.20 of radius 1 wavelength and a refractive index that differed by 20% from the surrounding medium.

While it is hard to evaluate quantitatively the two-dimensional reconstructions, it is certainly reasonable to conclude that only cylinders where the phase change across the object was less than or equal to 0.8π were adequately reconstructed. In general, the reconstruction for each cylinder where the phase change across the cylinder was greater than π shows severe artifacts near the center. This limitation in the phase change across the cylinder is consistent with the condition expressed in (51).

Finally, it is important to note that the reconstructions in Fig. 6.20 don't show the most severe limitation of the Born approximation, which is that the real and imaginary parts of a reconstruction can get mixed up. For objects that don't satisfy the 0.8π phase change limitation the Born approximation causes some of the real energy in the reconstruction to be rotated into the imaginary plane. This further limits the use of the Born approximation when it is necessary to separately image the real and imaginary components of the refractive index.

6.5.3 Evaluation of the Rytov Approximation

Fig. 6.22 shows the simulated results for 16 reconstructions using the Rytov approximation. To emphasize the insensitivity of the Rytov approximation to large objects the largest object simulated had a diameter of 100λ. Note that these reconstructions are an improvement over those published in [Sla84] due to decreased errors in the phase unwrapping algorithm used.[1] This was accomplished by using an adaptive phase unwrapping algorithm as described in [Tri77] and by reducing the sampling interval on the receiver line to 0.125λ.

It should be pointed out that the rounded edges of the 1λ reconstructions aren't due to any limitation of the Rytov approximation but instead are the result of a two-dimensional low pass filtering of the reconstructions. Recall that for a transmission experiment an estimate of the object's Fourier transform is only available up to frequencies less than $\sqrt{2}k_0$. Thus the reconstructions shown in Fig. 6.22 show the limitations of both the Rytov approximation and the Fourier Diffraction Theorem.

6.5.4 Comparison of the Born and Rytov Approximations

Reconstructions using exact scattered data show the similarity of the Born and the Rytov approximations. Within the limits of the Fourier Diffraction Theorem the reconstructions in Figs. 6.20 and 6.22 of a 1λ object with a small refractive index are similar. In both cases the reconstructed change in refractive index is close to that of the simulated object.

The two approximations differ for objects that have a large refractive index change or have a large radius. The Born reconstructions are good at a large refractive index as long as the phase shift of the incident field as predicted by (50) is less than π.

On the other hand, the Rytov approximation is very sensitive to the refractive index but produces excellent reconstructions for objects as large as

---

[1] Many thanks to M. Kaveh of the University of Minnesota for pointing this out to the authors.

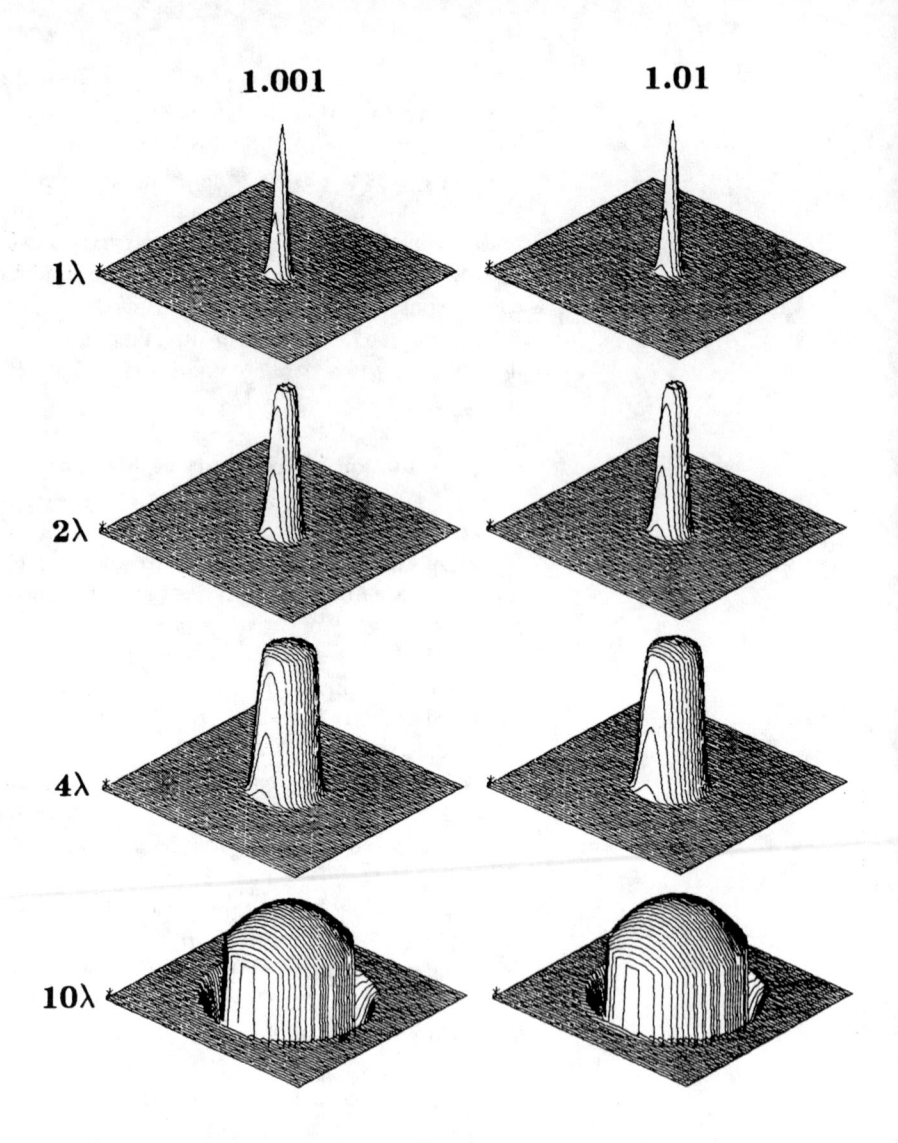

Fig. 6.20: *Reconstructions of 16 different cylinders are shown indicating the effect of cylinder radius and refractive index on the Born approximation. (From [Sla84].)*

100λ. Unfortunately, for objects with a refractive index larger than a few percent the Rytov approximation quickly deteriorates.

In addition to the qualitative studies a quantitative study of the error in the Born and Rytov reconstructions was also performed. As a measure of error we used the relative mean squared error in the reconstruction of the object function integrated over the entire plane. If the actual object function is $o(\vec{r})$ and the reconstructed object function is $o'(\vec{r})$, then the relative mean squared error (MSE) is

$$\iint \frac{[o(\vec{r}) - o'(\vec{r})]^2 \, d\vec{r}}{[o(\vec{r})]^2}. \tag{182}$$

250   COMPUTERIZED TOMOGRAPHIC IMAGING

1.10   **1.20**

1λ

2λ

4λ

10λ

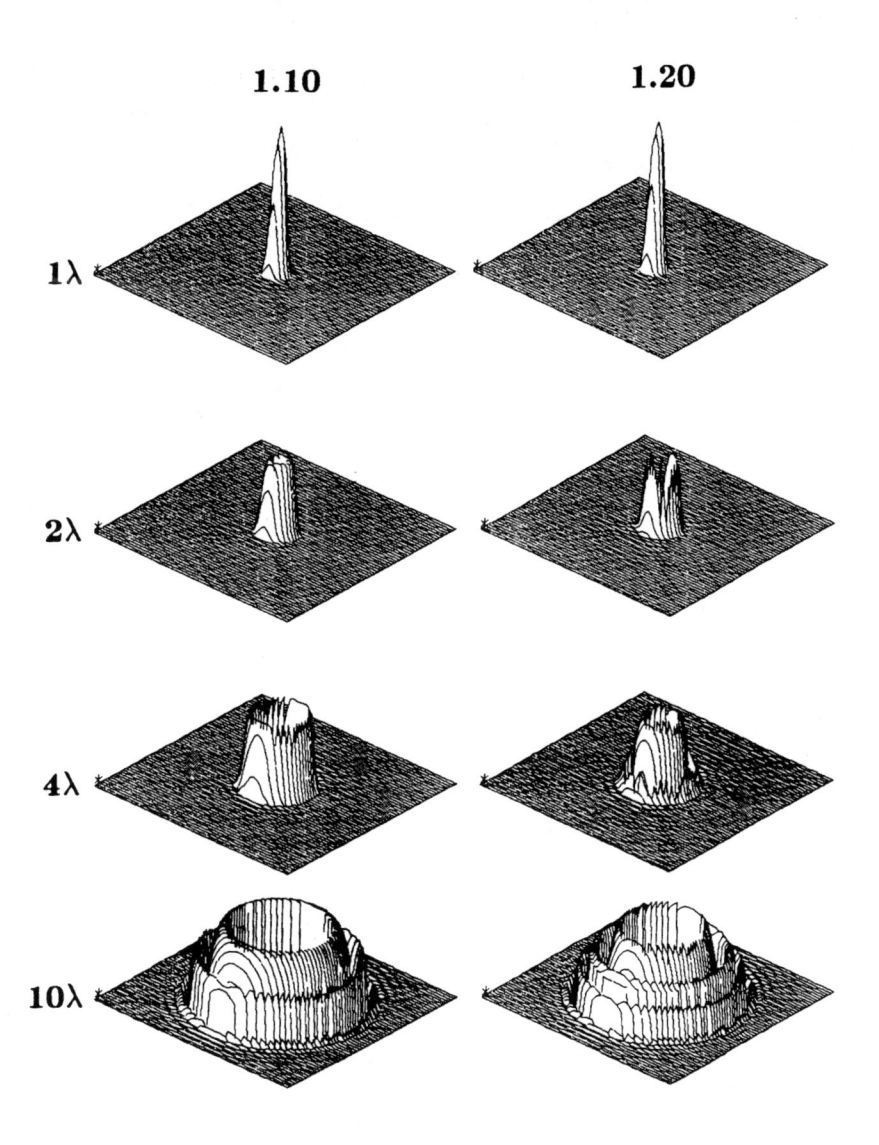

Fig. 6.20: *Continued.*

For this study 120 reconstructions were done of cylinders using the exact scattered data. In each case a 512-point receiver line was at a distance of 10λ from the center of the cylinder. Both the receiver line and the object reconstruction were sampled at 1/4λ intervals.

The plots of Fig. 6.23 present a summary of the mean squared error for cylinders of 1, 2, and 3λ in radius and for 20 refractive indexes between 1.01 and 1.20. In each case the error for the Born approximation is shown as a solid line while the Rytov reconstruction is shown as a broken line.

Many researchers [Kav82], [Kel69], [Sou83] have postulated that the Rytov approximation is superior to the Born but as the actual reconstructions in Fig. 6.23(a) show for a 1λ cylinder this is not necessarily true. While for

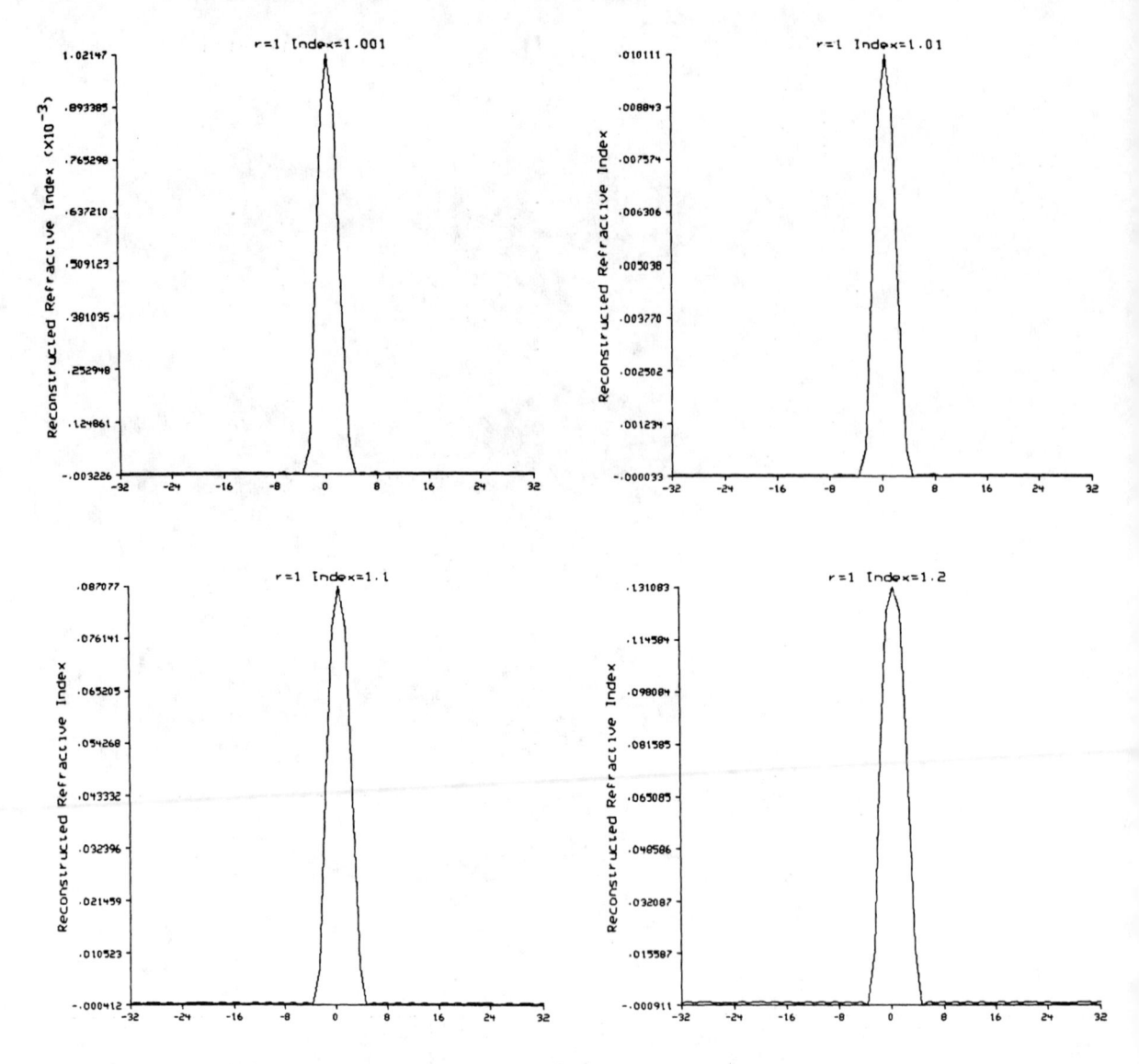

Fig. 6.21: *Cross sections of the cylinders shown in Fig. 6.20 are shown here.*

the cylinder of radius 2λ there is a region where the Rytov approximation shows less error than the Born reconstruction, this doesn't occur until the relative error is above 20%. What is clear is that both the Born and the Rytov approximations are only valid for small objects and that they both produce similar errors.

6.6 Evaluation of Reconstruction Algorithms

To study the approximations involved in the reconstruction process it is necessary to calculate scattered data assuming the forward approximations

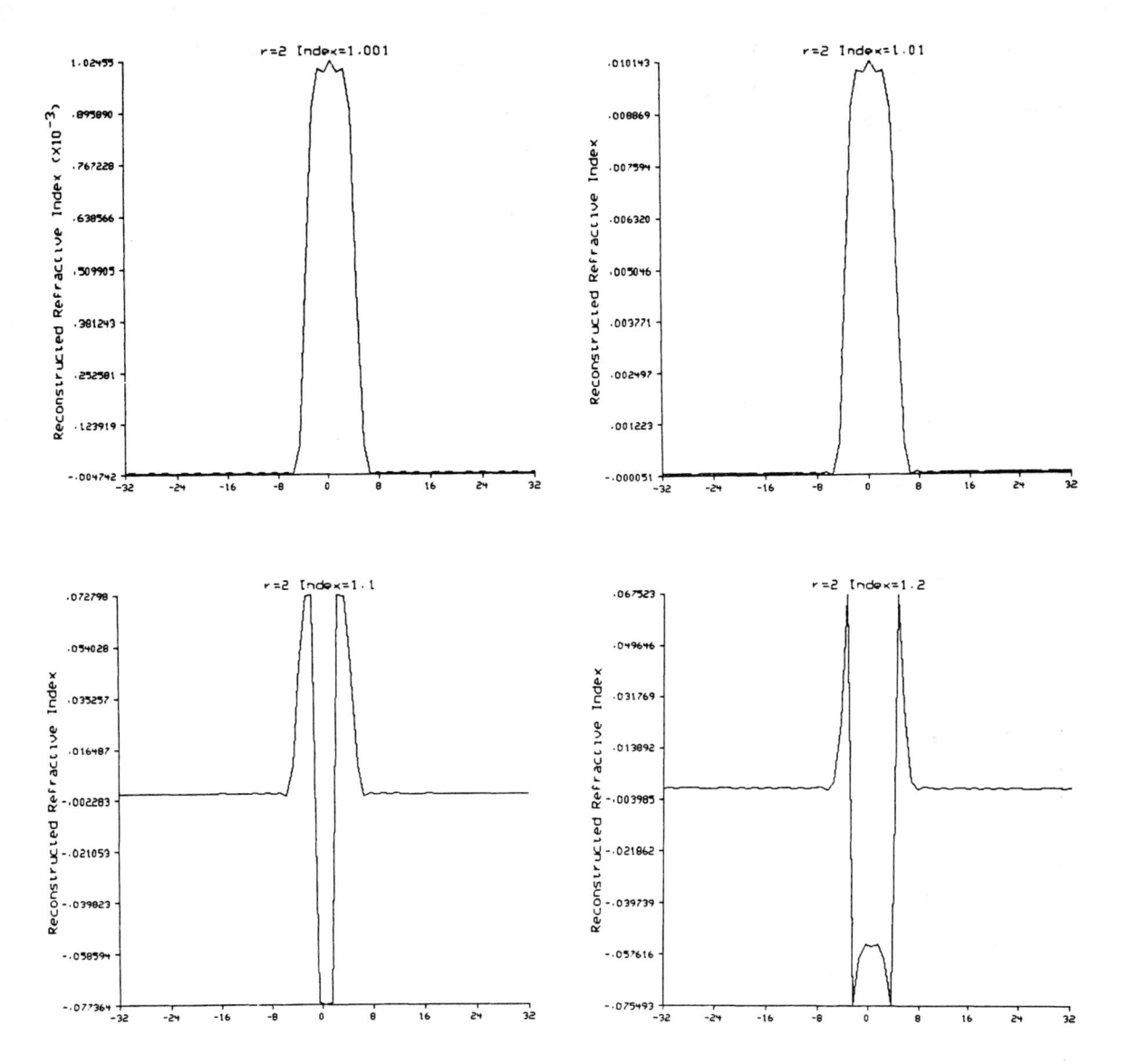

Fig. 6.21: *Continued.*

are valid. This can be done in one of two different ways. We have already discussed that the Born and Rytov approximations are valid for small objects and small changes in refractive index. Thus, if we calculate the exact scattered field for a small and weakly scattering object we can assume that either the Born or the Rytov approximation is exact.

A better approach is to recall the Fourier Diffraction Theorem, which says that the Fourier transform of the scattered field is proportional to the Fourier transform of the object along a semicircular arc. Since this theorem is the

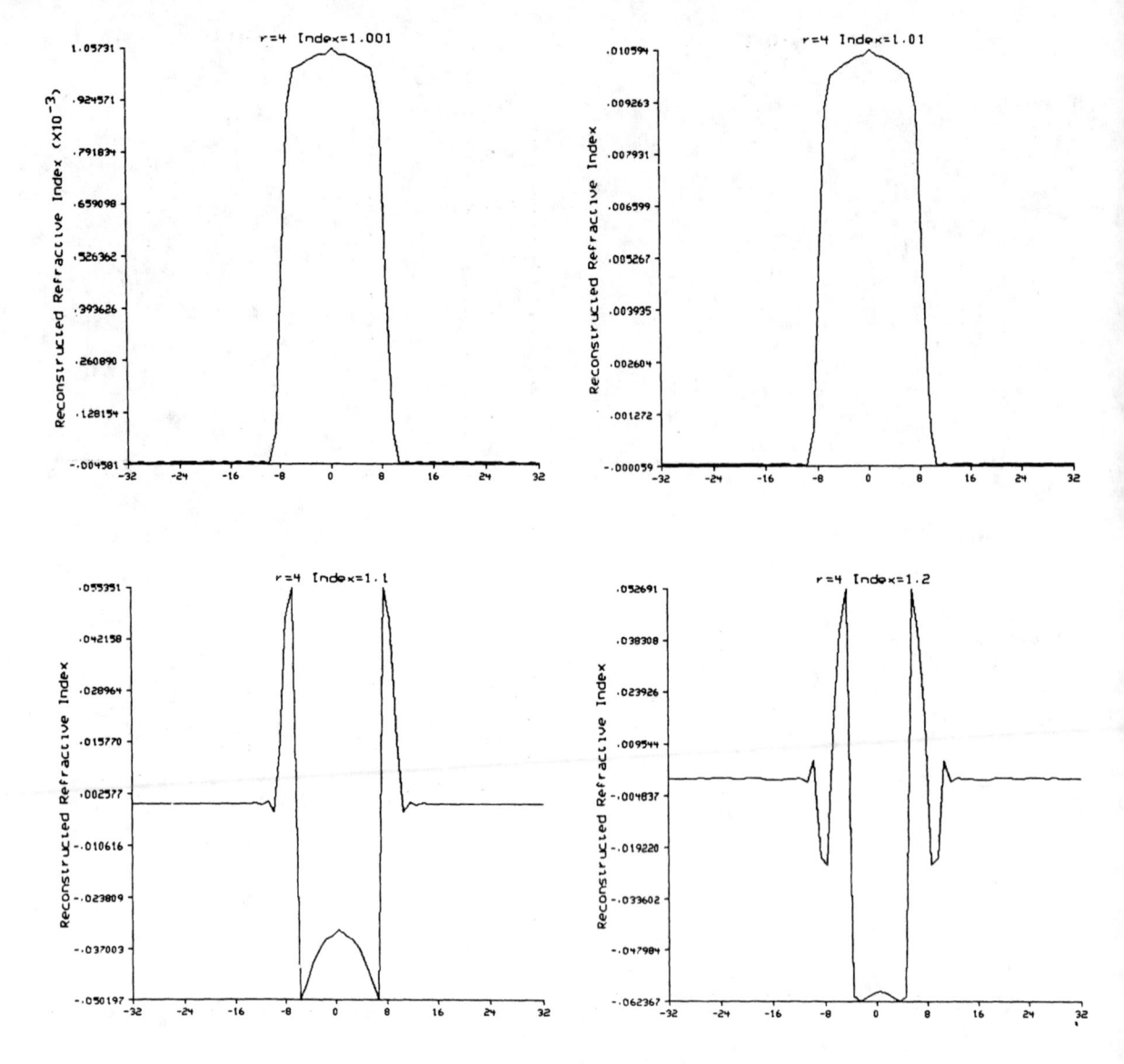

Fig. 6.21: *Continued.* basis for our inversion algorithm, if we assume it is correct we can study the approximations involved in the reconstruction process.

If we assume that the Fourier Diffraction Theorem holds, the exact scattered field can be calculated exactly for objects that can be modeled as ellipses. The analytic expression for the Fourier transform of the object along an arc is proportional to the scattered fields. This procedure is fast and allows us to calculate scattered fields for testing reconstruction algorithms and experimental parameters.

To illustrate the accuracy of the interpolation-based algorithms, we will

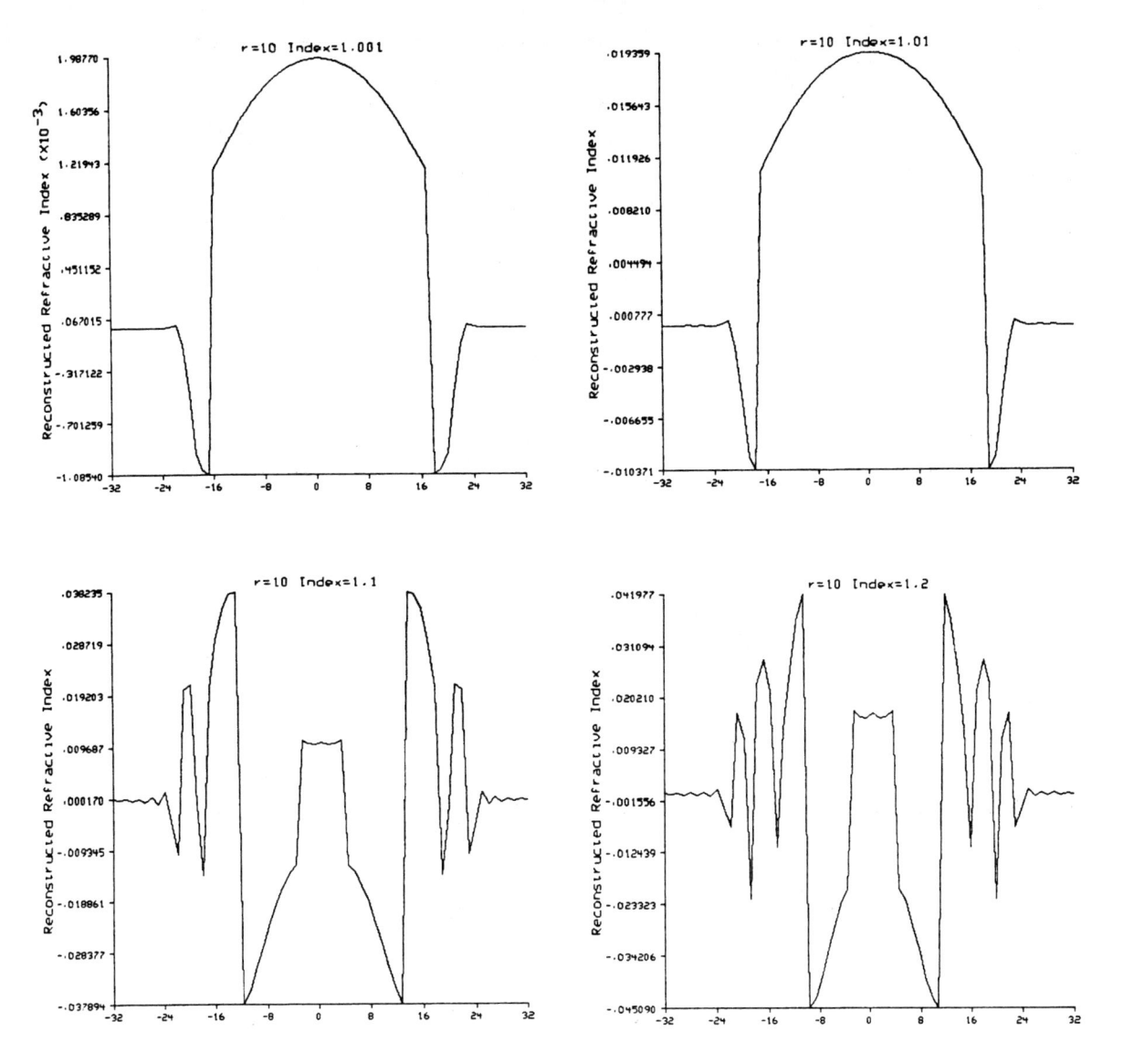

Fig. 6.21: *Continued.*

use the image in Fig. 6.24 as a test "object" for showing some computer simulation results. Fig. 6.24 is a modification of the Shepp and Logan "phantom" described in Chapter 3 to the case of diffraction imaging. The gray levels shown in Fig. 6.24 represent the refractive index values. This test image is a superposition of ellipses, with each ellipse being assigned a refractive index value as shown in Table 6.1.

A major advantage of using an image like that in Fig. 6.24 for computer simulation is that one can write analytical expressions for the transforms of the diffracted projections. The Fourier transform of an ellipse of semi-major

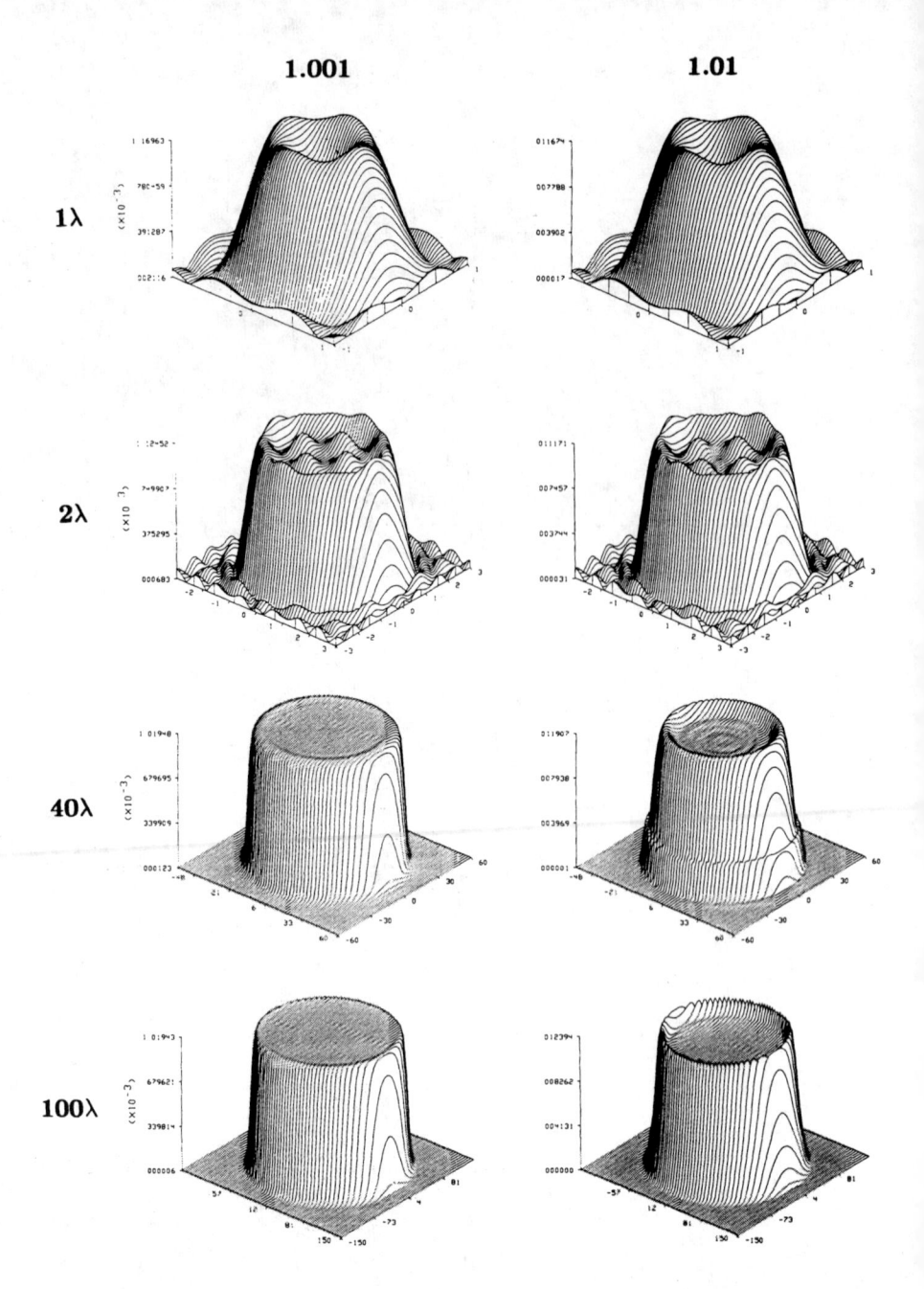

Fig. 6.22: *Reconstructions of 16 different cylinders are shown indicating the effect of cylinder radius and refractive index on the Rytov approximation. These reconstructions were calculated by sampling the scattered fields at 16,384 points along a line 100λ from the edge of the object. A sampling interval of 6(R + 100)/16,384 where R is the radius of the cylinder, was used to make it easier to unwrap the phase of the scattered fields. (Adapted from [Sla84].)*

256   COMPUTERIZED TOMOGRAPHIC IMAGING

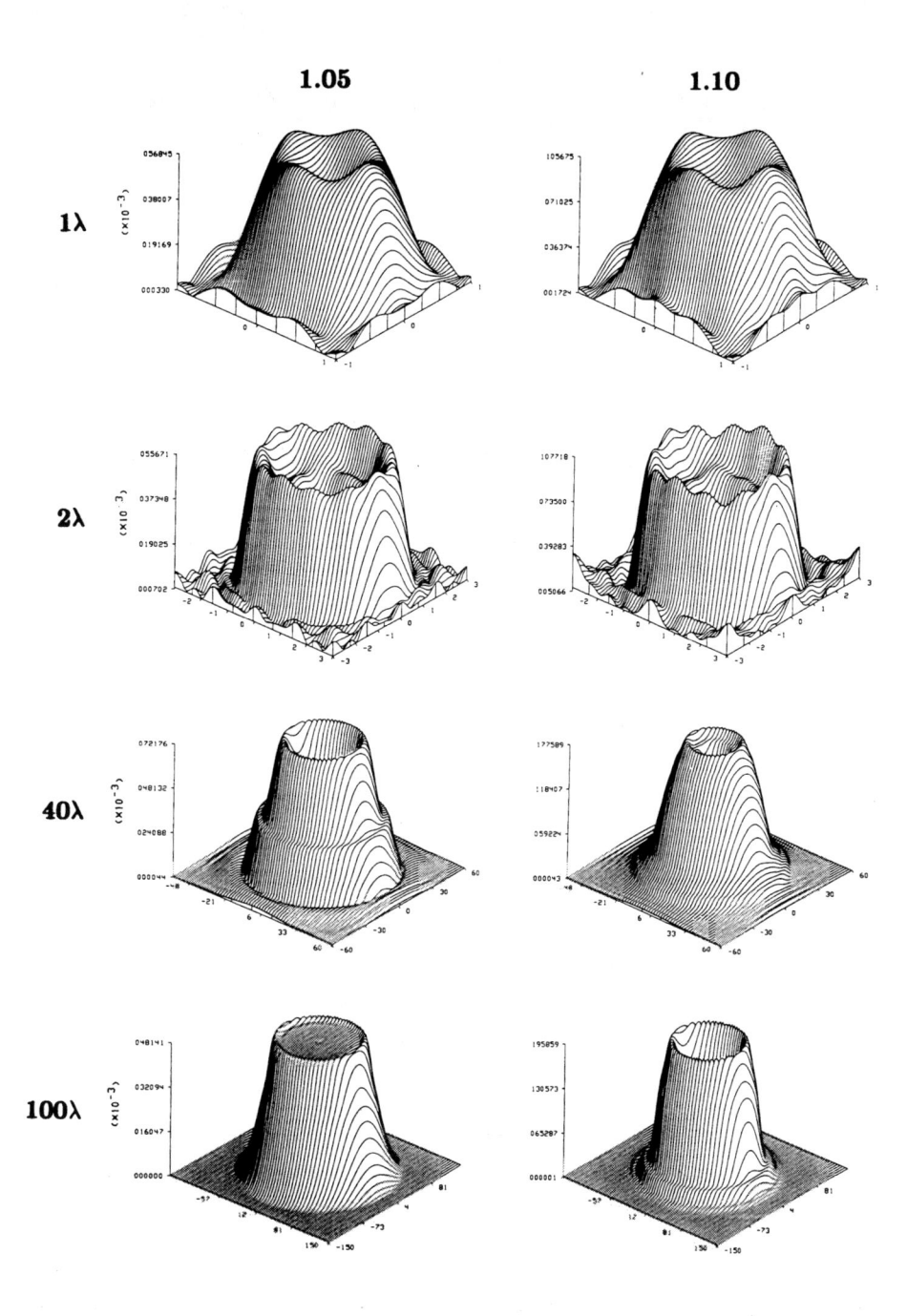

Fig. 6.22: *Continued.*

TOMOGRAPHIC IMAGING WITH DIFFRACTING SOURCES

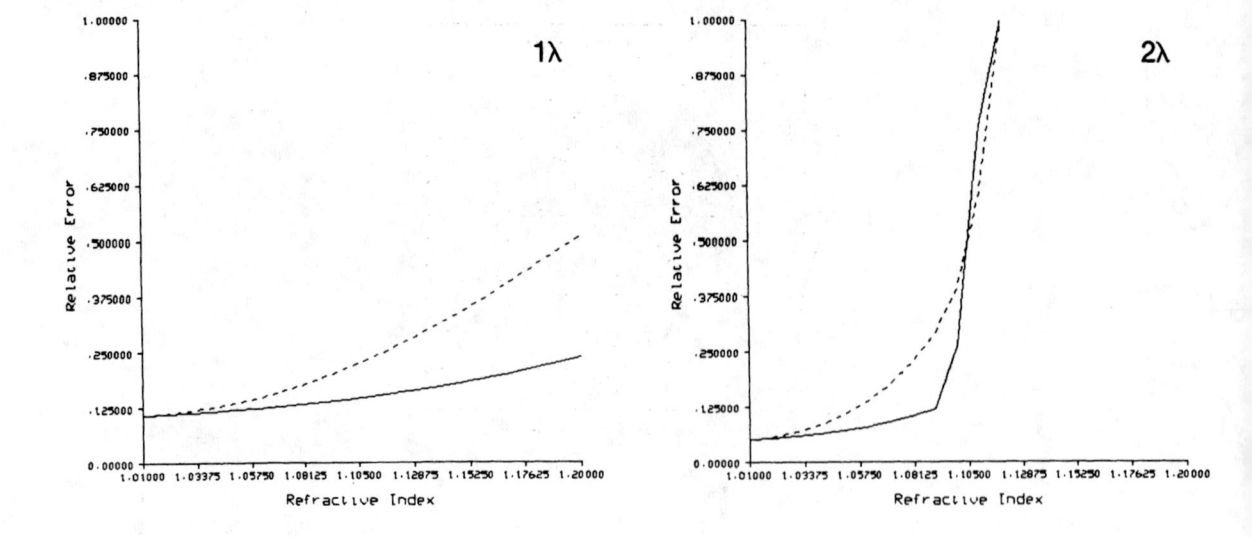

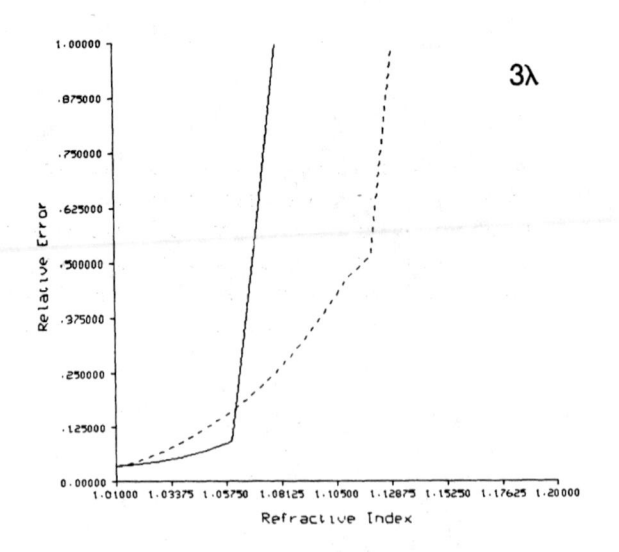

Fig. 6.23: *The relative mean squared errors for reconstructions with the Born (solid) and the Rytov (broken) approximations are shown here. Each plot is a function of the refractive index of the cylinder. The mean squared error is plotted for cylinders of radius 1λ, 2λ, and 3λ. (From [Sla84].)*

and semi-minor axes of lengths A and B, respectively, is given by

$$\frac{2\pi A J_1[B\sqrt{(uA/B)^2+v^2}]}{\sqrt{(uA/B)^2+v^2}} \tag{183}$$

where u and v are spatial angular frequencies in the x and y directions, respectively, and J_1 is a Bessel function of the first kind and order 1. When the center of this ellipse is shifted to the point (x_1, y_1), and the angle of the major axis tilted by α, as shown in Fig. 6.25(b), its Fourier transform

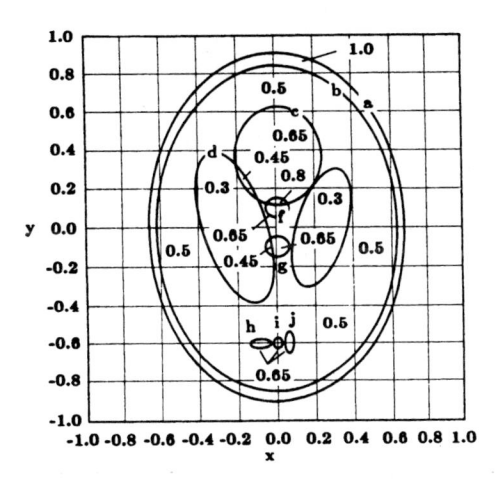

Fig. 6.24: *For diffraction tomographic simulations a slightly modified version of the Shepp and Logan head phantom is used. (From [Pan83].)*

becomes

$$e^{-j(ux_1+vy_1)}$$

$$\cdot \frac{2\pi A J_1\{B[((u\cos\alpha+v\sin\alpha)A/B)^2+(-u\sin\alpha+v\cos\alpha)^2]^{1/2}\}}{[((u\cos\alpha+v\sin\alpha)A/B)^2+(-u\sin\alpha+v\cos\alpha)^2]^{1/2}}.$$

(184)

Now consider the situation in which the ellipse is illuminated by a plane wave. By the Fourier Diffraction Theorem discussed previously, the Fourier transform of the transmitted wave fields measured on a line like TT' shown in Fig. 6.2(left), will be given by the values of the above function on a semicircular arc as shown in Fig. 6.2(right). If we assume weak scattering and therefore no interactions among the ellipses, the Fourier transform of the

Table 6.1: Summary of parameters for diffraction tomography simulations.

Center Coordinate	Major Axis	Minor Axis	Rotation Angle	Refractive Index
(0, 0)	0.92	0.69	90	1.0
(0, −0.0184)	0.874	0.6624	90	−0.5
(0.22, 0)	0.31	0.11	72	−0.2
(−0.22, 0)	0.41	0.16	108	−0.2
(0, 0.35)	0.25	0.21	90	0.1
(0, 0.1)	0.046	0.046	0	0.15
(0, −0.1)	0.046	0.046	0	0.15
(−0.08, −0.605)	0.046	0.023	0	0.15
(0, −0.605)	0.023	0.023	0	0.15
(0.06, −0.605)	0.046	0.023	90	0.15

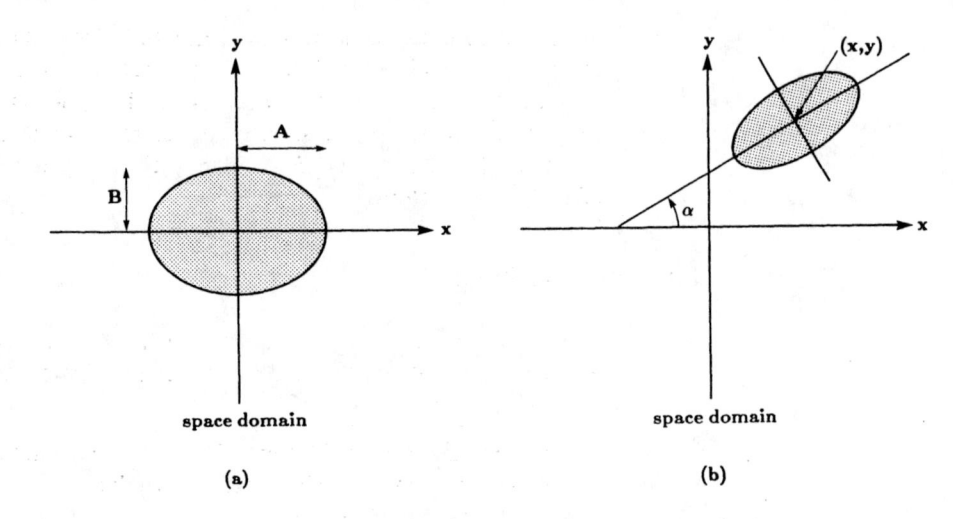

Fig. 6.25: *Assuming the Fourier Slice Theorem, the field scattered by an ellipse can be easily calculated. (From [Kak85].)*

total forward scattered field measured on the line TT' will be a sum of the values of functions like (184) over the semicircular arc. This procedure was used to generate the diffracted projection data for the test image.

We must mention that by generating the diffracted projection data for computer simulation by this procedure, we are only testing the accuracy of the reconstruction algorithm, without checking whether or not the "test object" satisfies the underlying assumption of weak scattering. In order to test this crucial assumption, we must generate exactly on a computer the forward scattered data of the object. For multicomponent objects, such as the one shown in Fig. 6.24, it is very difficult to do so due to the interactions between the components.

Pan and Kak [Pan83] presented the simulations shown in Fig. 6.26. Using a combination of increasing the sampling density by zero-padding the signal and bilinear interpolation, results were obtained in 2 minutes of CPU time on a VAX 11/780 minicomputer with a floating point accelerator (FPA). The reconstruction was done over a 128 × 128 grid using 64 views and 128 receiver positions. The number of operations required to carry out the interpolation and invert the object function is on the order of $N^2 \log N$. The resulting reconstruction is shown in Fig. 6.26(a).

Fig. 6.26(b) represents the result of backpropagating the data to 128 depths for each view, while Fig. 6.26(c) is the result of backpropagation to only a single depth centered near the three small ellipses at the bottom of the picture. The results were simulated on a VAX 11/780 minicomputer and the resulting reconstructions were done over a 128 × 128 grid. Like the previous image the input data consisted of 64 projections of 128 points each.

There was a significant difference in not only the reconstruction time but also the resulting quality. While the modified backpropagation only took 1.25 minutes, the resulting reconstruction is much poorer than that from the full backpropagation which took 30 minutes of CPU time. A comparison of the various algorithms is shown in Table 6.2. Note that the table doesn't explicitly show the extra CPU time required if zero-padding is used in the frequency domain to make space domain interpolation easier. To a very rough approximation space domain interpolation and modified backpropagation algorithms take $N^2 \log N$ steps while the full backpropagation algorithm takes $N^3 \log N$ steps.

6.7 Experimental Limitations

In addition to the limits on the reconstructions imposed by the Born and the Rytov approximations, there are also the following experimental limitations to consider:

- Limitations caused by ignoring evanescent waves
- Sampling the data along the receiver line
- Finite receiver length
- Limited views of the object.

Each of the first three factors can be modeled as a simple constant low pass filtering of the scattered field. Because the reconstruction process is linear the net effect can be modeled by a single low pass filter with a cutoff at the lowest of the three cutoff frequencies. The experiment can be optimized by adjusting the parameters so that each low pass filter cuts off at the same frequency.

The effect of a limited number of views also can be modeled as a low pass filter. In this case, though, the cutoff frequency varies with the radial direction.

6.7.1 Evanescent Waves

Since evanescent waves have a complex wavenumber they are severely attenuated over a distance of only a few wavelengths. This limits the highest received wavenumber to

$$k_{max} = \frac{2\pi}{\lambda}. \qquad (185)$$

This is a fundamental limit of the propagation process and can only be improved by moving the experiment to a higher frequency (or shorter wavelength).

6.7.2 Sampling the Received Wave

After the wave has been scattered by the object and propagated to the receiver line, it must be measured. This is usually done with a point receiver.

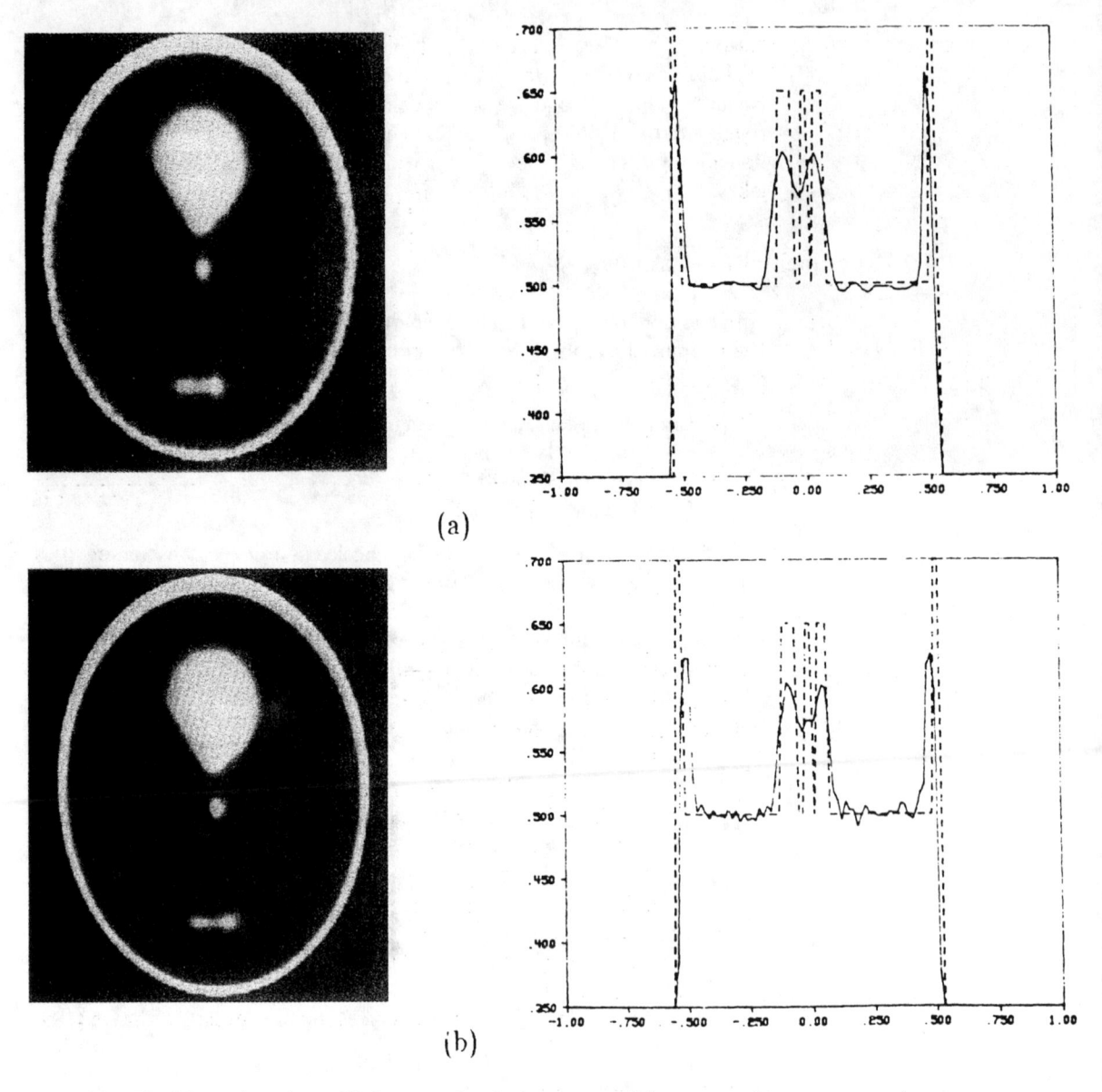

Fig. 6.26: *The images show the results of using the (a) interpolation, (b) backpropagation, and (c) modified backpropagation algorithms on reconstruction quality. The solid lines of the graphs represent the reconstructed value along a line through the three ellipses at the bottom of the phantom. (From [Pan83].)*

Unfortunately, it is not possible to sample at every point, so a nonzero sampling interval must be chosen. This introduces a measurement error into the process. By the Nyquist theorem this can be modeled as a low pass filtering operation, where the highest measured frequency is given by

$$k_{\text{meas}} = \frac{\pi}{T} \tag{186}$$

where T is the sampling interval.

262 COMPUTERIZED TOMOGRAPHIC IMAGING

(c)

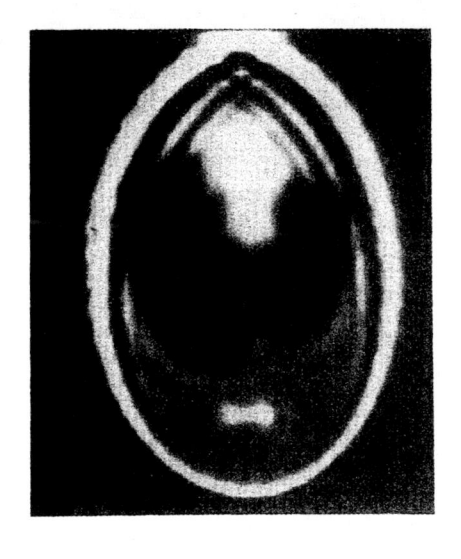

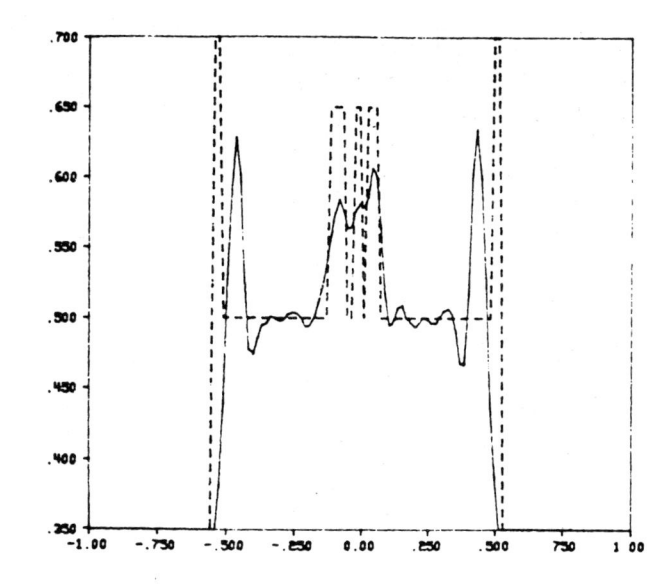

Fig. 6.26: *Continued.*

6.7.3 The Effects of a Finite Receiver Length

Not only are there physical limitations on the finest sampling interval but usually there is a limitation on the amount of data that can be collected. This generally means that samples of the received waveform will be collected at only a finite number of points along the receiver line. This is usually justified by taking data along a line long enough so that the unmeasured data can be safely ignored. Because of the wave propagation process this also introduces a low pass filtering of the received data.

Consider for a moment a single scatterer at some distance, l_0, from the receiver line. The wave propagating from this single scatterer is a cylindrical wave in two dimensions or a spherical wave in three dimensions. This effect is diagrammed in Fig. 6.27. It is easy to see that the spatial frequencies vary with the position along the receiver line. This effect can be analyzed using two different approaches.

It is easier to analyze the effect by considering the expanding wave to be

Table 6.2: Comparison of algorithms.

Algorithm	Complexity	CPU Time (minutes)
Frequency Domain Interpolation	$N^2 \log N$	2
Backpropagation	$N_d N_\phi N \log N$	30
Modified Backpropagation	$N_\phi N \log N$	1.25

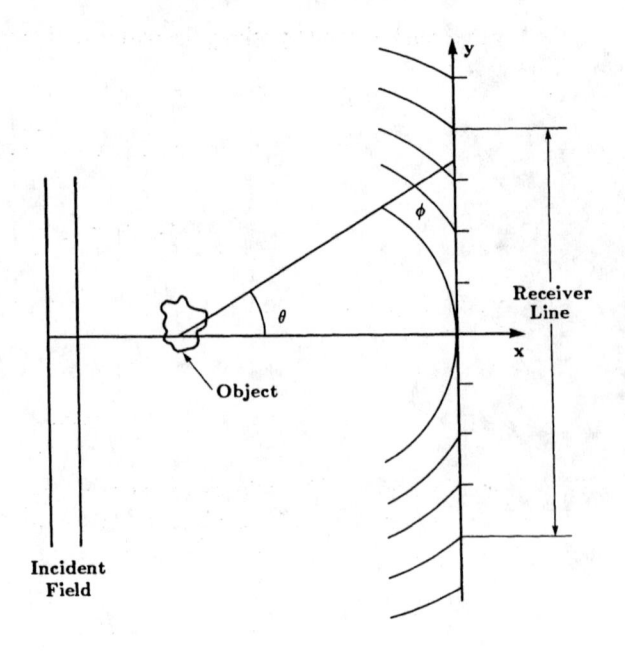

Fig. 6.27: *An object scatters a field which is measured with a finite receiver line. (From [Sla83].)*

locally planar at any point distant from the scatterer. At the point on the receiver line closest to the scatterer there is no spatial variation [Goo68]. This corresponds to receiving a plane wave or a received spatial frequency of zero.

Higher spatial frequencies are received at points along the receiver line that are farther from the origin. The received frequency is a function of the sine of the angle between the direction of propagation and a perpendicular to the receiver line. This function is given by

$$k(y) = k_{max} \sin \theta \qquad (187)$$

where θ is the angle and k_{max} is the wavenumber of the incident wave. Thus at the origin, the angle, θ, is zero and the received frequency is zero. Only at infinity does the angle become equal to 90° and the received spatial frequency approach the theoretical maximum.

This reasoning can be justified on a more theoretical basis by considering the phase function of the propagating wave. The received wave at a point ($x = l_0$, y) due to a scatterer at the origin is given by

$$u(x=l_0, y) = \frac{e^{jk_0\sqrt{x^2+y^2}}}{\sqrt{x^2+y^2}}. \qquad (188)$$

The instantaneous spatial frequency along the receiver line (y varies) of this wave can be found by taking the partial derivative of the phase with respect to y [Gag78].

$$\text{phase} = k_0 \sqrt{y^2 + x^2} \tag{189}$$

$$k_{\text{recv}} = \frac{k_0 y}{\sqrt{x^2 + y^2}} \tag{190}$$

where k_{recv} is the spatial frequency received at the point $(x = l_0, y)$. From Fig. 6.27 it is easy to see that

$$\sin \theta = \frac{y}{\sqrt{x^2 + y^2}} \tag{191}$$

and therefore (187) and (190) are equivalent.

This relation, (190), can be inverted to give the length of the receiver line for a given maximum received frequency, k_{max}. This becomes

$$y = \pm \frac{k_{\text{max}} x}{\sqrt{k_0^2 - k_{\text{max}}^2}}. \tag{192}$$

Since the highest received frequency is a monotonically increasing function of the length of the receiver line, it is easy to see that by limiting the sampling of the received wave to a finite portion of the entire line a low passed version of the entire scattered wave will be measured. The highest measured frequency is a simple function of the distance of the receiver line from the scatterer and the length of measured data. This limitation can be better understood if the maximum received frequency is written as a function of the angle of view of the receiver line. Thus substituting

$$\tan \theta = \frac{y}{x} \tag{193}$$

we find

$$k_{\text{recv}} = \frac{k_0 (y/x)}{\sqrt{(y/x)^2 + 1^2}} \tag{194}$$

and

$$k_{\text{recv}} = \frac{k_0 \tan \theta}{\sqrt{\tan^2 \theta + 1}}. \tag{195}$$

Thus k_{recv} is a monotonically increasing function of the angle of view, θ. It is easy to see that the maximum received spatial frequency can be increased either by moving the receiver line closer to the object or by increasing the length of the receiver line.

6.7.4 Evaluation of the Experimental Effects

The effect of a finite receiver length was simulated and results are shown in Fig. 6.28. The spatial frequency content of a wave, found by taking the FFT of the sampled points along the receiver line, was compared to the theoretical result as predicted by the Fourier transform of the object. The theory predicts that more of the high frequency components will be present as the length of the receiver line increases and this is confirmed by simulation.

While the above derivation only considered a single scatterer it is also approximately true for many scatterers collected at the origin. This is so because the inverse reconstruction process is linear and each point in the object scatters an independent cylindrical wave.

6.7.5 Optimization

Since each of the above three factors is independent of the other two, their effect in the frequency domain can be found by simply multiplying their frequency responses together. As has been described above, each of these effects can be modeled as a simple low pass filter so the combined effect is also a low pass filter but at the lowest frequency of the cutoff of the three effects.

First consider the effect of ignoring the evanescent waves. Since the maximum frequency of the received wave is limited by the propagation filter to

$$k_{max} = \frac{2\pi}{\lambda}, \qquad (196)$$

it is easy to combine this expression with the expression for the Nyquist frequency into a single expression for the smallest "interesting" sampling interval. This is given by

$$k_{max} = k_{meas} \qquad (197)$$

or

$$\frac{2\pi}{\lambda} = \frac{\pi}{T}. \qquad (198)$$

Therefore,

$$T = \frac{\lambda}{2}. \qquad (199)$$

Fig. 6.28: *These four reconstructions show the effect of a finite receiver line. Reconstructions of an object using 64 detectors spaced at (a) 0.5λ, (b) 1.0λ, (c) 1.5λ, and (d) 2.0λ are shown here. (From [Sla83].)*

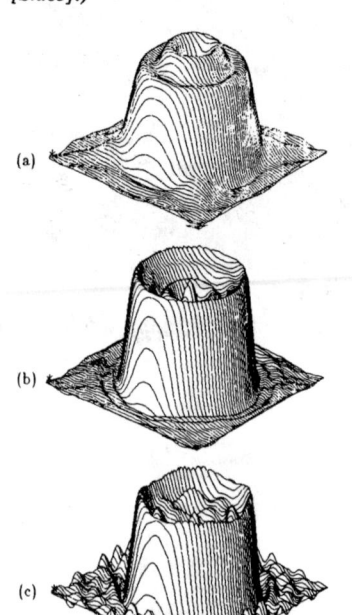

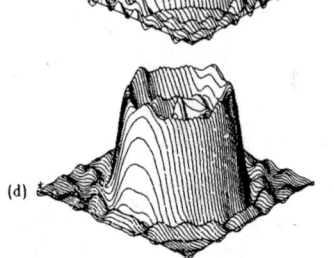

If the received waveform is sampled with a sampling interval of more than 1/2 wavelength, the measured data might not be a good estimate of the received waveform because of aliasing. On the other hand, it is not necessary to sample the received waveform any finer than 1/2 wavelength since this provides no additional information. Therefore, we conclude that the sampling interval should be close to 1/2 wavelength.

In general, the experiment will also be constrained by the number of data points (M) that can be measured along the receiver line. The distance from the object to the receiver line will be considered a constant in the derivation that follows. If the received waveform is sampled uniformly, the range of the receiver line is given uniquely by

$$y_{max} = \pm \frac{MT}{2}. \tag{200}$$

This is also shown in Fig. 6.27.

For a receiver line at a fixed distance from the object and a fixed number of receiver points, the choice of T is determined by the following two competing considerations: As the sampling interval is increased the length of the receiver line increases and more of the received wave's high frequencies are measured. On the other hand, increasing the sampling interval lowers the maximum frequency that can be measured before aliasing occurs.

The optimum value of T can be found by setting the cutoff frequencies for the Nyquist frequency equal to the highest received frequency due to the finite receiver length and then solving for the sampling interval. If this constraint isn't met, then some of the information that is passed by one process will be attenuated by the others. This results in

$$\frac{\pi}{T} = \frac{k_0 y}{\sqrt{y^2 + x^2}} \tag{201}$$

evaluated at

$$k_0 = \frac{2\pi}{\lambda} \tag{202}$$

and

$$y = \frac{MT}{2}. \tag{203}$$

Solving for T^2 we find that the optimum value for T is given by

$$\left(\frac{T}{\lambda}\right)^2 = \frac{\sqrt{64(x/\lambda)^2 + M^2} + M}{8M}. \tag{204}$$

If we make the substitution

$$\alpha = \frac{x}{\lambda M} \qquad (205)$$

we find that the optimum sampling interval is given by

$$\left(\frac{T}{\lambda}\right)^2 = \frac{\sqrt{64\alpha^2 + 1} + 1}{8}. \qquad (206)$$

This formula is to be used with the constraint that the smallest positive value for the sampling interval is 1/2 wavelength.

The optimum sampling interval is confirmed by simulations. Again using the method described above for calculating the exact scattered fields, four simulations were made of an object of radius 10 wavelengths using a receiver line that was 100 wavelengths from the object. In each case the number of receiver positions was fixed at 64. The resulting reconstructions for sampling intervals of 0.05, 1, 1.5, and 2 wavelengths are shown in Fig. 6.28. Equation (206) predicts an optimum sampling interval of 1.3 wavelengths and this is confirmed by the simulations. The best reconstruction occurs with a sampling interval between 1 and 1.5 wavelengths.

6.7.6 Limited Views

In many applications it is not possible to generate or receive plane waves from all directions. The effect of this is to leave holes where there is no estimate of the Fourier transform of the object.

Since the ideal reconstruction algorithm produces an estimate of the Fourier transform of the object for all frequencies within a disk, a limited number of views introduces a selective filter for areas where there are no data. As shown by Devaney [Dev84] for the VSP case, a limited number of views degrades the reconstruction by low pass filtering the image in certain directions. Devaney's results are reproduced in Figs. 6.29 and 6.30.

6.8 Bibliographic Notes

The paper by Mueller *et al.* [Mue79] was responsible for focusing the interest of many researchers on the area of diffraction tomography, although from a purely scientific standpoint the technique can be traced back to the now classic paper by Wolf [Wol69] and a subsequent article by Iwata and Nagata [Iwa75].

The small perturbation approximations that are used for developing the diffraction tomography algorithms have been discussed by Ishimaru [Ish78] and Morse and Ingard [Mor68]. A discussion of the theory of the Born and the Rytov approximations was presented by Chernov in [Che60]. A

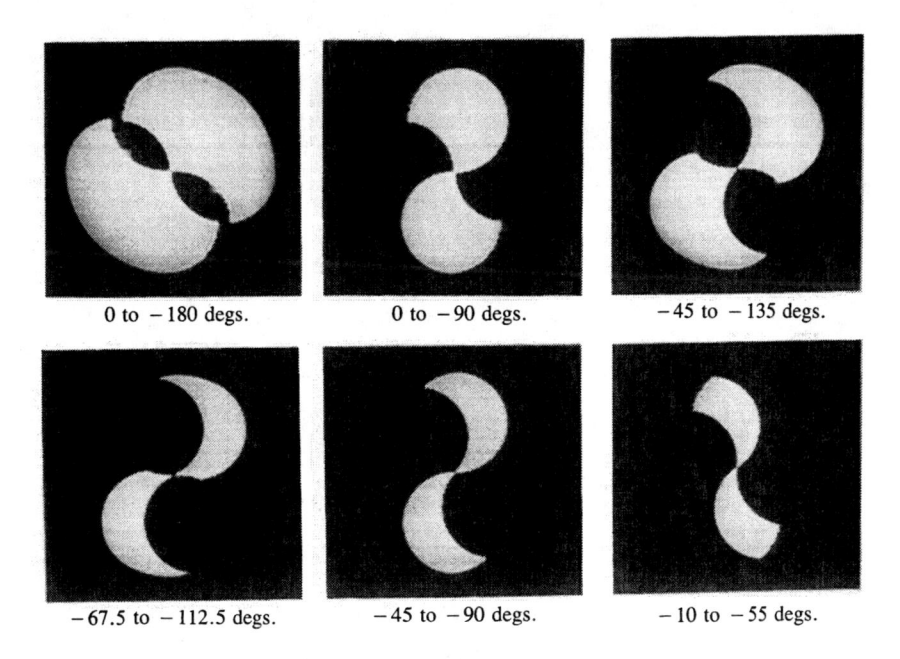

0 to −180 degs.	0 to −90 degs.	−45 to −135 degs.
−67.5 to −112.5 degs.	−45 to −90 degs.	−10 to −55 degs.

Fig. 6.29: *These figures show the coverage in the frequency domain for six different angular receiver limitations. (From [Dev84].)*

comparison of Born and Rytov approximations is presented in [Kel69], [Sla84], [Sou83]. The effect of multiple scattering on first-order diffraction tomography is described in [Azi83], [Azi85]. Another review of diffraction tomography is presented in [Kav86].

Diffraction tomography falls under the general subject of inverse scattering. The issues relating to the uniqueness and stability of inverse scattering solutions are addressed in [Bal78], [Dev78], [Nas81], [Sar81]. The mathematics of solving integral equations for inverse scattering problems is described in [Col83].

The filtered backpropagation algorithm for diffraction tomography was first advanced by Devaney [Dev82]. More recently, Pan and Kak [Pan83] showed that by using frequency domain interpolation followed by direct Fourier inversion, reconstructions of quality comparable to that produced by the filtered backpropagation algorithm can be obtained. Interpolation-based algorithms were first studied by Carter [Car70] and Mueller *et al.* [Mue80], [Sou84b]. An interpolation technique based on the known support of the object in the space domain is known as the unified frequency domain reconstruction (UFR) and is described in [Kav84]. Since the problems are related, the reader is referred to an excellent paper by Stark *et al.* [Sta81] that describes optimum interpolation techniques as applied to direct Fourier inversion of straight ray projections. The reader is also referred to [Fer79] to learn how in some cases it may be possible to avoid the interpolation, and still be able to reconstruct an object with direct 2-D Fourier inversion.

A diffraction tomography approach that requires only two rotational positions of the object has been advanced by Nahamoo *et al.* [Nah84] and

0 to −180 degs.   0 to −90 degs.   −45 to −135 degs.

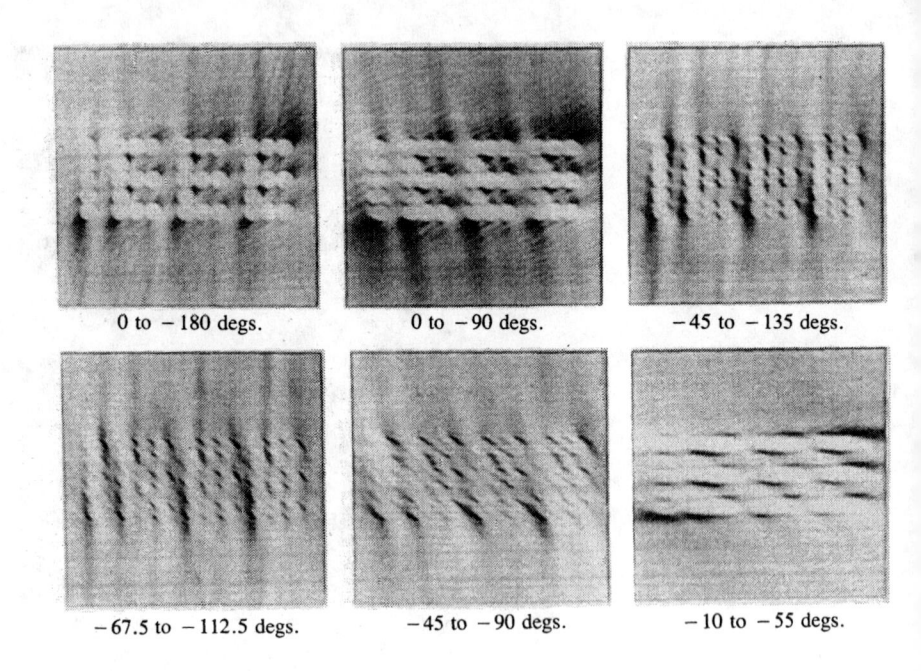

−67.5 to −112.5 degs.   −45 to −90 degs.   −10 to −55 degs.

Fig. 6.30: *Images due to the limited field of views as shown in Fig. 6.29. (From [Dev84].)*

Devaney [Dev83], and its computer implementation has been studied by Pan and Kak [Pan83]. Diffraction tomography based on the reflected data has been studied in great detail by Norton and Linzer [Nor81].

The first experimental diffraction tomography work was done by Carter and Ho using optical energy and is described in [Car70], [Car74], [HoP76]. More recently, Kaveh and Soumekh have reported experimental results in [Kav80], [Kav81], [Kav82], [Sou83].

Finally, more accurate techniques for imaging objects that don't fall within the domain of the Born and Rytov approximations have been reported in [Joh83], [Tra83], [Sla85], [Bey84], [Bey85a], [Bey85b].

6.9 References

[Azi83] M. Azimi and A. C. Kak, "Distortion in diffraction imaging caused by multiple scattering," *IEEE Trans. Med. Imaging,* vol. MI-2, pp. 176–195, Dec. 1983.

[Azi85] ——, "Multiple scattering and attenuation phenomena in diffraction imaging," TR-EE 85-4, School of Electrical Engineering, Purdue Univ., Lafayette, IN, 1985.

[Bal78] H. P. Baltes (Ed.), *Inverse Source Problems in Optics.* Berlin: Springer-Verlag, 1978.

[Bar78] V. Barthes and G. Vasseur, "An inverse problem for electromagnetic prospection," in *Applied Inverse Problems,* P. C. Sabatier, Ed. Berlin: Springer-Verlag, 1978.

[Bey84] G. Beylkin, "The inversion problem and applications of the generalized Radon transform," *Commun. Pure Appl. Math.,* vol. 37, pp. 579–599, 1984.

[Bey85a] ——, "Imaging of discontinuities in the inverse scattering problem by inversion of a causal generalized Radon transform," *J. Math. Phys.*, vol. 26-1, pp. 99-108, Jan. 1985.

[Bey85b] G. Beylkin and M. L. Oristaglio, "Distorted-wave Born and distorted-wave Rytov approximations," *Opt. Commun.*, vol. 53, pp. 213-216, Mar. 15, 1985.

[Car70] W. H. Carter, "Computational reconstruction of scattering objects from holograms," *J. Opt. Soc. Amer.*, vol. 60, pp. 306-314, Mar. 1970.

[Car74] W. H. Carter and P. C. Ho, "Reconstruction of inhomogeneous scattering objects from holograms," *Appl. Opt.*, vol. 13, pp. 162-172, Jan. 1974.

[Che60] L. A. Chernov, *Wave Propagation in a Random Medium*. New York, NY: McGraw-Hill, 1960.

[Col83] D. Colton and R. Kress, *Integral Equation Methods in Scattering Theory*. New York, NY: John Wiley and Sons, 1983.

[Dev78] A. J. Devaney, "Nonuniqueness in the inverse scattering problem," *J. Math. Phys.*, vol. 19, pp. 1525-1531, 1978.

[Dev82] ——, "A filtered backpropagation algorithm for diffraction tomography," *Ultrason. Imaging*, vol. 4, pp. 336-350, 1982.

[Dev83] ——, "A computer simulation study of diffraction tomography," *IEEE Trans. Biomed. Eng.*, vol. BME-30, pp. 377-386, July 1983.

[Dev84] ——, "Geophysical diffraction tomography," *IEEE Trans. Geological Science, Special Issue on Remote Sensing*, vol. GE-22, pp. 3-13, Jan. 1984.

[Fer79] A. F. Fercher, H. Bartelt, H. Becker, and E. Wiltschko, "Image formation by inversion of scattered data: Experiments and computational simulation," *Appl. Opt.*, vol. 18, pp. 2427-2439, 1979.

[Gag78] R. Gagliardi, *Introduction to Communications Engineering*. New York, NY: John Wiley and Sons, 1978.

[Goo68] J. W. Goodman, *Introduction to Fourier Optics*. San Francisco, CA: McGraw-Hill, 1968.

[Gre78] J. F. Greenleaf, S. K. Kenue, B. Rajagopalan, R. C. Bahn, and S. A. Johnson, "Breast imaging by ultrasonic computer-assisted tomography," in *Acoustical Imaging*, A. Metherell, Ed. New York, NY: Plenum Press, 1978.

[Hoc73] H. Hochstadt, *Integral Equations*. New York, NY: John Wiley and Sons, 1973.

[HoP76] P. C. Ho and W. H. Carter, "Structural measurement by inverse scattering in the first Born approximation," *Appl. Opt.*, vol. 15, pp. 313-314, Feb. 1976.

[Ish78] A. Ishimaru, *Wave Propagation and Scattering in Random Media*. New York, NY: Academic Press, 1978.

[Iwa75] K. Iwata and R. Nagata, "Calculation of refractive index distribution from interferograms using the Born and Rytov's approximations," *Japan. J. Appl. Phys.*, vol. 14, pp. 1921-1927, 1975.

[Joh83] S. A. Johnson and M. L. Tracy, "Inverse scattering solutions by a sinc basis, multiple source, moment method—Part I: Theory," *Ultrason. Imaging*, vol. 5, pp. 361-375, 1983.

[Kak85] A. C. Kak, "Tomographic imaging with diffracting and non-diffracting sources," in *Array Signal Processing*, S. Haykin, Ed. Englewood Cliffs, NJ: Prentice-Hall, 1985.

[Kav80] M. Kaveh, M. Soumekh, and R. K. Mueller, "Experimental results in ultrasonic diffraction tomography," in *Acoustical Imaging*, vol. 9, K. Wang, Ed. New York, NY: Plenum Press, 1980, pp. 433-450.

[Kav81] ——, "A comparison of Born and Rytov approximations in acoustic tomography," in *Acoustical Imaging*, vol. 11, J. P. Powers, Ed. New York, NY: Plenum Press, 1981, pp. 325-335.

[Kav82] ——, "Tomographic imaging via wave equation inversion," in *Proc. Int. Conf. on Acoustics, Speech and Signal Processing*, May 1982, pp. 1553-1556.

[Kav84] M. Kaveh, M. Soumekh, and J. F. Greenleaf, "Signal processing for diffraction tomography," *IEEE Trans. Sonics Ultrason.*, vol. SU-31, pp. 230-239, July 1984.

[Kav86] M. Kaveh and M. Soumekh, "Computer-assisted diffraction tomography," in *Image Recovery, Theory and Applications*, H. Stark, Ed. New York, NY: Academic Press, 1986.

[Kel69] J. B. Keller, "Accuracy and validity of the Born and Rytov approximations," *J. Opt. Soc. Amer.*, vol. 59, pp. 1003-1004, 1969.

[Ken82] S. K. Kenue and J. F. Greenleaf, "Limited angle multifrequency diffraction tomography," *IEEE Trans. Sonics Ultrason.*, vol. SU-29, pp. 213-217, July 1982.

[LuZ84] Z. Q. Lu, M. Kaveh, and R. K. Mueller, "Diffraction tomography using beam waves: Z-average reconstruction," *Ultrason. Imaging*, vol. 6, pp. 95-102, Jan. 1984.

[McG82] R. McGowan and R. Kuc, "A direct relation between a signal time series and its unwrapped phase," *IEEE Trans. Acoust. Speech Signal Processing*, vol. ASSP-30, pp. 719-726, Oct. 1982.

[Mor53] P. M. Morse and H. Feshbach, *Methods of Theoretical Physics*. New York, NY: McGraw-Hill, 1953.

[Mor68] P. M. Morse and K. U. Ingard, *Theoretical Acoustics*. New York, NY: McGraw-Hill, 1968.

[Mue79] R. K. Mueller, M. Kaveh, and G. Wade, "Reconstructive tomography and applications to ultrasonics," *Proc. IEEE*, vol. 67, pp. 567-587, 1979.

[Mue80] R. K. Mueller, M. Kaveh, and R. D. Iverson, "A new approach to acoustic tomography using diffraction techniques," in *Acoustical Imaging*, A. Metherall, Ed. New York, NY: Plenum Press, 1980, pp. 615-628.

[Nah81] D. Nahamoo, C. R. Crawford, and A. C. Kak, "Design constraints and reconstruction algorithms for transverse-continuous-rotate CT scanners," *IEEE Trans. Biomed. Eng.*, vol. BME-28, pp. 79-97, 1981.

[Nah82] D. Nahamoo and A. C. Kak, "Ultrasonic diffraction imaging," TR-EE 82-20, School of Electrical Engineering, Purdue Univ., Lafayette, IN, 1982.

[Nah84] D. Nahamoo, S. X. Pan, and A. C. Kak, "Synthetic aperture diffraction tomography and its interpolation-free computer implementation," *IEEE Trans. Sonics Ultrason.*, vol. SU-31, pp. 218-229, July 1984.

[Nas81] M. Z. Nashed, "Operato-theoretic and computational approaches to illposed problems with application to antenna theory," *IEEE Trans. Antennas Propagat.*, vol. AP-29, pp. 220-231, 1981.

[Nor81] S. J. Norton and M. Linzer, "Ultrasonic reflectivity imaging in three dimensions: Exact inverse scattering solutions for plane, cylindrical and spherical apertures," *IEEE Trans. Biomed. Eng.*, vol. BME-28, pp. 202-220, 1981.

[OCo78] B. T. O'Connor and T. S. Huang, "Techniques for determining the stability of two-dimensional recursive filters and their application to image restoration," TR-EE 78-18, School of Electrical Engineering, Purdue Univ., Lafayette, IN, pp. 6-24, 1978.

[Pan83] S. X. Pan and A. C. Kak, "A computational study of reconstruction algorithms for diffraction tomography: Interpolation vs. filtered-backpropagation," *IEEE Trans. Acoust. Speech Signal Processing*, vol. ASSP-31, pp. 1262-1275, Oct. 1983.

[Sar81] T. K. Sarkar, D. D. Weiner, and V. K. Jain, "Some mathematical considerations in dealing with the inverse problem," *IEEE Trans. Antennas Propagat.*, vol. AP-29, pp. 373-379, 1981.

[Sla83] M. Slaney and A. C. Kak, "Diffraction tomography," *Proc. S.P.I.E.*, vol. 413, pp. 2-19, Apr. 1983.

[Sla84] M. Slaney, A. C. Kak, and L. E. Larsen, "Limitations of imaging with first order diffraction tomography," *IEEE Trans. Microwave Theory Tech.*, vol. MTT-32, pp. 860-873, Aug. 1984.

[Sla85] M. Slaney and A. C. Kak, "Imaging with diffraction tomography," TR-EE 85-5, School of Electrical Engineering, Purdue Univ., Lafayette, IN, 1985.

[Sou83] M. Soumekh, M. Kaveh, and R. K. Mueller, "Algorithms and experimental results in acoustic tomography using Rytov's approximation," in *Proc. Int. Conf. on Acoustics, Speech and Signal Processing*, Apr. 1983, pp. 135-138.

[Sou84a] ——, "Fourier domain reconstruction methods with application to diffraction tomography," in *Acoustical Imaging*, vol. 13, M. Kaveh, R. K. Mueller, and J. F. Greenleaf, Eds. New York, NY: Plenum Press, 1984, pp. 17-30.

[Sou84b] M. Soumekh and M. Kaveh, "Image reconstruction from frequency domain data on arbitrary contours," in *Proc. Conf. on Acoustics, Speech and Signal Processing*, 1984, pp. 12A.2.1-12A.2.4.

[Sta81] H. Stark, J. W. Woods, I. Paul, and R. Hingorani, "Direct Fourier reconstruction in

[Tra83]   computer tomography," *IEEE Trans. Acoust. Speech Signal Processing,* vol. ASSP-29, pp. 237-244, 1981.

[Tra83]   M. L. Tracy and S. A. Johnson, "Inverse scattering solutions by a sinc basis, multiple source, moment method—Part II: Numerical evaluations," *Ultrason. Imaging,* vol. 5, pp. 376-392, 1983.

[Tri77]   J. M. Tribolet, "A new phase unwrapping algorithm," *IEEE Trans. Acoust. Speech Signal Processing,* vol. ASSP-25, pp. 170-177, Apr. 1977.

[Wee64]   W. L. Weeks, *Electromagnetic Theory for Engineering Applications.* New York, NY: John Wiley and Sons, Inc., 1964.

[Wol69]   E. Wolf, "Three-dimensional structure determination of semitransparent objects from holographic data," *Opt. Commun.,* vol. 1, pp. 153-156, 1969.

7 Algebraic Reconstruction Algorithms

An entirely different approach for tomographic imaging consists of assuming that the cross section consists of an array of unknowns, and then setting up algebraic equations for the unknowns in terms of the measured projection data. Although conceptually this approach is much simpler than the transform-based methods discussed in previous sections, for medical applications it lacks the accuracy and the speed of implementation. However, there are situations where it is not possible to measure a large number of projections, or the projections are not uniformly distributed over 180 or 360°, both these conditions being necessary requirements for the transform-based techniques to produce results with the accuracy desired in medical imaging. An example of such a situation is earth resources imaging using cross-borehole measurements discussed in Chapter 4. Problems of this type are sometimes more amenable to solution by algebraic techniques. Algebraic techniques are also useful when the energy propagation paths between the source and receiver positions are subject to ray bending on account of refraction, or when the energy propagation undergoes attenuation along ray paths as in emission CT. [Unfortunately, many imaging problems where refraction is encountered also suffer from diffraction effects (see Chap. 4).] As will be obvious from the discussion to follow, in algebraic methods it is essential to know ray paths that connect the corresponding transmitter and receiver positions. When refraction and diffraction effects are substantial (medium inhomogeneities exceed 10% of the average background value and the correlation length of these inhomogeneities is comparable to a wavelength), it becomes impossible to predict these ray paths. If algebraic techniques are applied under these conditions, we often obtain meaningless results.

If the refraction and diffraction effects are small (medium inhomogeneities are less than 2 to 3% of the average background value and the correlation width of these inhomogeneities is much greater than a wavelength), in some cases it is possible to combine algebraic techniques with digital ray tracing techniques [And82], [And84a], [And84b] and devise iterative procedures in which we first construct an image ignoring refraction, then trace rays connecting the corresponding transmitter and receiver locations through this distribution, and finally use these rays to construct a more accurate set of algebraic equations. Experimental verification of this iterative procedure for weakly refracting objects has been obtained [And84b].

Space limitations prevent us from discussing here the combined ray tracing and algebraic reconstruction algorithms. Our aim in this section is to merely introduce the reader to the algebraic approach for image reconstruction. First we will show how we may construct a set of linear equations whose unknowns are elements of the object cross section. The Kaczmarz method for solving these equations will then be presented. This will be followed by the various approximations that are used in this method to speed up its computer implementation.

7.1 Image and Projection Representation

In Fig. 7.1 we have superimposed a square grid on the image $f(x, y)$; we will assume that in each cell the function $f(x, y)$ is constant. Let f_j denote this constant value in the jth cell, and let N be the total number of cells. For algebraic techniques a ray is defined somewhat differently. A ray is now a "fat" line running through the (x, y)-plane. To illustrate this we have shaded the ith ray in Fig. 7.1, where each ray is of width τ. In most cases the ray width is approximately equal to the image cell width. A line integral will now be called a *ray-sum*.

Like the image, the projections will also be given a one-index representa-

Fig. 7.1: *In algebraic methods a square grid is superimposed over the unknown image. Image values are assumed to be constant within each cell of the grid. (From [Ros82].)*

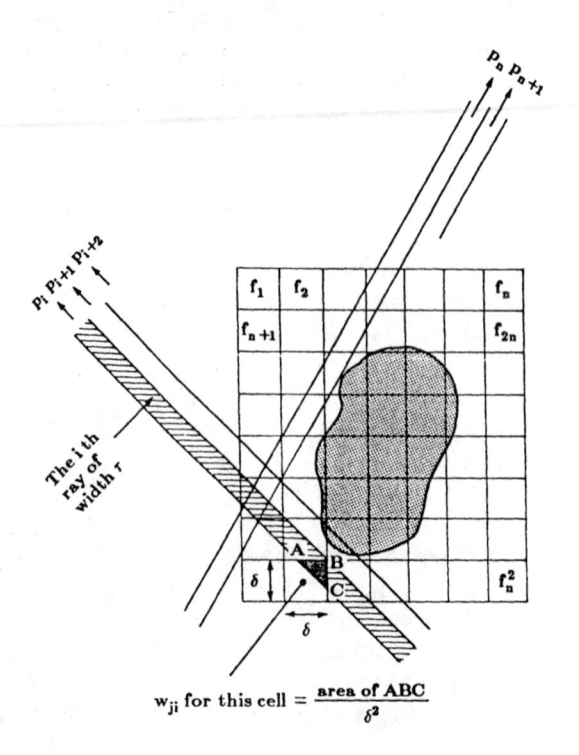

tion. Let p_i be the ray-sum measured with the ith ray as shown in Fig. 7.1. The relationship between the f_j's and p_i's may be expressed as

$$\sum_{j=1}^{N} w_{ij} f_j = p_i, \quad i = 1, 2, \cdots, M \quad (1)$$

where M is the total number of rays (in all the projections) and w_{ij} is the weighting factor that represents the contribution of the jth cell to the ith ray integral. The factor w_{ij} is equal to the fractional area of the jth image cell intercepted by the ith ray as shown for one of the cells in Fig. 7.1. Note that most of the w_{ij}'s are zero since only a small number of cells contribute to any given ray-sum.

If M and N were small, we could use conventional matrix theory methods to invert the system of equations in (1). However, in practice N may be as large as 65,000 (for 256 × 256 images), and, in most cases for images of this size, M will also have the same magnitude. For these values of M and N the size of the matrix $[w_{ij}]$ in (1) is 65,000 × 65,000 which precludes any possibility of direct matrix inversion. Of course, when noise is present in the measurement data and when $M < N$, even for small N it is not possible to use direct matrix inversion, and some least squares method may have to be used. When both M and N are large, such methods are also computationally impractical.

For large values of M and N there exist very attractive iterative methods for solving (1). These are based on the "method of projections" as first proposed by Kaczmarz [Kac37], and later elucidated further by Tanabe [Tan71]. To explain the computational steps involved in these methods, we first write (1) in an expanded form:

$$\begin{aligned} w_{11}f_1 + w_{12}f_2 + w_{13}f_3 + \cdots + w_{1N}f_N &= p_1 \\ w_{21}f_1 + w_{22}f_2 + \phantom{w_{13}f_3} + \cdots + w_{2N}f_N &= p_2 \\ &\vdots \\ w_{M1}f_1 + w_{M2}f_2 + \phantom{w_{13}f_3} + \cdots + w_{MN}f_N &= p_M. \end{aligned} \quad (2)$$

A grid representation with N cells gives an image N degrees of freedom. Therefore, an image, represented by $(f_1, f_2, \cdots, f_N)$, may be considered to be a single point in an N-dimensional space. In this space each of the above equations represents a hyperplane. When a unique solution to these equations exists, the intersection of all these hyperplanes is a single point giving that solution. This concept is further illustrated in Fig. 7.2 where, for the purpose of display, we have considered the case of only two variables f_1 and f_2 satisfying the following equations:

$$\begin{aligned} w_{11}f_1 + w_{12}f_2 &= p_1 \\ w_{21}f_1 + w_{22}f_2 &= p_2. \end{aligned} \quad (3)$$

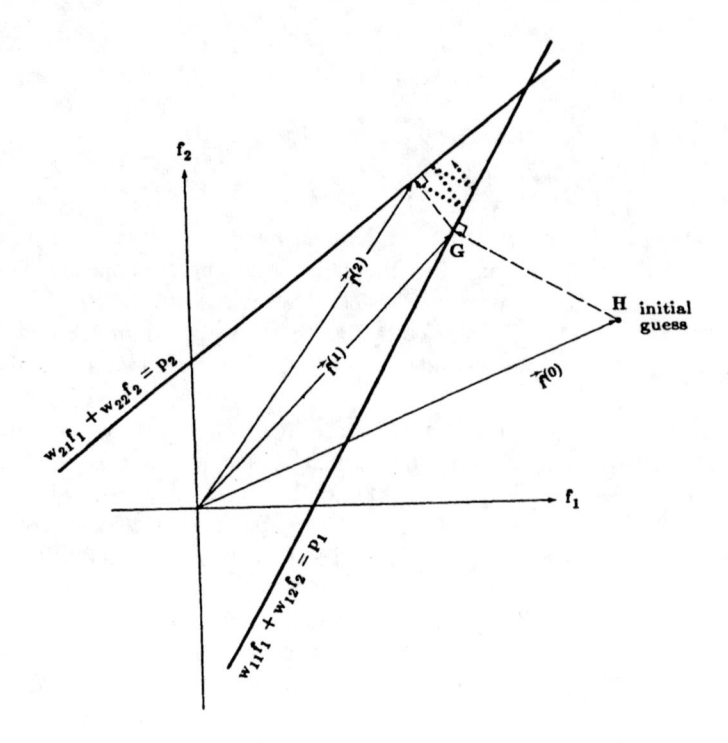

Fig. 7.2: *The Kaczmarz method of solving algebraic equations is illustrated for the case of two unknowns. One starts with some arbitrary initial guess and then projects onto the line corresponding to the first equation. The resulting point is now projected onto the line representing the second equation. If there are only two equations, this process is continued back and forth, as illustrated by the dots in the figure, until convergence is achieved. (From [Ros82].)*

The computational procedure for locating the solution in Fig. 7.2 consists of first starting with an initial guess, projecting this initial guess on the first line, reprojecting the resulting point on the second line, and then projecting back onto the first line, and so forth. If a unique solution exists, the iterations will always converge to that point.

For the computer implementation of this method, we first make an initial guess at the solution. This guess, denoted by $f_1^{(0)}, f_2^{(0)}, \cdots, f_N^{(0)}$, is represented vectorially by $\vec{f}^{(0)}$ in the N-dimensional space. In most cases, we simply assign a value of zero to all the f_i's. This initial guess is projected on the hyperplane represented by the first equation in (2) giving $\vec{f}^{(1)}$, as illustrated in Fig. 7.2 for the two-dimensional case. $\vec{f}^{(1)}$ is projected on the hyperplane represented by the second equation in (2) to yield $\vec{f}^{(2)}$ and so on. When $\vec{f}^{(i-1)}$ is projected on the hyperplane represented by the ith equation to yield $\vec{f}^{(i)}$, the process can be mathematically described by

$$\vec{f}^{(i)} = \vec{f}^{(i-1)} - \frac{(\vec{f}^{(i-1)} \cdot \vec{w}_i - p_i)}{\vec{w}_i \cdot \vec{w}_i} \vec{w}_i \qquad (4)$$

where $\vec{w}_i = (w_{i1}, w_{i2}, \cdots, w_{iN})$, and $\vec{w}_i \cdot \vec{w}_i$ is the dot product of $\vec{w}_i$ with itself. To see how (4) comes about we first write the first equation of (2) as

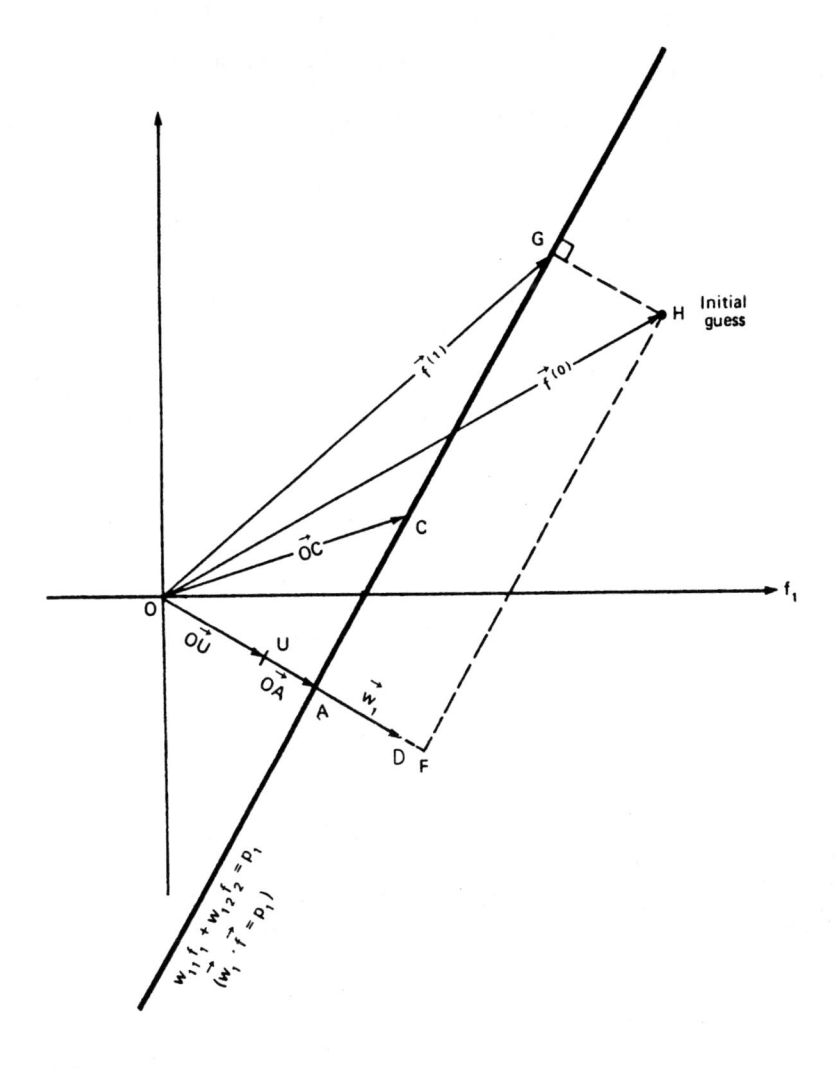

Fig. 7.3: *The hyperplane $\vec{w}_1 \cdot \vec{f} = p_1$ (represented by a line in this two-dimensional figure) is perpendicular to the vector $\vec{w}_1$. (From [Ros82].)*

follows:

$$\vec{w}_1 \cdot \vec{f} = p_1. \qquad (5)$$

The hyperplane represented by this equation is perpendicular to the vector $\vec{w}_1$. This is illustrated in Fig. 7.3, where the vector $\overrightarrow{OD}$ represents $\vec{w}_1$. This equation simply says that the projection of a vector $\overrightarrow{OC}$ (for any point C on the hyperplane) on the vector $\vec{w}_1$ is of constant length. The unit vector $\overrightarrow{OU}$ along $\vec{w}_1$ is given by

$$\overrightarrow{OU} = \frac{\vec{w}_1}{\sqrt{\vec{w}_1 \cdot \vec{w}_1}} \qquad (6)$$

and the perpendicular distance of the hyperplane from the origin, which is

ALGEBRAIC RECONSTRUCTION ALGORITHMS

equal to the length of $\overrightarrow{OA}$ in Fig. 7.3, is given by $\overrightarrow{OC} \cdot \overrightarrow{OU}$:

$$|\overrightarrow{OA}| = \overrightarrow{OU} \cdot \overrightarrow{OC} = \frac{1}{\sqrt{\vec{w}_1 \cdot \vec{w}_1}} (\vec{w}_1 \cdot \overrightarrow{OC})$$

$$= \frac{1}{\sqrt{\vec{w}_1 \cdot \vec{w}_1}} (\vec{w}_1 \cdot \vec{f}) = \frac{p_1}{\sqrt{\vec{w}_1 \cdot \vec{w}_1}}. \quad (7)$$

Now to get $\vec{f}^{(1)}$ we have to subtract from $\vec{f}^{(0)}$ the vector $\overrightarrow{HG}$:

$$\vec{f}^{(1)} = \vec{f}^{(0)} - \overrightarrow{HG} \quad (8)$$

where the length of the vector $\overrightarrow{HG}$ is given by

$$|\overrightarrow{HG}| = |\overrightarrow{OF}| - |\overrightarrow{OA}|$$
$$= \vec{f}^{(0)} \cdot \overrightarrow{OU} - |\overrightarrow{OA}|. \quad (9)$$

Substituting (6) and (7) in this equation, we get

$$|\overrightarrow{HG}| = \frac{\vec{f}^{(0)} \cdot \vec{w}_1 - p_1}{\sqrt{\vec{w}_1 \cdot \vec{w}_1}}. \quad (10)$$

Since the direction of $\overrightarrow{HG}$ is the same as that of the unit vector $\overrightarrow{OU}$, we can write

$$\overrightarrow{HG} = |\overrightarrow{HG}| \overrightarrow{OU} = \frac{\vec{f}^{(0)} \cdot \vec{w}_1 - p_1}{\vec{w}_1 \cdot \vec{w}_1} \vec{w}_1. \quad (11)$$

Substituting (11) in (8), we get (4).

As mentioned before, the computational procedure for algebraic reconstruction consists of starting with an initial guess for the solution, taking successive projections on the hyperplanes represented by the equations in (2), eventually yielding $\vec{f}^{(M)}$. In the next iteration, $\vec{f}^{(M)}$ is projected on the hyperplane represented by the first equation in (2), and then successively onto the rest of the hyperplanes in (2), to yield $\vec{f}^{(2M)}$, and so on. Tanabe [Tan71] has shown that if there exists a unique solution $\vec{f}_s$ to the system of equations (2), then

$$\lim_{k \to \infty} \vec{f}^{(kM)} = \vec{f}_s. \quad (12)$$

A few comments about the convergence of the algorithm are in order here. If in Fig. 7.2 the two hyperplanes are perpendicular to each other, the reader may easily show that given for an initial guess any point in the (f_1, f_2)-plane, it is possible to arrive at the correct solution in only two steps like (4). On the other hand, if the two hyperplanes have only a very small angle between them, k in (12) may acquire a large value (depending upon the initial guess) before the correct solution is reached. Clearly the angles between the hyperplanes considerably influence the rate of convergence to the solution. If the M hyperplanes in (2) could be made orthogonal with respect to one another, the correct solution would be arrived at with only one pass through the M equations (assuming a unique solution does exist). Although theoretically such orthogonalization is possible using, for example, the Gram-Schmidt procedure, in practice it is computationally not feasible. Full orthogonalization will also tend to enhance the effects of the ever present measurement noise in the final solution. Ramakrishnan *et al.* [Ram79] have suggested a pairwise orthogonalization scheme which is computationally easier to implement and at the same time considerably increases the speed of convergence. A simpler technique, first proposed in [Hou72] and studied in [Sla85], is to carefully choose the order in which the hyperplanes are considered. Since each hyperplane represents a distinct ray integral, it is quite likely that adjacent ray integrals (and thus hyperplanes) will be nearly parallel. By choosing hyperplanes representing widely separated ray integrals, it is possible to improve the rate of convergence of the Kaczmarz approach.

A not uncommon situation in image reconstruction is that of an overdetermined system in the presence of measurement noise. That is, we may have $M > N$ in (2) and $p_1, p_2, \cdots, p_m$ corrupted by noise. No unique solution exists in this case. In Fig. 7.4 we have shown a two-variable system represented by three "noisy" hyperplanes. The broken line represents the course of the solution as we successively implement (4). Now the "solution" doesn't converge to a unique point, but will oscillate in the neighborhood of the intersections of the hyperplanes.

When $M < N$ a unique solution of the set of linear equations in (2) doesn't exist, and, in fact, an infinite number of solutions are possible. For example, suppose we have only the first of the two equations in (3) to use for calculating the two unknowns f_1 and f_2; then the solution can be anywhere on the line corresponding to this equation. Given the initial guess $\vec{f}^{(0)}$ (see Fig. 7.3), the best one could probably do under the circumstances would be to draw a projection from $\vec{f}^{(0)}$ on this line, and call the resulting $\vec{f}^{(1)}$ a solution. Note that the solution obtained in this manner corresponds to that point on the line which is closest to the initial guess. This result has been rigorously proved by Tanabe [Tan71] who has shown that when $M < N$, the iterative approach described above converges to a solution, call it $\vec{f}_s'$, such that $|\vec{f}^{(0)} - \vec{f}_s'|$ is minimized.

Besides its computational efficiency, another attractive feature of the iterative approach presented here is that it is now possible to incorporate into the solution some types of a priori information about the image one is reconstructing. For example, if it is known a priori that the image $f(x, y)$ is nonnegative, then in each of the solutions $\vec{f}^{(k)}$, successively obtained by using (4), one may set the negative components equal to zero. One may similarly incorporate the information that $f(x, y)$ is zero outside a certain area, if this is known.

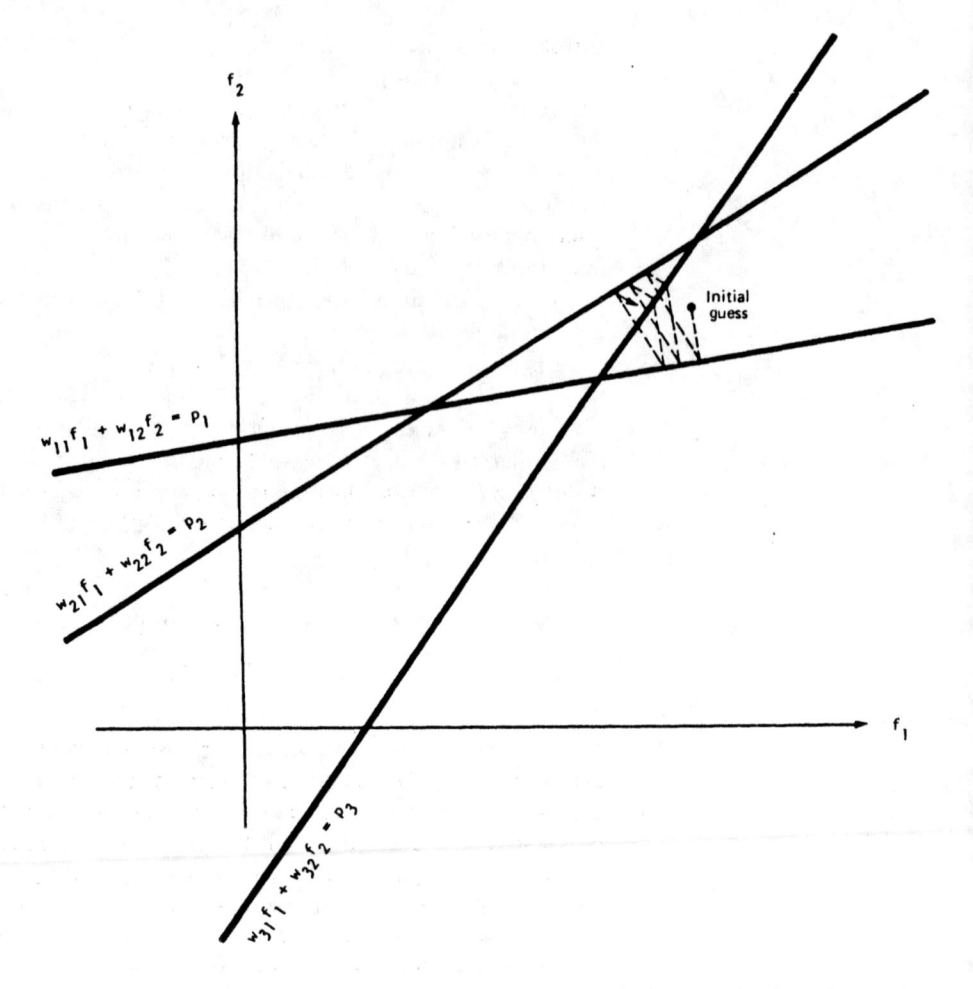

Fig. 7.4: *Illustrated here is the case when the number of equations is greater than the number of unknowns. The lines don't intersect at a single unique point, because the observations p_1, p_2, p_3 have been assumed to be corrupted by noise. No unique solution exists in this case, and the final solution will oscillate in the neighborhood of intersections of the three lines. (From [Ros82].)*

In applications requiring a large number of views and where large-sized reconstructions are made, the difficulty with using (4) can be in the calculation, storage, and fast retrieval of the weight coefficients w_{ij}. Consider the case where we wish to reconstruct an image on a 100×100 grid from 100 projections with 150 rays in each projection. The total number of weights, w_{ij}, needed in this case is 10^8, which is an enormous number and can pose problems in fast storage and retrieval in applications where reconstruction speed is important. This problem is somewhat eased by making approximations, such as considering w_{ij} to be only a function of the perpendicular distance between the center of the ith ray and the center of the jth cell. This perpendicular distance can then be computed at run time.

To get around the implementation difficulties caused by the weight coefficients, a myriad of other algebraic approaches have also been suggested, many of which are approximations to (4). To discuss some of the more implementable approximations, we first recast (4) in a slightly different form:

$$f_j^{(i)} = f_j^{(i-1)} + \frac{p_i - q_i}{\sum_{k=1}^{N} w_{ik}^2} w_{ij} \qquad (13)$$

where

$$q_i = \vec{f}^{(i-1)} \cdot \vec{w}_i \qquad (14)$$

$$= \sum_{k=1}^{N} f_k^{(i-1)} w_{ik}. \qquad (15)$$

These equations say that when we project the $(i-1)$th solution onto the ith hyperplane [ith equation in (2)] the gray level of the jth element, whose current value is $f_j^{(i-1)}$, is obtained by correcting its current value by $\Delta f_j^{(i)}$, where

$$\Delta f_j^{(i)} = f_j^{(i)} - f_j^{(i-1)} = \frac{p_i - q_i}{\sum_{k=1}^{N} w_{ik}^2} w_{ij}. \qquad (16)$$

Note that while p_i is the measured ray-sum along the ith ray, q_i may be considered to be the computed ray-sum for the same ray based on the $(i-1)$th solution for the image gray levels. The correction Δf_j to the jth cell is obtained by first calculating the difference between the measured ray-sum and the computed ray-sum, normalizing this difference by $\sum_{k=1}^{N} w_{ik}^2$, and then assigning this value to all the image cells in the ith ray, each assignment being weighted by the corresponding w_{ij}.

With the preliminaries presented above, we will now discuss three different computer implementations of algebraic algorithms. These are represented by the acronyms ART, SIRT, and SART.

7.2 ART (Algebraic Reconstruction Techniques)

In many ART implementations the w_{ik}'s in (16) are simply replaced by 1's and 0's, depending upon whether the center of the kth image cell is within the ith ray. This makes the implementation easier because such a decision can easily be made at computer run time. In this case the denominator in (16) is given by $\sum_{k=1}^{N} w_{ik}^2 = N_i$ which is the number of image cells whose centers are within the ith ray. The correction to the jth image cell from the ith equation in (2) may now be written as

$$\Delta f_j^{(i)} = \frac{p_i - q_i}{N_i} \qquad (17)$$

for all the cells whose centers are within the ith ray. We are essentially smearing back the difference $(p_i - q_i)/N_i$ over these image cells. In (17), q_i's are calculated using the expression in (15), except that one now uses the binary approximation for w_{ik}'s.

The approximation in (17), although easy to implement, often leads to artifacts in the reconstructed images, especially if N_i isn't a good approximation to the denominator. Superior reconstructions may be obtained if (17) is replaced by

$$\Delta f_j^{(i)} = \frac{p_i}{L_i} - \frac{q_i}{N_i} \qquad (18)$$

where L_i is the length (normalized by δ, see Fig. 7.1) of the ith ray through the reconstruction region.

ART reconstructions usually suffer from *salt and pepper noise*, which is caused by the inconsistencies introduced in the set of equations by the approximations commonly used for w_{ik}'s. The result is that the computed ray-sums in (15) are usually poor approximations to the corresponding measured ray-sums. The effect of such inconsistencies is exacerbated by the fact that as each equation corresponding to a ray in a projection is taken up, it changes some of the pixels just altered by the preceding equation in the same projection. The SIRT algorithm described briefly below also suffers from these inconsistencies in the forward process [appearing in the computation of q_i's in (16)], but by eliminating the continual and competing pixel update as each new equation is taken up, it results in smoother reconstructions.

It is possible to reduce the effects of this noise in ART reconstructions by relaxation, in which we update a pixel by $\alpha \cdot \Delta f_j^{(i)}$, where α is less than 1. In some cases, the relaxation parameter α is made a function of the iteration number; that is, it becomes progressively smaller with increase in the number of iterations. The resulting improvements in the quality of reconstruction are usually at the expense of convergence.

7.3 SIRT (Simultaneous Iterative Reconstructive Technique)

In this approach, which at the expense of slower convergence usually leads to better looking images than those produced by ART, we again use (17) or (18) to compute the change $\Delta f_j^{(i)}$ in the jth pixel caused by the ith equation in (2). However, the value of the jth cell isn't changed at this time. Before making any changes, we go through all the equations, and then only at the end of each iteration are the cell values changed, the change for each cell being the average value of all the computed changes for that cell. This constitutes one iteration of the algorithm. In the second iteration, we go back to the first equation in (2) and the process is repeated.

7.4 SART (Simultaneous Algebraic Reconstruction Technique)

We will now discuss a variation on the algebraic approaches discussed above that seems to combine the best of ART and SIRT. This technique, first reported in [And84a], yields reconstructions of good quality and numerical accuracy in only one iteration. Here are the main features of SART: First, to reduce errors in the approximation of ray integrals of a smooth image by finite sums, the traditional pixel basis is abandoned in favor of bilinear elements. Also, for a circular reconstruction region, only partial weights are assigned to the first and last picture elements on the individual rays. To further reduce the noise resulting from the unavoidable but now presumably considerably smaller inconsistencies with real projection data, the correction terms are simultaneously applied for all the rays in one projection; this is in contrast with the ray-by-ray updates in ART. In addition, a heuristic procedure is used to improve the quality of reconstructions: a longitudinal Hamming window is used to emphasize the corrections applied near the middle of a ray relative to those applied near its ends.

In what follows we will describe in more detail the individual steps outlined above. The contribution that each step makes in improving the overall accuracy of the proposed procedure will be illustrated with reconstructions of the test image of Fig. 7.5. Note that this image differs slightly from a similar image in Chapter 3 by the presence of a "subdural hematoma," which is a small ellipse right next to the "skull" in the lower right-hand part. All these reconstructions were carried out on a 128 × 128 sampling lattice with 100 projections of 127 rays each.

Fig. 7.5: *(a) The Shepp and Logan head phantom with a subdural hematoma. (b) The gray level distribution of the Shepp and Logan phantom. (From [Kak84].)*

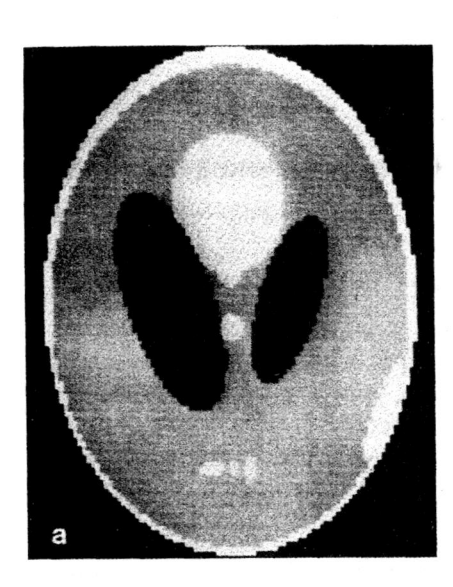

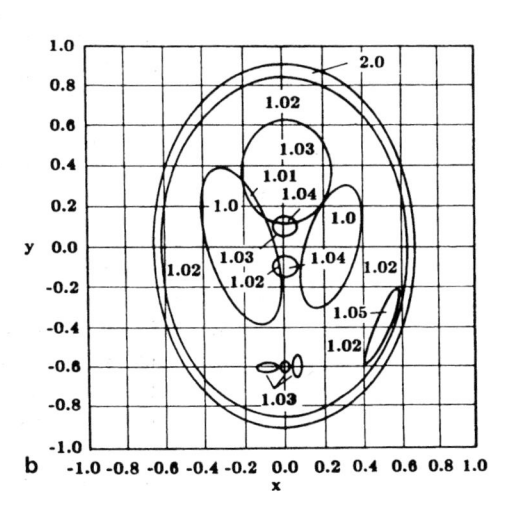

7.4.1 Modeling the Forward Projection Process

In (1), projection data were modeled by

$$p_i = \sum_{j=1}^{N} w_{ij} f_j, \quad i = 1, 2, \cdots, M. \tag{19}$$

This is a good model for the projection process if for w_{ij}'s we use the theoretically dictated values—which, as mentioned before, is hard to do for various reasons.

To seek alternative methods for modeling the projection process, the relationship between a continuous image and the discrete projection data can be expressed by the following general form

$$p_i = R_i f(x, y) = \int_{-\infty}^{\infty} \int_{-\infty}^{\infty} f(x, y) \delta(r_i(x, y)) \, dx \, dy \tag{20}$$

where

$$r_i(x, y) = 0 \tag{21}$$

is the equation of the ith ray and R_i is the projection operator along the ray. The integral on the right-hand side serves as the definition of the projection operator.

Now suppose we assume that in an expansion for the image $f(x, y)$, we use basis functions $b_j(x, y)$ and that a good approximation to $f(x, y)$ is obtained by using N of them. This assumption can be represented mathematically by

$$f(x, y) \approx \hat{f}(x, y) \equiv \sum_{j=1}^{N} g_j b_j(x, y) \tag{22}$$

where g_j's are the coefficients of expansion; they form a finite set of numbers which describe the image $f(x, y)$ relative to the chosen basis set $b_j(x, y)$.

Substituting (22) in (20), we can write for the forward process

$$p_i = R_i f(x, y) \approx R_i \hat{f}(x, y) = \sum_{j=1}^{N} g_j R_i b_j(x, y) = \sum_{j=1}^{N} g_j a_{ij} \tag{23}$$

where a_{ij} represents the line integral of $b_j(x, y)$ along the ith ray. This equation has the same basic form as (1), yet it is more general in the sense that g_j's aren't constrained to be image gray level values over an array of points. Of course, the form here reduces to (1) if for b_j's we use the following pixel basis that is obtained by dividing the image frame into N identical subsquares; these are referred to as pixels and identified by the index j for $1 \leq j \leq N$:

$$b_j(x, y) = \begin{cases} 1 & \text{inside the } j\text{th pixel} \\ 0 & \text{everywhere else.} \end{cases} \tag{24}$$

In keeping with the nature of f_j's in (1), g_j's with these basis functions represent the average of $f(x, y)$ over the jth pixel and $R_i b_j(x, y)$ represents the length of the intersection of the ith ray with the jth pixel. Although (20) implies rays of zero width, if we now associate a finite width with each ray, the elements of the projection matrix will represent the areas of intersection of these ray strips with the pixels.

In SART, superior reconstructions are obtained by using a model of the forward projection process that is more accurate than what can be obtained by the choice of pixel basis functions—this is done by using bilinear elements which are the simplest higher order basis functions. The basis functions obtained from bilinear elements are pyramid shaped, each with a support extending over a square region the size of four pixels. It can be shown that the g_j's appearing in (22) for the case of bilinear elements are the sample values of the image function $f(x, y)$ on a square lattice. It can further be shown that whereas the pixel basis leads to a discontinuous image representation, the bilinear elements allow a continuous form of $\hat{f}(x, y)$ to be regenerated for computation. However, finding the exact ray integrals across such bilinear elements [as called for by $R_i b_j(x, y)$ in (23)] for a large number of rays is a time-consuming task and we will use an approximation.

Rather than try to find separately the individual coefficients a_{ij} for a particular ray, we approximate the overall ray integral $R_i \hat{f}(x, y)$ by a finite sum involving a set of M_i equidistant points $\{\hat{f}(s_{im})\}$, for $1 \leq m \leq M_i$ [Lyt80] (see Fig. 7.6):

$$p_i \approx \sum_{m=1}^{M_i} \hat{f}(s_{im}) \Delta s. \qquad (25)$$

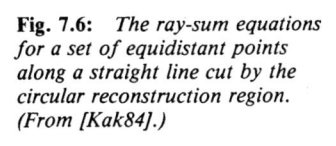

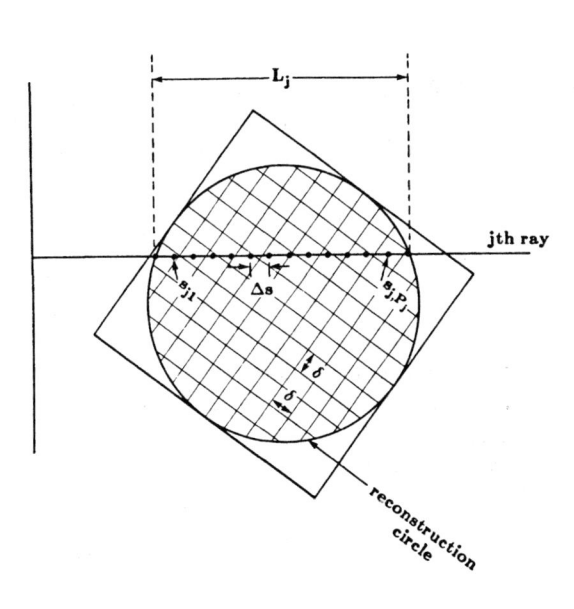

Fig. 7.6: *The ray-sum equations for a set of equidistant points along a straight line cut by the circular reconstruction region. (From [Kak84].)*

The value $\hat{f}(s_{im})$ is determined from the values g_j of $f(x, y)$ on the four neighboring points of the sampling lattice, i.e., by bilinear interpolation. We write

$$\hat{f}(s_{im}) = \sum_{j=1}^{N} d_{ijm} g_j \quad \text{for } m = 1, 2, \cdots, M_i. \tag{26}$$

The coefficient d_{ijm} is therefore the contribution that is made by the jth image sample to the mth point on the ith ray. Combining (25) and (26), we obtain an approximation to the ray integral p_i as a linear function of the image samples g_j:

$$p_i = \sum_{m=1}^{M_i} \sum_{j=1}^{N} d_{ijm} g_j \Delta s \tag{27}$$

$$= \sum_{j=1}^{N} \sum_{m=1}^{M_i} d_{ijm} g_j \Delta s \quad \text{for } 1 \leq i \leq J \tag{28}$$

$$= \sum_{j=1}^{N} a_{ij} g_j \tag{29}$$

where the coefficients a_{ij} represent the net effect of the linear transformations. They are determined as the sum of the contributions from different points along the ray:

$$a_{ij} = \sum_{m=1}^{M_i} d_{ijm} \Delta s. \tag{30}$$

Therefore, a_{ij} is proportional to the sum of contributions made by the jth image sample to all the points on the ith ray. It is important to the overall accuracy of the model that for $m = 1$ and for $m = M_i$, i.e., for the first and last points of the ray within the reconstruction circle, the weights are adjusted so that $\sum_{j=1}^{N} a_{ij}$ equals the actual physical length L_i.

One certainly has latitude about selecting the step size Δs; setting it equal to half the spacing of the sampling lattice provides a good trade-off between the accuracy of representation and computational cost.

7.4.2 Implementation of the Reconstruction Algorithm

As mentioned before, the results of SART implementation will be shown on 128 × 128 matrices using 100 projections, each with 127 rays. In the model of (29), this corresponds to $N = 16,384$ picture elements and an overall number of rays $I = 12,700$. Note that the system of equations is underdetermined by about 25%, but then the reconstruction circle covers only about 75% of the area of the square sampling lattice.

With the a_{ij}'s determined by the method just described, the reader will now be taken through a series of steps that are part of the SART implementation.

First, it will be shown that even with the superior forward projection modeling by the use of bilinear elements, one doesn't want to carry out a sequential implementation of the reconstruction algorithm.

A sequential implementation can be carried out by using the update formula of (4), reexpressed here in terms of SART symbols:

$$\vec{g}^{(k+1)} = \vec{g}^{(k)} + \vec{a}_i \frac{p_i - \vec{a}_i^T \vec{g}^{(k)}}{\vec{a}_i^T \vec{a}_i} \quad (31)$$

where $\vec{a}_i$ denotes the ith row vector of the array a_{ij}. As described before, the estimate $\vec{g}^{(k)}$ of the image vector is updated after each ray has been considered. We set the initial estimate $\vec{g}^{(0)}$ to zero, and we say that one iteration of the algebraic reconstruction technique is completed when all I rays, i.e., all I ray-sum equations, have been used exactly once. Owing to reasons discussed in Section 7.1, for sequential processing the projection data are ordered in such a manner that the angle between the projections considered successively is kept large; for the reconstructions shown here that were obtained with sequential updating, this angle was 73.8°.

Fig. 7.7(a) illustrates the reconstruction of the test image for one iteration of the sequential implementation. In order to avoid streak artifacts in the final image, the correction terms for the first few projections are de-emphasized relative to those for projections considered later on. The image has been thresholded to the gray level range 0.95–1.05 to illustrate the finer detail. Note that even the larger structures are buried in the salt and pepper noise present when no form of relaxation or smoothing is used. Fig. 7.7(b) shows a line plot through the three small tumors of the phantom (the profile shown is along the line $y = -0.605$). We observe that the amplitude variations of the noise largely exceed the density differences characterizing these structures.

Fig. 7.7: *Reconstruction from one iteration of sequential ART. (a) Image. (b) Line plot through the three small tumors (for $y = -0.605$). (From [And84a].)*

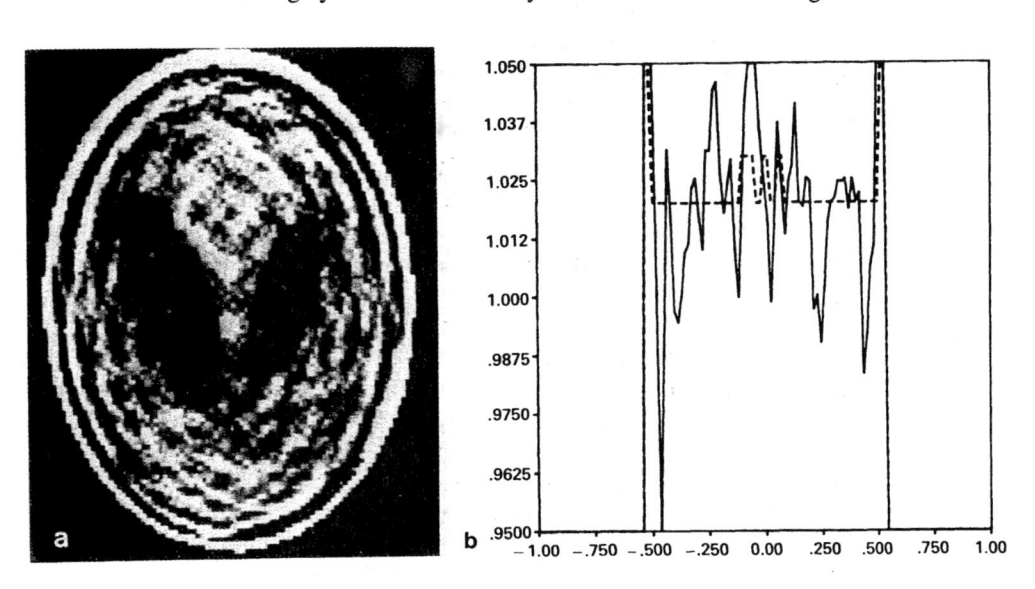

ALGEBRAIC RECONSTRUCTION ALGORITHMS

It will now be shown that superior results are obtained if instead of sequentially updating pixels on a ray-by-ray basis we simultaneously apply to a pixel the average of the corrections generated by all the rays in a projection. Stated in a bit more detail, this is what we want to do: For the first ray in a projection we compute as before the corrections to be made at every pixel. Instead of actually applying these corrections, we store them in a separate array to be called the correction array (the size of which is the same as that of the image array). Then we take up the next ray and add the pixel updates generated by this ray to the correction array. And then the next ray, and so on. After we are through all the rays in a projection, we add the correction array (or some fraction thereof) to the image array. This entire process is repeated with every projection. Fig. 7.8(a) illustrates the reconstruction obtained with this method. The precise formula that was used in the reconstruction in Fig. 7.8 for updating the pixel values can be stated as follows:

$$g_j^{(k+1)} = g_j^{(k)} + \frac{\sum_i \left[a_{ij} \frac{p_i - \vec{a}_i^T \vec{g}^{(k)}}{\sum_{j=1}^N a_{ij}} \right]}{\sum_i a_{ij}} \tag{32}$$

where the summation with respect to i is over the rays intersecting the jth image element for a given scan direction.

Compared to the reconstruction of Fig. 7.7 for the sequential scheme, the simultaneous method offers a reduction in the amplitude of the noise. In addition, the noise in the reconstructed image has become more slowly

Fig. 7.8: *Reconstruction from one iteration of SART. (a) Image. (b) Line plot through the three small tumors (for y = −0.605). (From [And84a].)*

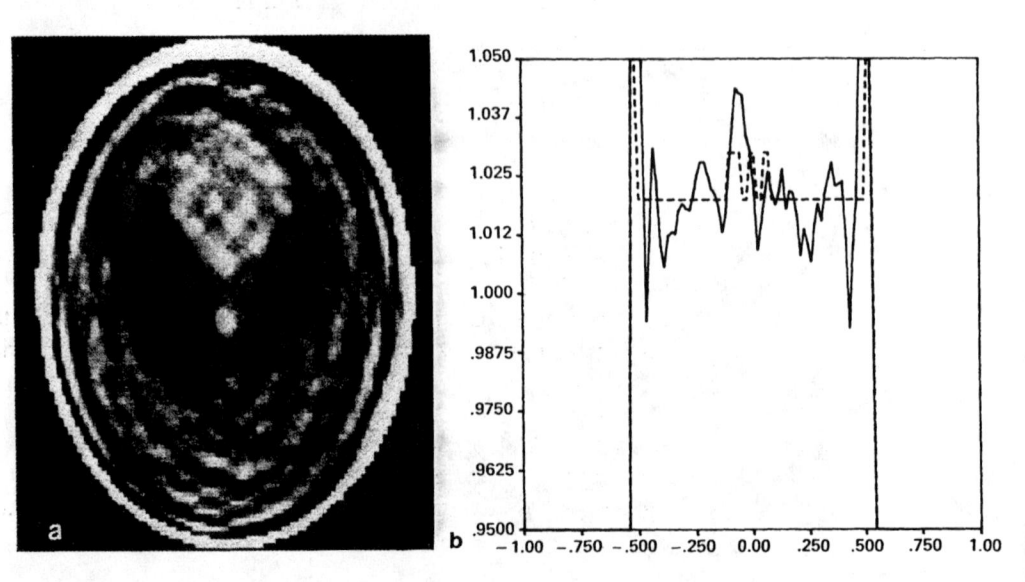

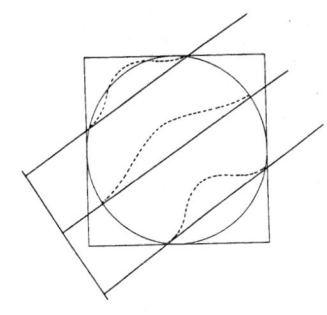

Fig. 7.9: *The longitudinal Hamming window for a set of straight rays. (From [And84a].)*

undulating compared to the previous salt and pepper appearance. This technique maintains the rapid convergence of ART-type algorithms while at the same time it has the noise suppressing features of SIRT. As with SIRT, the simultaneous implementation does require the storage of an additional array for the correction terms.

The last step, heuristic in nature, in SART consists of modifying the back-distribution of correction terms by a longitudinal Hamming window. The idea of the window is illustrated in Fig. 7.9. The uniform back-distribution according to the coefficients a_{ij} is replaced by a weighted version. This corresponds to replacing the correction term

$$a_{ij} \frac{p_i - \vec{a}_i^T \vec{g}^{(k)}}{\sum_{j=1}^{N} a_{ij}} \qquad (33)$$

in (32) by a weighted correction term

$$t_{ij} \frac{p_i - \vec{a}_i^T \vec{g}^{(k)}}{\sum_{j=1}^{N} a_{ij}} \qquad (34)$$

where the weighting coefficients t_{ij} are given by [compare with (30)]

$$t_{ij} = \sum_{m=1}^{M_i} h_{im} d_{ijm} \Delta s. \qquad (35)$$

The sequence h_{im}, for $1 \leq m \leq M_i$, is a Hamming window of length M_i. Note that the length of the window varies according to the number of points M_i describing the part of the ray inside the reconstruction circle.

The weighted back-distribution of corrections emphasizes the central portions of rays in relation to portions closer to the periphery. Fig. 7.10 illustrates a reconstruction of the test image after one iteration with the longitudinal window in conjunction with the simultaneous scheme previously described. We see an improvement over the reconstructions of Figs. 7.7 and 7.8: the noise is practically gone and all the structures can be fairly well distinguished. If we hadn't applied the corrections in a simultaneous scheme but incorporated the longitudinal Hamming window only for the sequential implementation, we would have arrived at the noisy reconstruction illustrated in Fig. 7.11.

An important question that remains to be answered is: What happens when we go through iterations with, say, the simultaneous implementation; meaning that after we have made a reconstruction by going through all the projections once, we go through them all once again using the reconstruction of Fig. 7.10 as our initial solution; and then continue iterating in like fashion?

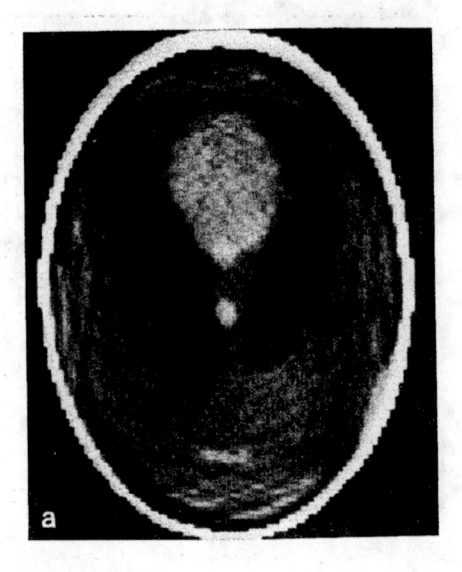

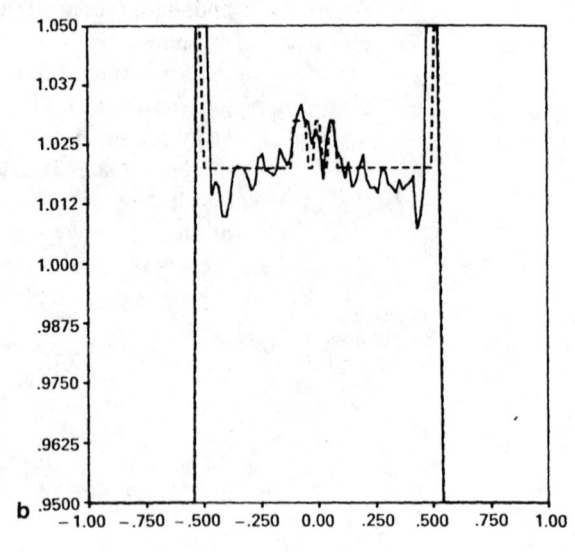

Fig. 7.10: *Reconstruction from one iteration of SART with a longitudinal Hamming window. (a) Image. (b) Line plot through the three small tumors (for y = −0.605). (From [And84a].)*

In Figs. 7.12 and 7.13, we have shown the reconstructions obtained with two and three iterations, respectively. As is evident from the reconstructions, we do gain more contrast, although at the cost of increased salt and pepper noise. All reconstructions shown represent the raw output from the algorithms with no postprocessing applied to suppress noise.

For the purpose of comparison, we have included in Fig. 7.14 the reconstruction obtained by using a convolution-backprojection algorithm. Comparing this with Fig. 7.10, we see that the SART reconstruction with one iteration is quite similar, although with further iterations, as displayed in Figs. 7.12 and 7.13, we see an increased amplitude of the salt and pepper noise, which is probably an indication of remaining inconsistencies in the model used for the forward projection process.

7.5 Bibliographic Notes

The earliest expositions on algebraic reconstruction were by Gordon *et al.* [Gor70], [Gor71], [Gor74], Herman *et al.* [Her71], [Her73], [Her77], and Budinger and Gullberg [Bud74]. The reader is also referred to the book by Herman [Her80] for an exhaustive treatment of the subject.

When binary values are chosen for the weights w_{ij} in (16) in ART, i.e., w_{ij} is set equal to 1 if the center of the *j*th pixel falls within the strip of the *i*th ray and 0 if not, it becomes necessary to adjust the width of each ray according to the orientation of the projection [Gor74], [Her73], [Opp75].

Attempts have been made to reduce the salt and pepper noise associated with ART-type reconstructions by increasing the number of rays per view [Smi77]. When the number of rays per view is increased, many pixels are

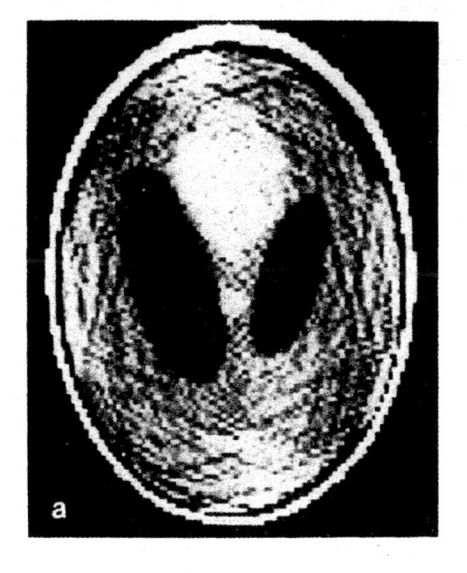

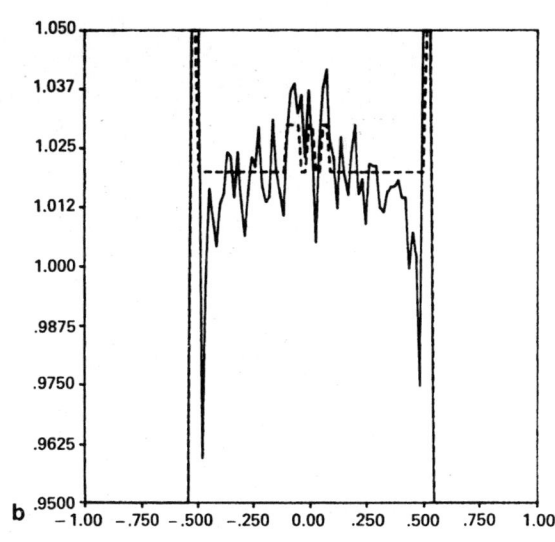

Fig. 7.11: *Reconstruction from one iteration of sequential ART with a longitudinal Hamming window. (a) Image. (b) Line plot through the three small tumors (for y = −0.605). (From [And84a].)*

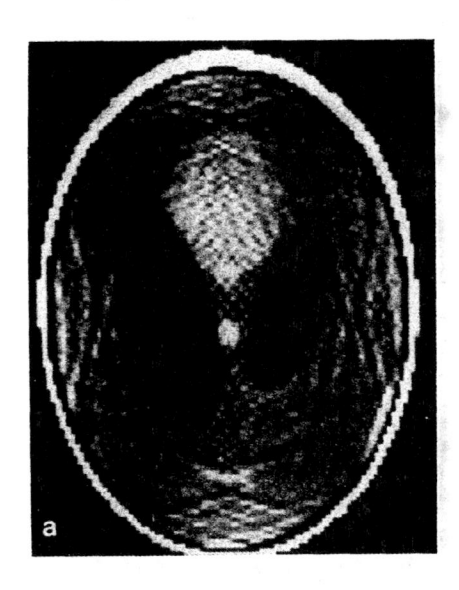

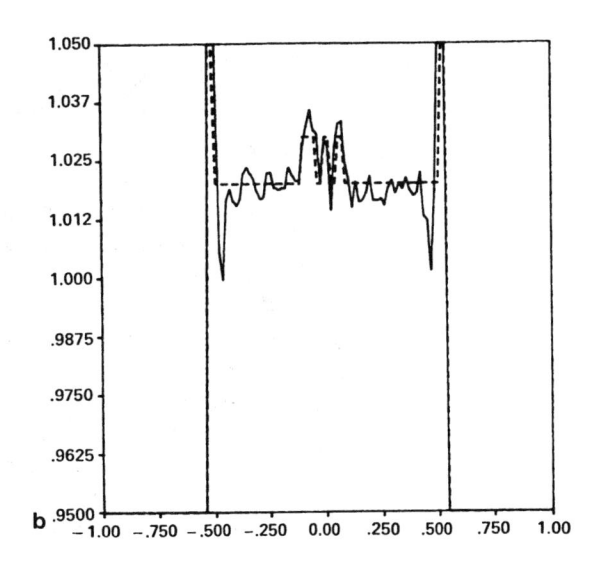

Fig. 7.12: *Reconstruction from two iterations of SART with a longitudinal Hamming window. (a) Image. (b) Line plot through the three small tumors (for y = −0.605). (From [And84a].)*

intersected by several rays in each projection. This results in the averaging of possible errors committed in the correction procedure such as the one given by (4). Common practice is to have a system with about four times as many equations as unknown pixel values [Her80], [Her78], [She74]. The computational cost, however, is increased directly with the number of rays processed. An additional method has been to use a relaxation factor $\lambda < 1$ [Gor74], [Her80], [Her76], [Her78], [Hou72], [Swe73] which, although reducing the salt and pepper noise, increases the number of iterations required for convergence.

The SART algorithm was first reported in [And84a]. In contrast with the bilinear elements used for SART, the pixel basis is common to much

ALGEBRAIC RECONSTRUCTION ALGORITHMS 293

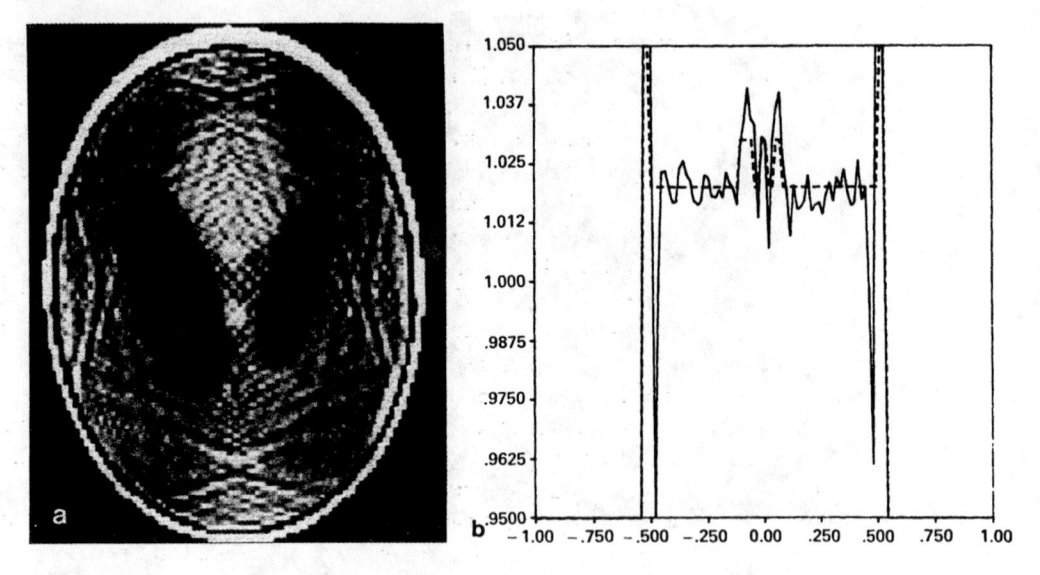

Fig. 7.13: *Reconstruction from three iterations of SART with a longitudinal Hamming window. (a) Image. (b) Line plot through the three small tumors (for y = −0.605). (From [And84a].)*

Fig. 7.14: *Convolution-backprojection reconstruction of the test image. (a) Image. (b) Line plot through the three small tumors (for y = −0.605). (From [And84a].)*

literature published on algebraic techniques [Din79], [Gil72], [Gor74], [Gor70], [Her80], [Her76], [Her78], [Her73], [Hou72], [Opp75], [She74].

The error-correcting procedure of the basic ART algorithm as given by (4) is discussed in [Gor74], [Gor70], [Her80], [Her76], [Her78], [Her73], [Hou72].

As first shown by Hounsfield [Hou72], in order to improve the convergence of a sequential algebraic algorithm one should order the projections in such a manner that successive projections are well separated. This he justified on the basis of high correlation between the information in neighboring projections. Later the scheme was demonstrated to have a deeper

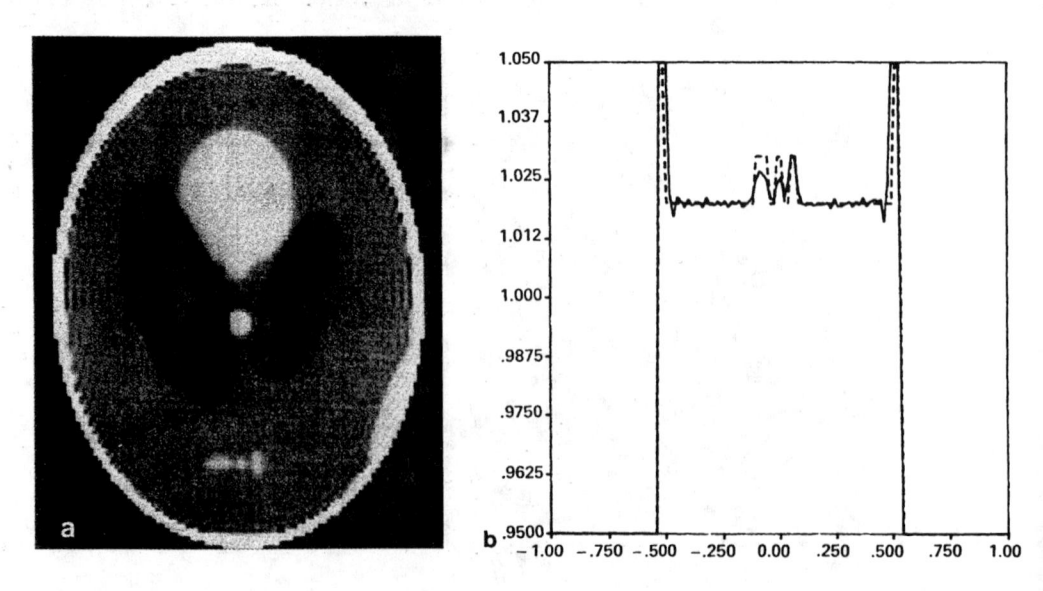

294   COMPUTERIZED TOMOGRAPHIC IMAGING

mathematical foundation as a tool for speeding up the convergence of ART-type algorithms. (The proof relies on a continuous formulation of ART, as shown by Hamaker and Solmon [Ham78].) Ramakrishnan *et al.* [Ram79] have shown how by orthogonalization of the algebraic equations we can increase the speed of convergence of a reconstruction algorithm.

The SIRT algorithm was first proposed by Gilbert [Gil72]. A simplified form of the simultaneous technique was used by Oppenheim in [Opp75]. However, the scope of the implementation as described by (32) is much wider. The method can be used advantageously in the general image reconstruction problem for curved rays with overlapping and nonoverlapping ray strips as well as in conjunction with any image representation, provided the forward process can be expressed in the form of (23).

A combination of algebraic reconstruction and digital ray tracing appears ideal for imaging lightly refracting objects [Cha79], [Cha81]. A survey of digital ray tracing and ray linking for this purpose is presented in [And82]. If a refracting object has special symmetries, then as shown by Vest [Ves75] it may be possible to reconstruct the object without ray tracing. The reader is referred to [And84b] for experimental demonstrations of how algebraic reconstruction can be combined with digital ray tracing for the cross-sectional imaging of lightly refracting objects.

7.6 References

[And82]   A. H. Andersen and A. C. Kak, "Digital ray tracing in two-dimensional refractive fields," *J. Acoust. Soc. Amer.*, vol. 72, pp. 1593-1606, Nov. 1982.

[And84a]   ———, "Simultaneous algebraic reconstruction technique (SART): A superior implementation of the art algorithm," *Ultrason. Imaging*, vol. 6, pp. 81-94, Jan. 1984.

[And84b]   ———, "The application of ray tracing towards a correction for refracting effects in computed tomography with diffracting sources," TR-EE 84-14, School of Electrical Engineering, Purdue Univ., Lafayette, IN, 1984.

[Bud74]   T. F. Budinger and G. T. Gullberg, "Three-dimensional reconstruction in nuclear medicine emission imaging," *IEEE Trans. Nucl. Sci.*, vol. NS-21, pp. 2-21, 1974.

[Cha79]   S. Cha and C. M. Vest, "Interferometry and reconstruction of strongly refracting asymmetric-refractive-index fields," *Opt. Lett.*, vol. 4, pp. 311-313, 1979.

[Cha81]   ———, "Tomographic reconstruction of strongly refracting fields and its application to interferometric measurements of boundary layers," *Appl. Opt.*, vol. 20, pp. 2787-2794, 1981.

[Din79]   K. A. Dines and R. J. Lytle, "Computerized geophysical tomography," *Proc. IEEE*, vol. 67, pp. 1065-1073, 1979.

[Gil72]   P. Gilbert, "Iterative methods for the reconstruction of three dimensional objects from their projections," *J. Theor. Biol.*, vol. 36, pp. 105-117, 1972.

[Gor70]   R. Gordon, R. Bender, and G. T. Herman, "Algebraic reconstruction techniques (ART) for three dimensional electron microscopy and X-ray photography," *J. Theor. Biol.*, vol. 29, pp. 471-481, 1970.

[Gor71]   R. Gordon and G. T. Herman, "Reconstruction of pictures from their projections," *Commun. Assoc. Comput. Mach.*, vol. 14, pp. 759-768, 1971.

[Gor74]   R. Gordon, "A tutorial on ART (algebraic reconstruction techniques)," *IEEE Trans. Nucl. Sci.*, vol. NS-21, pp. 78-93, 1974.

[Ham78]   C. Hamaker and D. C. Solmon, "The angles between the null spaces of X rays," *J. Math. Anal. Appl.*, vol. 62, pp. 1-23, 1978.

[Her71]   G. T. Herman and S. Rowland, "Resolution in ART: An experimental investigation of the resolving power of an algebraic picture reconstruction," *J. Theor. Biol.*, vol. 33, pp. 213–233, 1971.

[Her73] G. T. Herman, A. Lent, and S. Rowland, "ART: Mathematics and applications: A report on the mathematical foundations and on applicability to real data of the algebraic reconstruction techniques," *J. Theor. Biol.*, vol. 43, pp. 1–32, 1973.

[Her76] G. T. Herman and A. Lent, "Iterative reconstruction algorithms," *Comput. Biol. Med.*, vol. 6, pp. 273–294, 1976.

[Her77] G. T. Herman and A. Naparstek, "Fast image reconstruction based on a Radon inversion formula appropriate for rapidly collected data," *SIAM J. Appl. Math.*, vol. 33, pp. 511–533, Nov. 1977.

[Her78] G. T. Herman, A. Lent, and P. H. Lutz, "Relaxation methods for image reconstruction," *Commun. A.C.M.*, vol. 21, pp. 152–158, 1978.

[Her80] G. T. Herman, *Image Reconstructions from Projections*. New York, NY: Academic Press, 1980.

[Hou72] G. N. Hounsfield, "A method of and apparatus for examination of a body by radiation such as x-ray or gamma radiation," Patent Specification 1283915, The Patent Office, 1972.

[Kac37] S. Kaczmarz, "Angenaherte auflosung von systemen linearer gleichungen," *Bull. Acad. Pol. Sci. Lett. A*, vol. 6-8A, pp. 355–357, 1937.

[Kak84] A. C. Kak, "Image reconstructions from projections," in *Digital Image Processing Techniques*, M. P. Ekstrom, Ed. New York, NY: Academic Press, 1984.

[Lyt80] R. J. Lytle and K. A. Dines, "Iterative ray tracing between boreholes for underground image reconstruction," *IEEE Trans. Geosciences and Remote Sensing*, vol. GE-18, pp. 234–240, 1980.

[Opp75] B. E. Oppenheim, "Reconstruction tomography from incomplete projections," in *Reconstruction Tomography in Diagnostic Radiology and Nuclear Medicine*, M. M. Ter Pogossian *et al.*, Eds. Baltimore, MD: University Park Press, 1975.

[Ram79] R. S. Ramakrishnan, S. K. Mullick, R. K. S. Rathore, and R. Subramanian, "Orthogonalization, Bernstein polynomials, and image restoration," *Appl. Opt.*, vol. 18, pp. 464–468, 1979.

[Ros82] A. Rosenfeld and A. C. Kak, *Digital Picture Processing*, 2nd ed. New York, NY: Academic Press, 1982.

[She74] L. S. Shepp and B. F. Logan, "The Fourier reconstruction of a head section," *IEEE Trans. Nucl. Sci.*, vol. NS-21, pp. 21–43, 1974.

[Sla85] M. Slaney and A. C. Kak, "Imaging with diffraction tomography," TR-EE 85-5, School of Electrical Engineering, Purdue Univ., Lafayette, IN, 1985.

[Smi77] K. T. Smith, D. C. Solmon, and S. L. Wagner, "Practical and mathematical aspects of the problem of reconstructing objects from radiographs," *Bull. Amer. Math. Soc.*, vol. 83, pp. 1227–1270, 1977.

[Swe73] D. W. Sweeney and C. M. Vest, "Reconstruction of three-dimensional refractive index fields from multi-directional interferometric data," *Appl. Opt.*, vol. 12, pp. 1649–1664, 1973.

[Tan71] K. Tanabe, "Projection method for solving a singular system," *Numer. Math.*, vol. 17, pp. 203–214, 1971.

[Ves75] C. M. Vest, "Interferometry of strongly refracting axisymmetric phase objects," *Appl. Opt.*, vol. 14, pp. 1601–1606, 1975.

8 Reflection Tomography

8.1 Introduction

The tomographic images up to this point have generally been formed by illuminating an object with some form of energy (x-rays, microwaves, or ultrasound) and measuring the energy that passes through the object to the other side. In the case of straight ray propagation, the measurement can be of either the amplitude or the time of arrival of the received signal; an estimate is then formed of a line integral of the object's attenuation coefficient or refractive index. Even when the energy doesn't travel in a straight line it is often possible to use either algebraic techniques or diffraction tomography to form an image.

Transmission tomography is sometimes not possible because of physical constraints. For example, when ultrasound is used for cardiovascular imaging, the transmitted signal is almost immeasurable because of large impedance discontinuities at tissue–bone and air–tissue interfaces and other attenuation losses. For this reason most medical ultrasonic imaging is done using reflected signals. In the most straightforward approach to reflection imaging with ultrasound, the echoes are recorded as in radar; in medical areas this approach goes by the name of B-scan imaging.

The basic aim of reflection tomography is to construct a quantitative cross-sectional image from reflection data. One nice aspect of this form of imaging, especially in comparison with transmission tomography, is that it is not necessary to encircle the object with transmitters and receivers for gathering the "projection" data; transmission and reception are now done from the same side. The same is of course true of B-scan imaging where a small beam of ultrasonic energy illuminates the object and an image is formed by displaying the reflected signal as a function of time and direction of the beam.

While in transmission tomography it is possible to use both narrow band and broadband signals, in reflection tomography only the latter type is acceptable. As will become evident by the discussion in this chapter, with short pulses (broadband signals) it is possible to form line integrals of some object parameter over lines of constant propagation delays.

Since researchers in reflection tomography are frequently asked to compare B-scan imaging with reflection tomography, in this chapter we will first give a very brief introduction to B-scan imaging, taking great liberties with conceptual detail; for a rigorous treatment of the subject, the reader is referred to [Fat80]. We will then illustrate how reflection tomography can be carried out with plane wave transducers and some of the fundamental limitations of this type of imaging. Our discussion of reflection tomography with plane wave transducers will include a demonstration of the relationship that exists between reflection tomography and the diffraction tomography formalism presented in Chapter 6. Finally, we will describe how reflection tomographic imaging can be carried out with point transducers producing spherical waves.

8.2 B-Scan Imaging

To explain B-scan imaging, assume that the object inhomogeneities can be modeled by an isotropic scattering function $f(x, y)$, a function of position. In the rest of this chapter, $f(x, y)$ will be referred to as the object reflectivity function. Within certain restrictions, it is a measure of the portion of the local transmitted field that is reflected back toward the receiver. Note that we are taking liberties with rigorous theory, since the scattering process is also a function of the direction of the illumination and the direction in which the reflection is measured. For a more precise analysis the reader is referred to [Fat80].

As shown in Fig. 8.1, a B-scan is a simple example of radar imaging. For illustration, we will assume that within the object the beam is confined to a narrow region along a line as shown in Fig. 8.1(a) and that the amplitude of the field along this line isn't decaying so that it can be written as a function of only one variable, the distance along the line. If the illuminating wave has a very short time duration, there will be a direct mapping between the time at which a portion of the reflected wave is received and the distance into the object.

Mathematically, the received waveform is a convolution of the input waveform, $p_t(t)$, and the object's reflectivity. The incident field can be written as

$$\psi_i(x, y) = p_t\left(t - \frac{x}{c}\right) \quad \text{for } y = 0 \tag{1}$$

and

$$\psi_i(x, y) = 0 \quad \text{elsewhere} \tag{2}$$

where c is the propagation speed of the wave. This function models a pulse, $p_t(t)$, propagating down the x-axis, assumed perpendicular to the face of the transducer, with speed c. This is pictorially illustrated in Fig. 8.1(b). At a point (x, y) in the object a portion of the incident field, $\psi_i(x, y)$, will be scattered back toward the transducer. Therefore the amplitude of the scattered

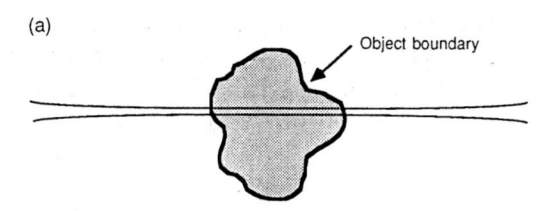

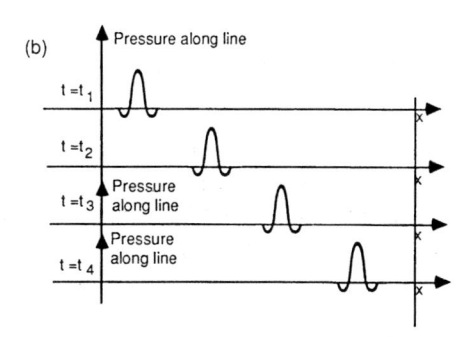

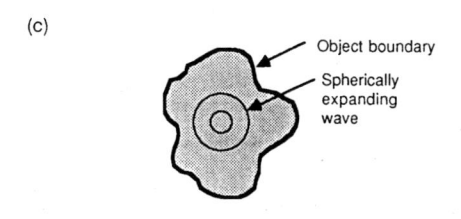

Fig. 8.1: *In B-scan imaging an object is illuminated by a narrow beam of energy. A short (temporal) pulse is transmitted and will propagate through the object. (a) shows a portion of the object illuminated by a "pencil" beam of energy, (b) shows the pulse at different times within the object, and (c) shows the spherically expanding wave caused by a single scatterer within the object.*

field at the scatterer is given approximately by

$$\psi(x, y=0) = f(x, y=0) p_t\left(t - \frac{x}{c}\right). \tag{3}$$

In traveling back to the receiver, the reflected pulse will be delayed by x/c due to the propagation distance involved and attenuated because the reflected field is diverging as depicted in Fig. 8.1(c). To maintain conservation of energy (in two dimensions here) the amplitude attenuation due to spreading is proportional to $1/\sqrt{x}$. That means the energy density will decay as $1/x$ and, when integrated over the boundary of a circle enclosing the scattering site, the total energy outflow will always be the same regardless of the radius of the circle. Thus the field received due to reflection at x is given by

$$\psi_s|_{\text{scattered at } x} = p_t\left(t - \frac{x}{c} - \frac{x}{c}\right) f(x, y=0) \frac{1}{\sqrt{x}}. \tag{4}$$

Integrating this with respect to all the reflecting sites along the transmitter

REFLECTION TOMOGRAPHY

line, the total field at the receiver is given by

$$\psi_s(t) = \int p_t\left(t - 2\frac{x}{c}\right) \frac{f(x, y=0)}{\sqrt{x}} \, dx. \qquad (5)$$

With the above expression for the scattered field due to a narrow incident beam it is relatively straightforward to find a reconstruction process for the object's reflectivity. Certainly the simplest approach is to illuminate the object with a pulse, $p_t(t)$, that looks like an impulse. The scattered field can then be approximated by

$$\psi_s(t) = \int \delta\left(t - 2\frac{x}{c}\right) \frac{f(x, y=0)}{\sqrt{x}} \, dx = \sqrt{\frac{c}{2t}} f\left(\frac{tc}{2}, y=0\right). \qquad (6)$$

This expression shows that there is a direct relation between the scattered field at t and the object's reflectivity at $x = tc/2$. This is shown in Fig. 8.2. With this expression it is easy to see that a reconstruction can be formed using

$$\tilde{f}(x, y=0) = \sqrt{\frac{4x}{c^2}} \psi_s\left(\frac{2x}{c}\right) \qquad (7)$$

where $\tilde{f}$ is the estimate of the reflectivity function f. The term $4x/c^2$ that multiplies the scattered field is known as time gain compensation and it compensates for the spreading of the fields after they are scattered by the object.

In B-scan imaging, a cross-sectional image of the object's reflectivity variation is mapped out by a combination of scanning the incident beam and measuring the reflected field over a period of time. Recall that in B-scan imaging the object is illuminated by a very narrow beam of energy. Equation (7) then gives an estimate of the object's reflectivity along the line of the object illuminated by the field. To reconstruct the entire object it is then necessary to move the transducer in such a manner that all parts of the object are scanned. There are many ways this can be accomplished, the simplest

Fig. 8.2: *When an object is illuminated by a pulse there is a direct relationship between the backscattered field and the object's reflectivity along a line.*

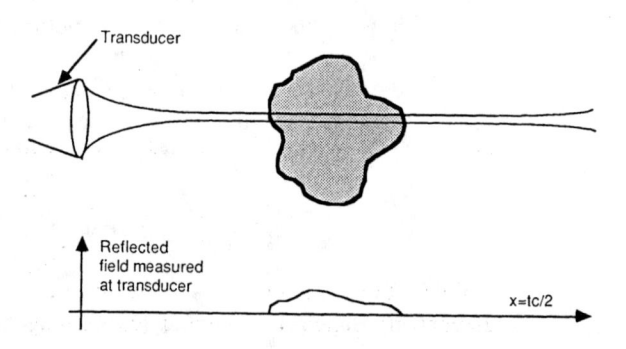

300   COMPUTERIZED TOMOGRAPHIC IMAGING

being to spin the transducer and let each position of the transducer illuminate one line of a fan. This is the type of scan shown in Fig. 8.3.

Clearly, the resolution in a B-scan image is a function of two parameters: the duration of the incident pulse and the width of the beam. Resolution as determined by the duration of the pulse is often called the range resolution and the resolution controlled by the width of the beam is referred to as the lateral resolution. The range resolution can be found by considering the system response for a single point scatterer. From (5) the field measured at the point (0, 0) due to a single scatterer of "unit strength" at $x = x_0$ will be equal to

$$\psi_s(t) = \frac{p_t\left(t - \frac{2x_0}{c}\right)}{\sqrt{x_0}}. \tag{8}$$

Substituting this in (7), our expression for estimating the reflectivity, we obtain the following form for the image of the object's reflectivity:

$$\tilde{f}(x, y=0) = \sqrt{\frac{4x}{c^2}} \psi_s\left(\frac{2x}{c}\right) = \frac{\sqrt{\frac{4x}{c^2}} p_t\left(\frac{2x}{c} - \frac{2x_0}{c}\right)}{\sqrt{x_0}}. \tag{9}$$

From this it is easy to see that an incident pulse of width t_p seconds will lead to an estimate that is $t_p c$ units wide.

It is interesting to examine in the frequency domain the process by which the object reflectivity function may be recovered from the measured data. In the simple model described here, the frequency domain techniques can be used by merging the $1/\sqrt{x}$ factor with the reflectivity function; this can be done by defining a modified reflectivity function

$$f'(x, y) = \frac{f(x, y)}{\sqrt{x}}. \tag{10}$$

Now the scattered field at the point (0, 0) can be written as the convolution

$$\psi_s(t) = \int p_t\left(t - 2\frac{x}{c}\right) f'(x, y=0) \, dx \tag{11}$$

and can be expressed in the Fourier domain as

$$\tilde{\psi}_s(\omega) = P_t(\omega) F'\left(2\frac{\omega}{c}, y=0\right). \tag{12}$$

Given the scattered field in this form it is easy to derive a procedure to estimate the reflectivity of the object. Ideally it is only necessary to divide the

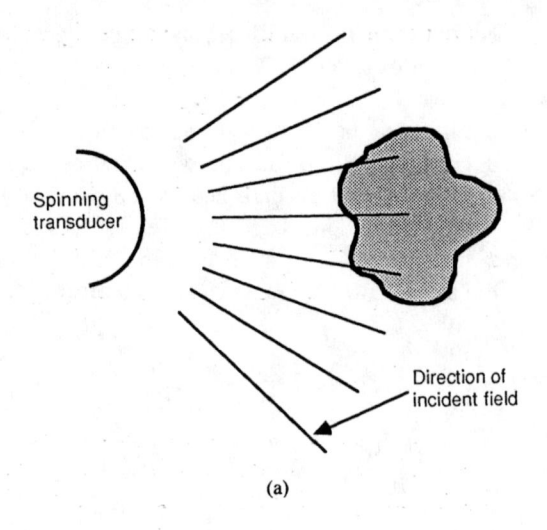

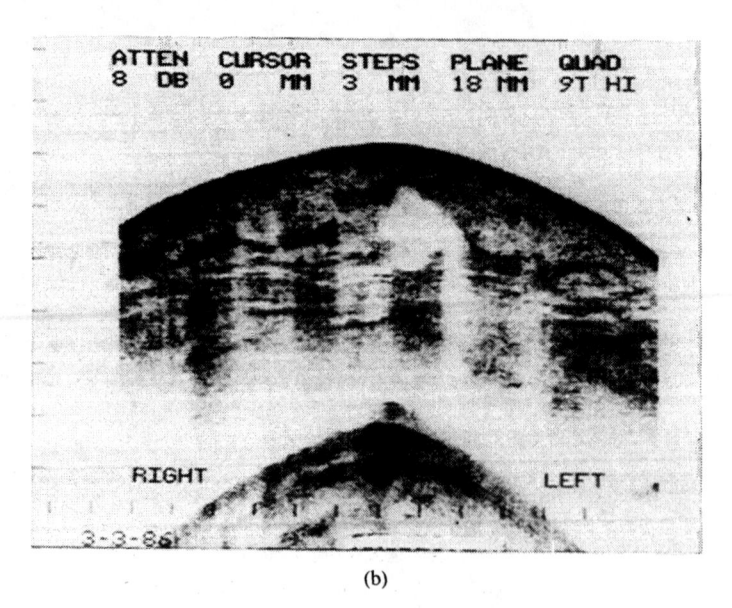

Fig. 8.3: Often, in commercial B-scan imaging a focused beam of energy is moved past the object. An image is formed by plotting the received field as a function of time and transducer position. (a) shows this process schematically. (b) is a transverse 7.5-MHz sonogram of a carcinoma in the upper half of the right breast. (This image is courtesy of Valerie P. Jackson, M.D., Associate Professor of Radiology, Indiana University School of Medicine.) (c) is a drawing of the tissue shown in (b). The mass near the center of the sonogram is lobulated, has some irregular borders and low-level internal echoes, and there is an area of posterior shadowing at the medial aspect of the tumor. These findings are compatible with malignancy.

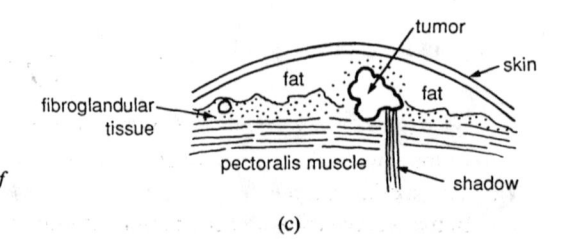

302   COMPUTERIZED TOMOGRAPHIC IMAGING

Fourier transform of the received field by $P_t(\omega)$ to find

$$F'\left(2\frac{\omega}{c}, y=0\right) = \frac{\tilde{\psi}_s(\omega)}{P_t(\omega)}. \tag{13}$$

Unfortunately, in most cases this simple implementation doesn't work because there can be frequencies where $P_t(\omega)$ is equal to zero, which can cause instabilities in the division, especially if there is noise present at those frequencies in the measured data. A more noise insensitive implementation can be obtained via Wiener filtering [Fat80].

8.3 Reflection Tomography

Reflection tomography is based on the measurement of line integrals of the object reflectivity function. Consider a single point transducer illuminating an object with a very wide fan-shaped beam. If the incident field is just an impulse in the time domain, then the received signal at time t represents the total of all reflections at a distance of tc from the transducer. The locus of all points at the same distance from the transmitter/receiver is a circle; thus this mode of reflection tomography measures line integrals over circular arcs. (See Fig. 8.4.) Then by moving the transducer over a plane, or alternatively on a sphere wrapped around the object, it is possible to collect enough line integrals to reconstruct the entire object. This approach to tomographic imaging was described first by Norton and Linzer [Nor79a], [Nor79b].

In principle, reconstruction from such data is similar to the following case that is easier to describe: Instead of using a point transducer, we will use a plane wave transducer. As we will show below, for the two-dimensional case the lines of equal propagation delay now become straight lines through the object and thus the reconstruction algorithms are exactly like those for conventional parallel beam tomography. First, though, we will describe the field generated and received by a plane transducer.

8.3.1 Plane Wave Reflection Transducers

Before deriving a reconstruction procedure using plane waves we first must define what a plane wave transducer measures. In the transmit mode, the field produced by an ideal plane wave transducer when excited by the waveform $p_t(t)$ is equal to

$$\psi_i(x, y, t) = p_t\left(t - \frac{x}{c}\right), \quad x > 0 \tag{14}$$

where we have assumed that the transducer is flush with the plane $x = 0$. Note that the field is only defined in the positive x half space and is a function of one spatial variable.

In the receive mode the situation is slightly more complicated. If $\psi_r(x, y, t)$

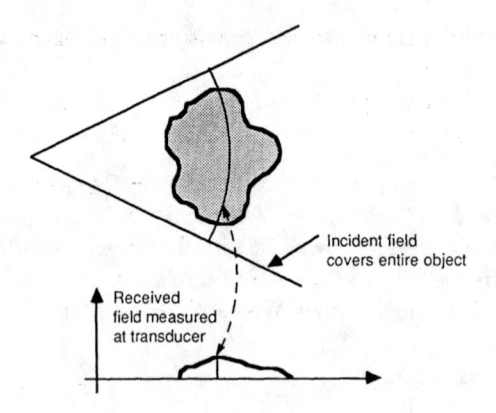

Fig. 8.4: *If a transducer with a wide beam illuminates the object, then it will measure line integrals over circular arcs of the object's reflectivity.*

is the scattered field, the signal generated at the electrical terminals of the transducer is proportional to the integral of this field. We will ignore the constant of proportionality and write the electrical received signal, $p_r(t)$, as

$$p_r(t) = \int \psi_r(0, y, t) \, dy. \tag{15}$$

In order to derive an expression for the received waveform given the field at points distant from the transducer it is necessary to consider how the waves propagate back to the transducer. First assume that there is a line of reflectors at $x = x_0$ that reflect a portion, $f(x = x_0, y)$, of the field. As described above we can write the scattered field at the line $x = x_0$ as the product of the incident field and the reflectivity parameter or

$$\psi_s(x=x_0, y, t) = \psi_i(x=x_0, y, t) f(x=x_0, y)$$

$$= p_t\left(t - \frac{x}{c}\right) f(x=x_0, y). \tag{16}$$

To find the field at the transducer face it is necessary to find the Fourier transform of the field and then propagate each plane wave to the transducer face. This is done by first finding the spatial and temporal Fourier transform of the field at the line of reflectors

$$\tilde{\psi}_s(k_y, \omega) = \int_{-\infty}^{\infty} \int_{-\infty}^{\infty} \psi_s(x=x_0, y, t) e^{-jk_y y} e^{j\omega t} \, dy \, dt. \tag{17}$$

The function $\tilde{\psi}_s(k_y, \omega)$ therefore represents the amplitude of the plane wave propagating with direction vectors $(-\sqrt{(\omega/c)^2 - k_y^2}, k_y)$. It is important to realize that the above equation represents the field along the line as a function of two variables. For any temporal frequency, ω, there is an entire spectrum of plane waves, each with a unique propagation direction.

Recall that we are using the convention for the Fourier transform defined in Chapter 6. Thus the forward transform has a phase factor of $e^{-jk_y y}$ in the spatial domain, as is conventional, while the temporal Fourier transform uses

$e^{+j\omega t}$ for the forward transform. The signs are reversed for the inverse transform.

With this plane wave expansion for the field it is now easy to propagate each plane wave to the transducer face. Consider an arbitrary plane wave

$$\psi(x, y) = e^{j(k_x x + k_y y)} \tag{18}$$

where k_x will be negative indicating a wave traveling back toward the transducer. Using (15), the electrical signal produced is quickly seen to be equal to zero for all plane waves when $k_y \neq 0$. This is due to the fact that

$$\int_{-\infty}^{\infty} e^{jk_y y} dy = \delta(k_y). \tag{19}$$

Those plane waves traveling perpendicular to the face of the transducer ($k_y = 0$) will experience a delay due to the propagation distance x_0. In the frequency domain this represents a factor of $e^{j\omega(x_0/c)}$. The electrical response due to a unit amplitude plane wave is then seen to be

$$P_r(\omega, k_y) = \delta(k_y) e^{j\omega(x_0/c)}. \tag{20}$$

By summing each of the plane waves at frequency ω in (17), the total electrical response due to the scattered fields from the plane $x = x_0$ is given by

$$\tilde{P}_r(\omega) = \tilde{\psi}_s(k_y = 0, \omega) e^{j\omega(x_0/c)} \tag{21}$$

or back in the time domain it is simply equal to

$$p_r(t) = \frac{1}{2\pi} \int_{-\infty}^{\infty} \tilde{\psi}_s(k_y = 0, \omega) e^{j\omega(x_0/c)} e^{-j\omega t} d\omega. \tag{22}$$

Now substituting (14), (17), and (16) into this expression, the received signal can be written

$$p_r(t) = \frac{1}{2\pi} \int_{-\infty}^{\infty} e^{-j\omega t} d\omega \int_{-\infty}^{\infty} \int_{-\infty}^{\infty} \psi_s(x = x_0, y, t')$$

$$\cdot e^{j\omega(x_0/c)} e^{-jk_y y} e^{j\omega t'} dy \, dt' \Big|_{k_y = 0} \tag{23}$$

which is the same as

$$p_r(t) = \frac{1}{2\pi} \int_{-\infty}^{\infty} e^{-j\omega t} d\omega \int_{-\infty}^{\infty} \int_{-\infty}^{\infty} \psi_i(x = x_0, y, t')$$

$$\cdot f(x = x_0, y) e^{j\omega(x_0/c)} e^{j\omega t'} dy \, dt' \tag{24}$$

which reduces to

$$p_r(t) = \frac{1}{2\pi} \int_{-\infty}^{\infty} e^{-j\omega t} \, d\omega \int_{-\infty}^{\infty} \int_{-\infty}^{\infty} p_t\left(t' - \frac{x_0}{c}\right)$$
$$\cdot f(x=x_0, y) e^{j\omega(x_0/c)} e^{j\omega t'} \, dy \, dt'. \quad (25)$$

Interchanging the order of integrations yields

$$p_r(t) = p_t\left(t - 2\frac{x_0}{c}\right) \int_{-\infty}^{\infty} f(x=x_0, y) \, dy. \quad (26)$$

The above equation represents the measured signal due to a single line of scatterers at $x = x_0$. Let the total (integrated) reflectivity of the object along the line $x = x_0$ be denoted by $f_1(x_0)$. The received signal for all parts of the object can be written as the sum of each individual line (since we are assuming that the backscattered fields satisfy the Born approximation and thus the system is linear) and the total measured signal can be written

$$p_r(t) = \int_{-\infty}^{\infty} p_t\left(t - 2\frac{x}{c}\right) f_1(x) \, dx. \quad (27)$$

This signal is similar to that of B-scan imaging. Like B-scan the transmitted pulse is convolved with the reflectivity of the object but in each case the reflectivity is summed over the portion of the object illuminated by the incident field. In B-scan the object is illuminated by a narrow beam so each portion of the received signal represents a small area of the object. With reflection tomography the beam is very wide and thus each measurement corresponds to a line integral through the object.

Like B-scan imaging the reflectivity of the object can be found by first deconvolving the effects of the incident pulse. If the incident pulse can be approximated by an impulse, then the object's reflectivity over line integrals is equal to

$$f_1(x) = p_r\left(2\frac{x}{c}\right); \quad (28)$$

otherwise a deconvolution must be done and the line integrals recovered using

$$F_1(\omega) = \frac{P_r(\omega)}{P_t\left(2\frac{\omega}{c}\right)} \quad (29)$$

where $F_1(\omega)$, $P_r(\omega)$, and $P_t(\omega)$ represent the Fourier transform of the corresponding time or space domain signal. (In practice, of course, one may have to resort to techniques such as Wiener filtering for implementing the frequency domain inversion.)

The line integral data in the equation above are precisely the information needed to perform a reconstruction using the Fourier Slice Theorem. As described in Chapter 3, the object's reflectivity can be found using the relationship

$$\hat{f}(x, y) = \int_0^{2\pi} \int_{-\infty}^{\infty} S_\theta(\omega) |\omega| e^{j\omega t} \, d\omega \, d\theta \tag{30}$$

where S_θ represents the Fourier transform of the projection data measured with the transducer face at an angle of θ to the horizontal and

$$t = x \cos\theta + y \sin\theta. \tag{31}$$

8.3.2 Reflection Tomography vs. Diffraction Tomography

It is interesting to compare reflection tomography as just described using plane wave transducers to the methods of diffraction tomography presented in Chapter 6. To see the similarities, consider the following imaging experiment. Instead of using a plane wave transducer, let's use a line array to illuminate the object, as shown in Fig. 8.5.

To perform a reflection tomography experiment of the type described in the preceding subsection, we need to be able to generate a plane wave with the array; this can be done easily by applying the same broadband signal $p(t)$ to every transducer in the array. For reception, if we simply add the electrical signals generated by the transducer elements in the array, we will obtain a close approximation to the receiving characteristics of a plane wave transducer.

Now imagine that instead of summing all the received electrical signals, we record each one separately—call each such signal $s(t, y)$. If we take the Fourier transform of each received waveform $s(t, y)$ with respect to time, we obtain

$$S(\omega, y) = \int_{-\infty}^{\infty} s(t, y) e^{j\omega t} \, dt. \tag{32}$$

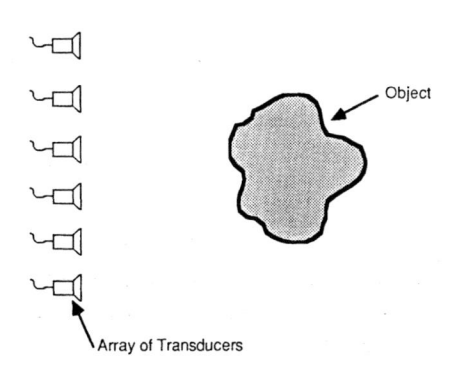

Fig. 8.5: By using a common signal source and combining all the electrical signals, an array of transducers can be used to generate a plane wave for reflection tomography. However, by recording the information separately for each transducer, they can also be used for the more general form of reflection tomography.

If the original signal has a spectrum given by

$$P_t(\omega) = \int_{-\infty}^{\infty} p_t(t) e^{j\omega t} \, dt, \tag{33}$$

then the scattered fields can be normalized by dividing the received spectrum by the transmitted spectrum to find

$$S'(\omega, y) = \frac{S(\omega, y)}{P_t(\omega)}. \tag{34}$$

Again, as described before, this represents an idealized approach and in practice a more robust filter must be used.

Because of the normalization at the array element at location y, the data $S'(\omega, y)$ represent a single plane wave component of the scattered field that is at a temporal frequency of ω. If we take a Fourier transform of $S'(\omega, y)$ with respect to the variable y, by using the techniques of Chapter 6 we can derive the following relationship:

$$S'(\omega, k_y) = \int_{-\infty}^{\infty} S'(\omega, y) e^{-jk_y y} \, dy = F(-\sqrt{k_0^2 - k_y^2} - k_0, k_y) \tag{35}$$

which shows that the Fourier transform[1] $S'(\omega, k_y)$ provides us with an estimate of the Fourier transform of the object reflectivity function along a circular arc, as illustrated in Fig. 8.6 for a number of different frequencies.

This means that a cross-sectional image of the object could be reconstructed by rotating the object in front of the array, since via such a rotation we should be able to fill out a "disk with a hole in the center" shaped region in the frequency domain. The reconstruction can be carried out by taking an inverse Fourier transform of this region. Clearly, since the center part of the disk would be missing, the reconstructed image would be a "high pass" version of the actual reflectivity distribution.

Reflection tomography using plane wave transducers, as described in the preceding subsection, is a special case of the more general form presented here. This can be shown as follows: If the signals $s(t, y)$ received by the transducers are simply summed over y, the resulting signal as a function of time represents not only the output from an idealized plane wave receiver but also the Fourier transform of the received field at a spatial frequency of $k_y = 0$. We can, for example, show that the Fourier transform of the summed signal

$$\int_{-\infty}^{\infty} s(t, y) \, dy \tag{36}$$

Fig. 8.6: *The Fourier transform of the field received by a plane wave transducer gives samples of the two-dimensional Fourier transform of the object along the line indicated by the cross marks. For each spatial frequency, k_0, the backscattered field gives information along an arc. A plane wave transducer only measures the dc component; thus the measured signal contains information about only one point of each arc. By rotating the transducer around the object a complete reconstruction can be formed.*

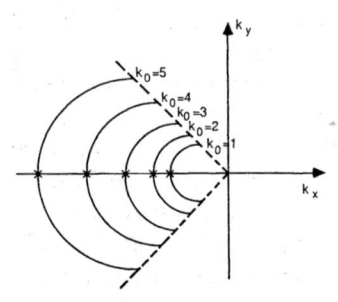

[1] Note that the expression defined in (32) represents the received signal, S, as a function of temporal frequency, ω, and spatial position, y, while (35) represents the normalized signal as a function of both spatial (k_y) and temporal (ω) frequency.

is given by

$$\int_{-\infty}^{\infty}\int_{-\infty}^{\infty} s(t,y)\,dy\,e^{j\omega t}\,dt = P_t(\omega)[F(-\sqrt{k_0^2-k_y^2}-k_0,k_y)]_{k_y=0} \qquad (37)$$

$$= P_t(\omega)F(-2k_0,0) \qquad (38)$$

$$= P_t(\omega)F\left(-2\frac{\omega}{c},0\right) \qquad (39)$$

which shows that the Fourier transform of the summed signal gives the Fourier transform of the object along the straight lines as given by

$$F\left(-2\frac{\omega}{c},0\right) \quad \text{for } 0<\omega<\infty. \qquad (40)$$

These data points are shown as crosses in Fig. 8.6.

8.3.3 Reflection Tomography Limits

Limitations of reflection tomography are similar to those of transmission tomography described in Chapter 6. In both cases the interactions of the field and the object are modeled using first-order approximations.

Barry Roberts at Purdue University performed a number of simulations to study the limitations of plane wave reflection tomography. The simulations were done to model an ideal plane wave tomography experiment using a large bandwidth and a very large transducer.

The data used to study the quality of the reflection tomographic algorithms were calculated by assuming that the incident field is the sum of a number of discrete frequencies between K_{0L} and K_{0H}. For each frequency, a unit amplitude plane wave was scattered off a cylinder with a constant refractive index. The backscattered field was then integrated over the receiver line to find $S(\omega, k_y = 0)$.

Fig. 8.7 shows the reflection tomographic reconstructions using an ideal transducer with infinite frequency response. Even in this case it is not possible to measure the object's response for a wave at $k_0 = 0$ (temporal frequency is zero). Thus the value for the $k_0 = 0$ term was interpolated and there was some shift in the dc value of the reconstruction.

The reconstructions shown here are similar to the ones shown in Chapter 6 for the Born approximation in the forward direction. For small objects and refractive indexes the reflection reconstructions are good, but for large objects the high frequency part of the reconstruction is distorted. This is because the high frequency components, or those with the shortest wavelengths, are first to undergo a 180° phase change. Thus in the $10\lambda_c$ reconstructions the edges are distorted until finally, as the refractive index

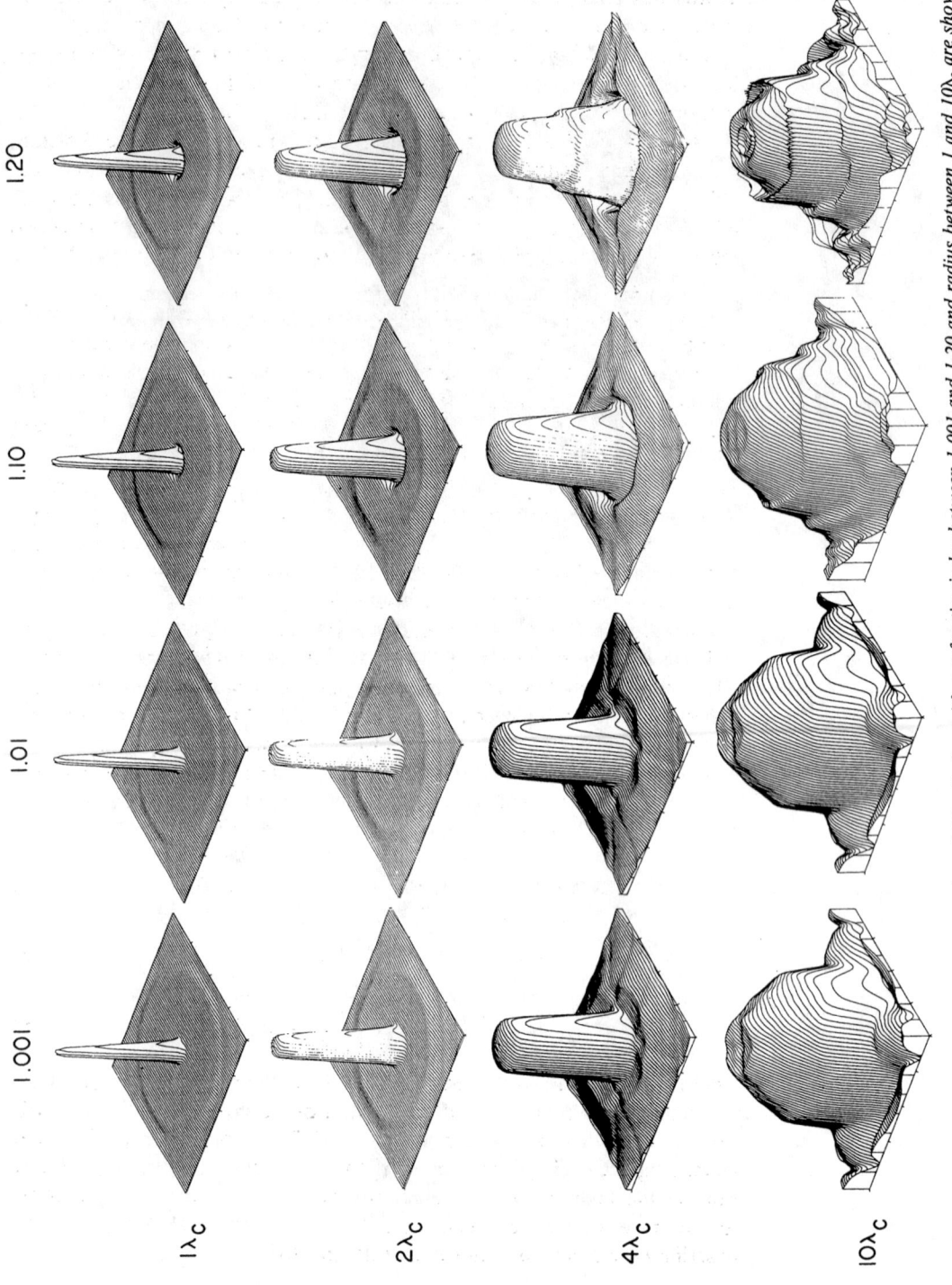

Fig. 8.7: Plane wave reflection reconstruction of 16 cylinders with a refractive index between 1.001 and 1.20 and radius between 1 and $10\lambda_c$ are shown here. The incident field includes wavelengths between $(20/32)\lambda_c$ and $(20/8)\lambda_c$ and represents nearly an ideal case since very low frequencies (high wavelengths) are included. The dc component of these reconstructions was calculated by interpolation. (Courtesy of Barry Roberts, Purdue University, Lafayette, IN.)

approaches 1.20, there are some small high frequency ripples. (λ_c refers to the wavelength at the center frequency of the transducer bandwidth.)

Using a more practical frequency range the reconstructions shown in Fig. 8.8 are obtained. Here the data simulate what might be measured with a transducer with a center frequency of 1 MHz and a bandwidth of 1.2 MHz. As would be expected, the reconstructions aren't as good as those shown in Fig. 8.7 because some of the low and high frequency information about the object is missing. Thus there is very little information in the reconstructions other than the location of the edges of the cylinders. The average refractive index of each cylinder isn't reconstructed because that is contained in the low frequencies.

A big problem with reflection tomography is that it doesn't provide information about the object at low frequencies. To a certain extent this problem can be rectified by extrapolating the measured object spectrum into the low frequency band where the information is missing. A popular algorithm for such an extrapolation is the Gerchberg–Papoulis algorithm [Ger74], [Pap75].

The Gerchberg–Papoulis algorithm is an iterative procedure to combine information about the Fourier transform of a function (as might be produced by a reflection tomography experiment) with independent space domain constraints. Typically, the spatial constraint might be the known support of the object or the fact that it is always positive.

Assume that a reflection tomography experiment has yielded $F_0(u, v)$ as an estimate of the Fourier transform of an object's cross section; its inverse Fourier transform $f_0(x, y)$ is then the image that would be the result of the experiment. From the preceding arguments $F_0(u, v)$ is known in a doughnut-shaped region of the (u, v) space; we will denote this region by D_f. In general, the experiment itself wouldn't reveal anything about the object outside the doughnut-shaped region. If $f(x, y)$ denotes the true cross section and $F(u, v)$ the corresponding transform, we can write

$$F(u, v) = \begin{cases} F_0(u, v) & (u, v) \text{ in } D_f \\ ? & \text{elsewhere.} \end{cases} \quad (41)$$

We will invoke the constraint that the object is known to be spatially limited:

$$f(x, y) = \begin{cases} ? & (x, y) \text{ in } D_s \\ 0 & \text{elsewhere} \end{cases} \quad (42)$$

where we have used D_s to denote the maximum a priori known object size.

Typically, the inverse Fourier transform of the known data $F_0(u, v)$ will lead to a reconstruction that is not spatially limited. The goal of the Gerchberg–Papoulis algorithm is to find a reconstruction $f^*(x, y)$ that satisfies the space constraint and whose Fourier transform $F^*(u, v)$ is equal to that measured by reflection tomography in region D_f. We will now describe how this algorithm can be implemented.

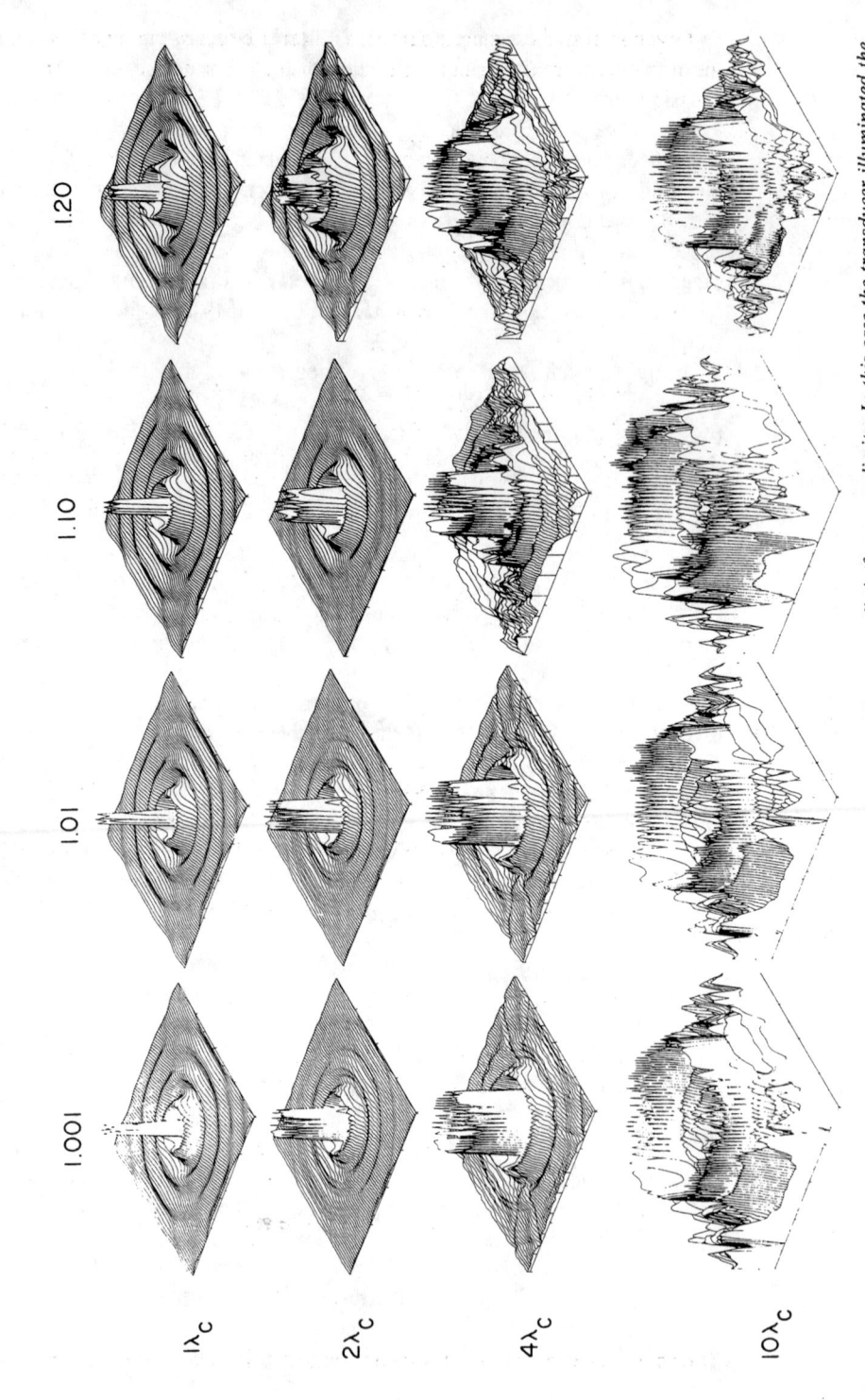

Fig. 8.8: Reconstructions similar to those in Fig. 8.7 are shown here with more realistic frequency limits. In this case the transducer illuminated the object with a pulse at a center frequency of 1 MHz and a bandwidth of 1.2 MHz. The radius of the cylinders is shown as a function of the wavelength of the center frequency (1 MHz). (Courtesy of Barry Roberts, Purdue University, Lafayette, IN.)

312　COMPUTERIZED TOMOGRAPHIC IMAGING

Given an initial estimate $F_0(u, v)$, a better estimate of the object is found by finding the inverse Fourier transform of $F_0(u, v)$ and setting the first iteration to be

$$f_1(x, y) = \begin{cases} \text{IFT} \{F_0(u, v)\} & (x, y) \text{ in } D_s \\ 0 & \text{elsewhere.} \end{cases} \quad (43)$$

The next iteration is obtained by Fourier transforming $f_1(x, y)$ and then constructing a composite function in the frequency domain as follows:

$$F_1(u, v) = \begin{cases} F_0(u, v) & (u, v) \text{ in } D_f \\ \text{FT} \{f_1(x, y)\} & \text{elsewhere} \end{cases} \quad (44)$$

(FT = Fourier transform). We now construct the next iterate $f_2(x, y)$, which is an improvement over $f_1(x, y)$, by first inverse Fourier transforming $F_1(u, v)$ and setting to zero any values that are outside the region D_s. This iterative process may be continued to yield f_3, f_4, and so on, until the difference between two successive approximations is below a prespecified bound. This is shown schematically in Fig. 8.9.

The result of applying 150 iterations of the Gerchberg-Papoulis algorithm to the reconstructions of Fig. 8.7 is shown in Fig. 8.10. The reader is referred to [Rob85] for further details on the application of this algorithm to reflection tomography.

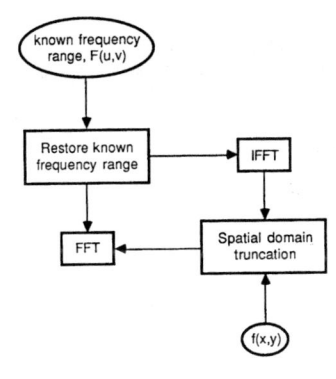

Fig. 8.9: *In the Gerchberg-Papoulis algorithm an estimate of a portion of the object's Fourier transform is combined with knowledge of its spatial support. The method iterates until an estimate of the object is found that is consistent with the known frequency domain data and the spatial extant of the object. (From [Rob85].)*

8.4 Reflection Tomography with Point Transmitter/Receivers

As mentioned before, reflection tomography using point transducers leads to line integrals of the object reflectivity function over circular arcs. We will now show that it is possible to reconstruct the reflectivity function by carrying out a backprojection over circular arcs. The derivation here will follow that of Norton and Linzer [Nor79a], [Nor79b]. A more rigorous derivation can be found in [Nor81].

8.4.1. Reconstruction Algorithms

Assume that the object is illuminated by spherical waves produced by a point source at $\vec{r} = (0, 0)$. Such a field can be expressed as

$$\psi_i(t, \vec{r}) = p_t\left(t - \frac{|\vec{r}|}{c}\right). \quad (45)$$

The field scattered by a single scattering site at position $\vec{r}$ can be expressed as

$$\psi_s(t, \vec{r}) = f(\vec{r}) p_t\left(t - \frac{|\vec{r}|}{c}\right). \quad (46)$$

(For simplicity we will continue to assume that both the illuminating field and

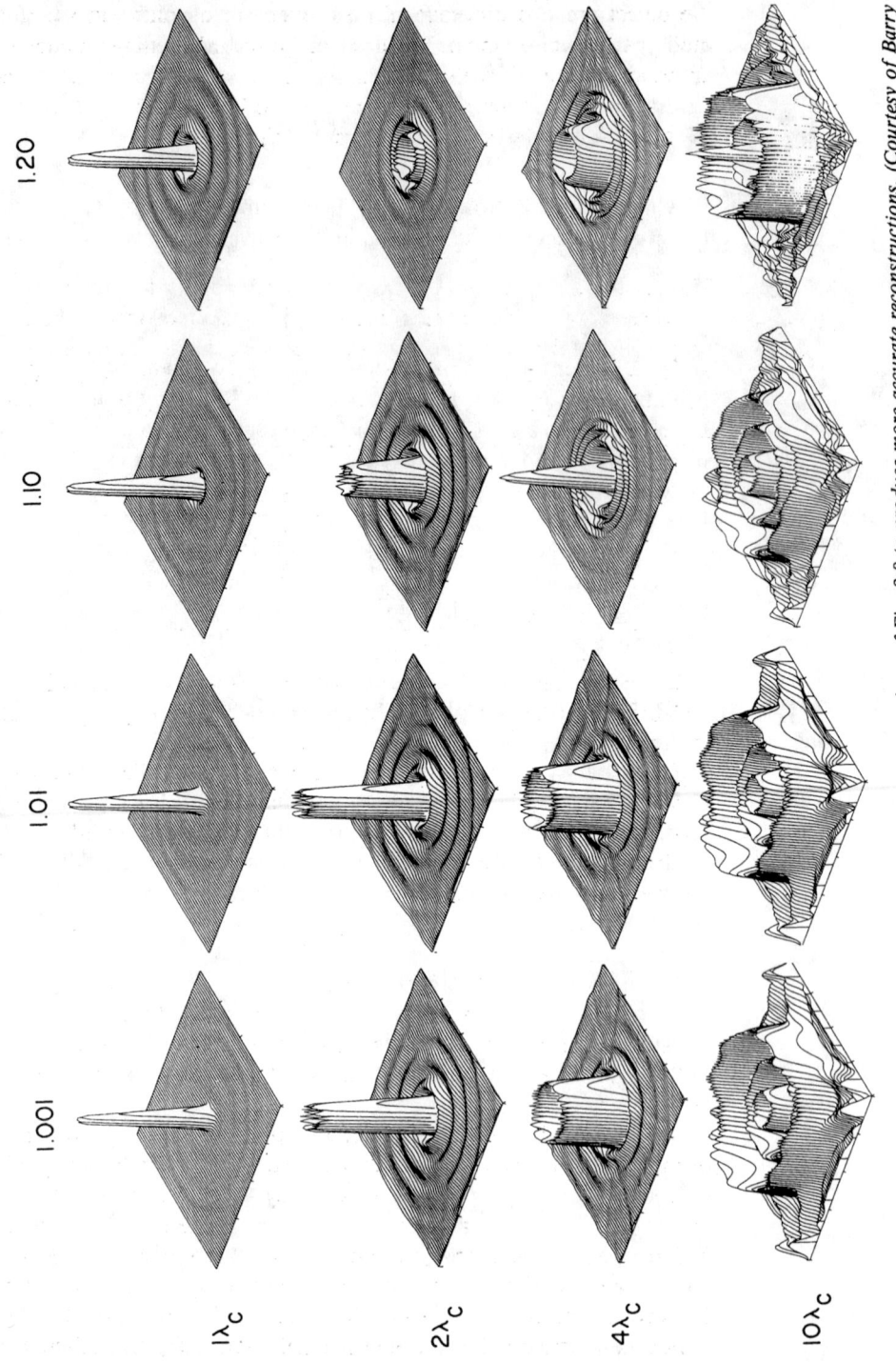

Fig. 8.10: *The Gerchberg–Papoulis algorithm is used on the reconstructions of Fig. 8.8 to produce more accurate reconstructions. (Courtesy of Barry Roberts, Purdue University, Lafayette, IN.)*

314   COMPUTERIZED TOMOGRAPHIC IMAGING

the object are two dimensional.) Since we are operating in the reflection mode, we use the same point transducer to record whatever scattered fields arrive at that site. Since the illuminating field is omnidirectional, the scattered field measured at the point transducer will be given by the following integration over the half space in front of the transducer:

$$\psi_s(t) = \int f(\vec{r}) p_t\left(t - 2\frac{|\vec{r}|}{c}\right) |\vec{r}|^{-1/2} d\vec{r}. \tag{47}$$

The reason for the factor $|\vec{r}|^{-1/2}$ is the same as that for the factor $1/\sqrt{x}$ in our discussion on B-scan imaging and the extra factor of $|\vec{r}|/c$ represents the propagation delay from the point scatterer back to the transducer. Again, as was done for the B-scan case, the effect of the transmitted pulse can now be deconvolved, at least in principle, and the following estimate for the line integral of the reflection data, $g(r)$, can be made:

$$g(r) = \text{IFT}\left[\frac{\text{FT}\{\psi_s(t)\}}{\text{FT}\{p_t(t)\}}\right] r^{1/2} \tag{48}$$

where FT{ } indicates a Fourier transform with respect to t and IFT{ } represents the corresponding inverse Fourier transform. The function $g(r)$ is therefore a measure of line integrals through the object where the variable r indicates the distance from the transducer to the measurement arc. The variable r is related to t by $r = ct/2$, where c is the velocity of propagation in the medium.

This type of reflection imaging makes a number of assumptions. Most importantly, for (47) to be valid it is necessary for the Born approximation to hold. This means that not only must the scattered fields be small compared to the incident fields, but the absorption and velocity change of the field must also be small. Second, the scatterers in the object must be isotropic scatterers so that the field scattered by any point is identical no matter from what direction the incident field arrives.

These line integrals of reflectivity can be measured from different directions by surrounding the object with a ring of point transducers. The line integrals measured by different transducers can be labeled as $g_\phi(r)$, ϕ indicating the "direction" (and location) of the point transducer in the ring, as shown in Fig. 8.11.

By analogy with the straight ray case it seems appropriate to form an image of the object by first filtering each line integral and then backprojecting the data over the same lines on which they were measured. Because the backprojection operation is linear we can ignore the filter function for now and derive a point spread function for the backprojection operator over circular arcs. With this information an optimum filter function $h(r)$ will then be derived that looks surprisingly like that used in straight ray tomography.

For now assume that the line integral data, $g_\phi(r)$, are filtered by the

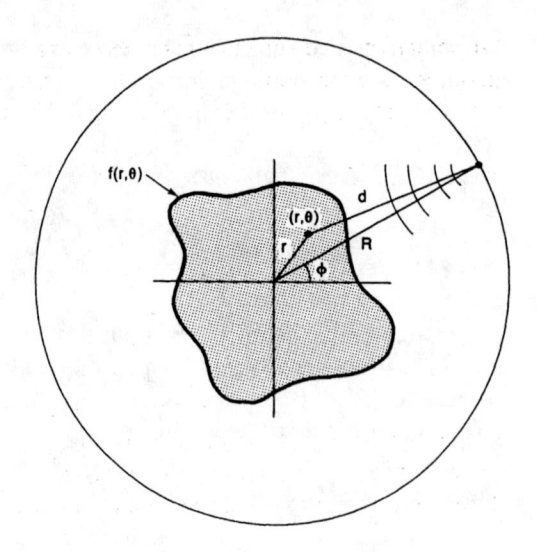

Fig. 8.11: *In reflection tomography with a point source the transducer rotates around the object at a radius of R and its position is indicated by (R, φ). The measured signal, $g_\phi(r)$, represents line integrals over circular arcs centered at the transducer.*

function $h(r)$ to find

$$g'_\phi(r) = g_\phi(r) * h(r). \tag{49}$$

The backprojection operation over circular arcs can now be written

$$\hat{f}(r, \phi) = \frac{1}{2\pi} \int_0^{2\pi} g'_\phi [\rho(\phi; r, \theta)] \, d\phi \tag{50}$$

where the distance from the transducer at (R, ϕ) to the reconstruction point at (r, θ) is given by

$$\rho(\phi; r, \theta) = \sqrt{R^2 + r^2 - 2Rr \cos(\theta - \phi)}. \tag{51}$$

In order to determine $h(r)$ we will now use (50) to reconstruct the image of a single scatterer; this image is called the point spread function of the backprojection process. For a single scatterer at (r, θ_0) the filtered projection is

$$p_{r,\phi}(r - \rho(\phi; r, \theta)) = p_t(r - \rho(\phi; r, \theta)) * h(r) \tag{52}$$

since $p_{r,\phi}$, p_t, and h are all functions of distance. The function $p_{r,\phi}$ represents a filtered version of the transmitted pulse; in an actual system the filter could be applied before the pulse is transmitted so that simple backprojection would produce an ideal reconstruction.

The reconstruction image is then given by

$$\hat{f}(r, \theta) = \frac{1}{2\pi} \int_0^{2\pi} p_{r,\phi}[\rho(\phi; r, \theta) - \rho(\phi; r_0, \theta_0)] \, d\phi. \tag{53}$$

We want $h(r)$ to be such that $\hat{f}$ is as close to a Dirac delta function as possible. In order to find an optimum $h(r)$ in this manner, a number of approximations are necessary. First we expand the argument for $g'_\phi(r)$ in the equation above

$$\rho(\phi; r, \theta) - \rho(\phi; r_0, \theta_0) = [R^2 + r^2 - 2Rr \cos(\theta - \phi)]^{1/2}$$
$$- [R^2 + r_0^2 - 2Rr_0 \cos(\theta_0 - \phi)]^{1/2}. \quad (54)$$

Each term on the right-hand side can be expanded by using

$$\sqrt{1+x} = 1 + \frac{1}{2}x - \frac{1}{8}x^2 + \frac{1}{48}x^3 + \cdots. \quad (55)$$

We will now assume that the measurement circle is large enough so that $(r/R)^2$ and $(r_0/R)^2$ are both sufficiently small; as a consequence, the terms that contain powers of r/R and r_0/R_0 greater than 2 can be dropped. Therefore the difference in distances between the two points can be written as

$$\rho(\phi; r, \theta) - \rho(\phi; r_0, \theta_0) \approx -r \cos(\theta - \phi) + r_0 \cos(\theta_0 - \phi) + \frac{r^2 - r_0^2}{4R}$$
$$- \frac{r^2}{4R} \cos 2(\theta - \phi) + \frac{r_0^2}{4R} \cos 2(\theta_0 - \phi). \quad (56)$$

This can be further simplified to

$$\rho(\phi; r, \theta) - \rho(\phi; r_0, \theta_0) = X \cos(\phi - Y) + \gamma_1 + \gamma_2 \cos 2(\phi - \alpha) \quad (57)$$

where

$$X = \sqrt{r_0^2 + r^2 - 2r_0 r \cos(\theta - \theta_0)} \quad (58)$$

$$\tan Y = \frac{r_0 \sin \theta_0 - r \sin \theta}{r_0 \cos \theta_0 - r \cos \theta} \quad (59)$$

$$\gamma_1 = \frac{1}{4R}(r^2 - r_0^2) \quad (60)$$

$$\gamma_2 = \frac{1}{4R}[r_0^4 + r^4 - 2r^2 r_0^2 \cos 2(\theta - \theta_0)]^{1/2} \quad (61)$$

$$\tan \alpha = \frac{r_0^2 \sin 2\theta_0 - r^2 \sin 2\theta}{r_0^2 \cos 2\theta_0 - r^2 \cos 2\theta}. \quad (62)$$

Now (53) can be written as

$$\hat{f}(r, \theta) = \frac{1}{2\pi} \int_0^{2\pi} p_{r,\phi}[X \cos(\phi - Y) + \gamma_1 + \gamma_2 \cos 2(\phi - \alpha)] \, d\phi. \quad (63)$$

Let $P_{r,\phi}(\omega)$ denote the Fourier transform of the line integral $p_{r,\phi}(r)$, that is,

$$p_{r,\phi}(r) = \frac{1}{2\pi} \int_{-\infty}^{\infty} P_{r,\phi}(\omega) e^{j\omega r} \, d\omega. \tag{64}$$

In terms of the Fourier transform of the filtered line integral data, $\hat{f}$ can be written as

$$\hat{f}(r, \theta) = \int_0^{2\pi} d\phi \int_{-\infty}^{\infty} d\omega \, P_{r,\phi}(\omega) e^{j\omega[\gamma_1 + \gamma_2 \cos 2(\phi - \alpha)]} e^{j\omega X \cos(\phi - Y)}. \tag{65}$$

This result can be further simplified if the measurement radius, R, is large compared to both the radii r and r_0 and the distance between the point scatterer and the point of interest in the reconstruction. With this assumption it can be shown that both γ_1 and γ_2 are small and the point spread function can be written [Nor79a]

$$\hat{f}(r, \theta) = \frac{1}{2\pi} \int_0^{2\pi} d\phi \int_{-\infty}^{\infty} d\omega \, P_{r,\phi}(\omega) e^{j\omega X \cos(\phi - Y)}. \tag{66}$$

When the scattering center is located at the origin, the point spread function is obtained by using

$$\rho(\phi; r, \theta) - \rho(\phi; 0, 0) = r \cos(\phi - \theta) \tag{67}$$

and is given by

$$\hat{f}(r, \theta) = \frac{1}{2\pi} \int_0^{2\pi} d\phi \int_{-\infty}^{\infty} d\omega \, P_{r,\phi}(\omega) e^{j\omega r \cos(\phi - \theta)}. \tag{68}$$

This result can be further simplified by using the Bessell identity

$$J_0(r) = \frac{1}{2\pi} \int_0^{2\pi} d\phi \, e^{jr \cos(\phi - q)} \tag{69}$$

(where q is an arbitrary constant) and rearranging the order of integration to find

$$\hat{f}(r, \theta) = \int_{-\infty}^{\infty} P_{r,\phi}(\omega) J_0(\omega r) \, d\omega \tag{70}$$

where we have assumed that $P_{r,\phi}$ is independent of ϕ for a scatterer located at the origin.

With an expression for the point spread function it is possible to set it equal to a delta function and solve for the optimum filter function. The optimum impulse response $\delta(x, y)$ can be written in polar form as

$$\delta(x, y) = \frac{\delta(r)}{|r|\pi} \qquad (71)$$

when the scattering center is located at the origin. The optimum filter function is then found by noting the identity

$$\int_0^\infty J_0(r\omega)\omega\, d\omega = \frac{1}{r}\delta(r). \qquad (72)$$

Rewriting the point spread function to put it into this form and using the fact that $J_0(\cdot)$ is an even function, it is easy to show that the optimum form for the filtered line integral data is

$$P_{r,\phi}(\omega) = \frac{|\omega|}{2\pi}. \qquad (73)$$

Since $P_{r,\phi}(\omega)$ is equal to

$$P_{r,\phi}(\omega) = H(\omega) P_{t,\phi}(\omega) \qquad (74)$$

the optimum point spread response will occur when the product of the Fourier transform of the transmitted pulse and the reconstruction filter is equal to

$$P_{t,\phi}(\omega) H(\omega) = \frac{|\omega|}{2\pi}. \qquad (75)$$

If the spectrum of the transmitted pulse is equal to

$$P_{t,\phi}(\omega) = \frac{|\omega|}{2\pi}, \qquad (76)$$

then backprojection, without any additional filtering, will produce the optimum reconstruction.

This filter function is not practical since it emphasizes the high frequencies. Generally, a more realistic filter will be a low pass filtered version of the optimum filter or

$$H(\omega) = \frac{|\omega|}{2\pi} \quad \text{for } |\omega| < \omega_c \qquad (77)$$

$$H(\omega) = 0 \quad \text{elsewhere.} \qquad (78)$$

Using this filter function the point spread function for the reconstruction procedure becomes

$$\hat{f}(r, \theta) = \frac{\omega_c J_1(2\omega_c X)}{X}. \qquad (79)$$

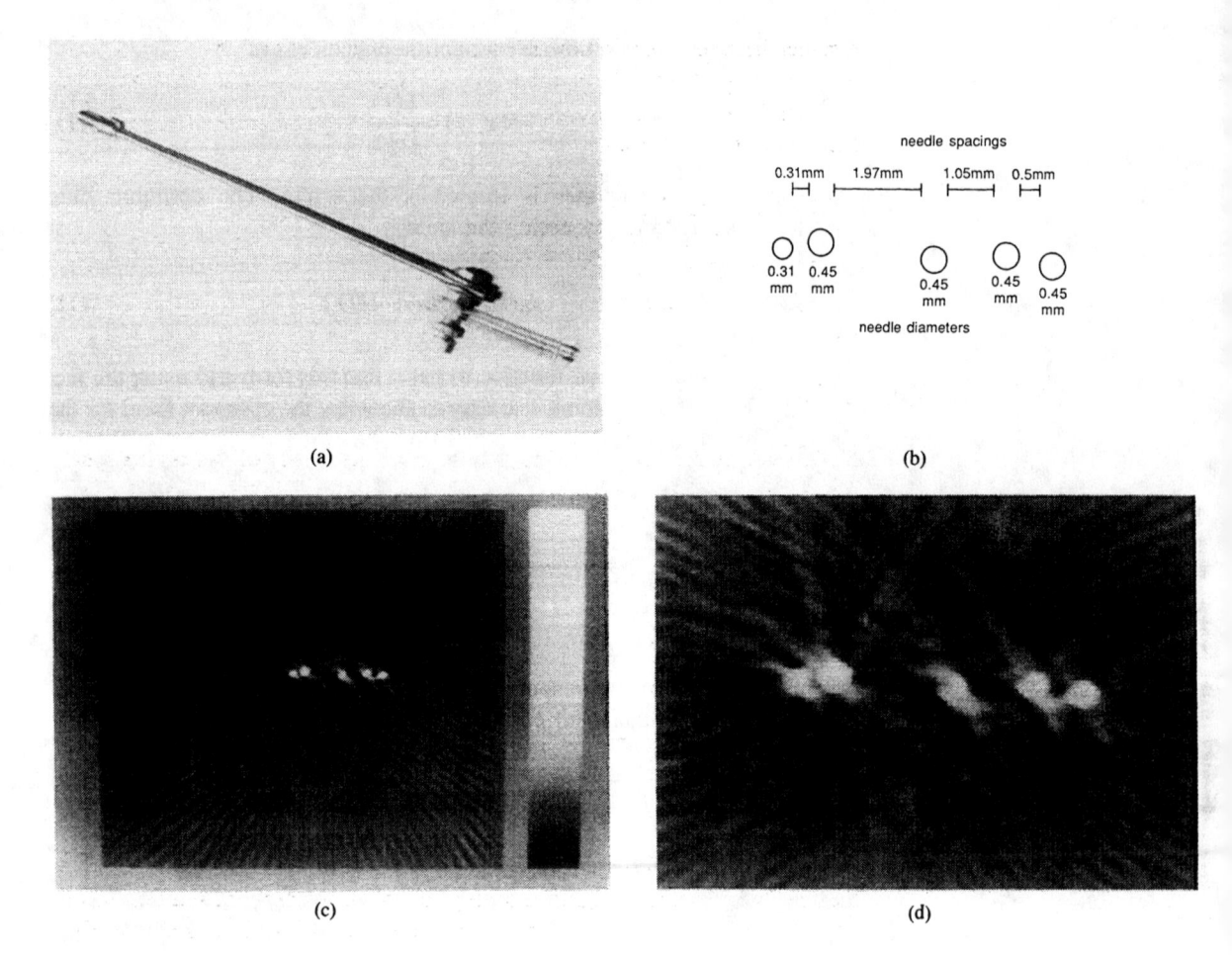

Fig. 8.12: *A broadband reflection tomogram of five needles is shown here. In this experiment a pixel size of 0.1 mm, an image size of 300 × 300 pixels, 120 projections, and 256 samples per projection were used. This figure shows (a) the needle array, (b) a diagram of a needle array cross section showing sizes and spacing, (c) a reflection tomogram of an array cross section, and (d) a magnified (zoomed) view of (c). (These images are courtesy of Kris Dines, XDATA Corp., Indianapolis, IN, based on work sponsored by National Institute of Health Grant #1 R43 CA36673-01.)*

Thus the width of the main sidelobe is given by

$$X_0 \approx 0.30 \frac{2\pi}{\omega_c} = 0.30 \lambda_c \qquad (80)$$

where λ_c is the wavelength of the wave corresponding to the cutoff frequency ω_c.

The reconstruction procedure can be summarized as follows. First use (48) to transform the measured data into measures of line integrals over circular arcs. The data should then be filtered with (49) and then backprojected using (50).

8.4.2 Experimental Results

We would now like to mention experimental results obtained by Kris Dines of XDATA Corporation, Indianapolis, IN. In these reconstructions the distance between the point transducer and the object was large enough so that the line integrals over circular arcs could be approximated as straight lines; the transducer was 200 mm from the center of a 10-mm object. By assuming the integration path can be approximated by a straight line the maximum error in the integration path is 0.25 mm.

The reconstruction of Fig. 8.12(c) shows the resolution that is possible with this method. The five needles suspended in water represent nearly the ideal case since there is no phase shift caused by the object. More experimental work is needed to show the viability of this method in human patients.

8.5 Bibliographic Notes

There is a large body of work that describes the theory of B-scan imaging; for a sampler the reader is referred to [Fat80], [Fla81], [Fla83]. This technique is in wide use by the medical community and the reader's attention is drawn to the well-known book by Wells [Wel77] for an exhaustive treatment of the subject.

One of the first approaches to reflection tomography was by Johnson et al. [Joh78] who employed a ray tracing approach to synthetic aperture imaging. This approach attempts to correct for refraction and attenuation but ignores diffraction. In 1979, Norton and Linzer [Nor79a], [Nor79b] published a backprojection-based method for reconstructing ultrasonic reflectivity. A more rigorous treatment and a further generalization of this approach were then presented in [Nor81] where different possible scanning configurations were also discussed.

More recently, Dines [Din85] has shown experimental results that establish the feasibility of this imaging modality, although much work remains to be done for improving the quality of the reconstructed image. Also, recently, computer simulation results that show the usefulness of spectral extrapolation techniques to reflection tomography were presented in [Rob85].

8.6 References

[Din85]   K. A. Dines, "Imaging of ultrasonic reflectivity," presented at the Symposium on Computers in Ultrasound, Philadelphia, PA, 1985.

[Fat80]   M. Fatemi and A. C. Kak, "Ultrasonic B-scan imaging: Theory of image formation and a technique for restoration," *Ultrason. Imaging*, vol. 2, pp. 1–47, Jan. 1980.

[Fla81]   S. W. Flax, G. H. Glover, and N. J. Pelc, "Textural variations in B-mode ultrasonography: A stochastic model," *Ultrason. Imaging*, vol. 3, pp. 235-257, 1981.

[Fla83]   S. W. Flax, N. J. Pelc, G. H. Glover, F. D. Gutmann, and M. McLachlan, "Spectral characterization and attenuation measurements in ultrasound," *Ultrason. Imaging*, vol. 5, pp. 95–116, 1983.

[Ger74]   G. Gerchberg, "Super-resolution through error energy reduction," *Opt. Acta*, vol. 21, pp. 709-720, 1974.

[Joh78]   S. A. Johnson, J. F. Greenleaf, M. Tanaka, B. Rajagopalan, and R. C. Bahn,

	"Quantitative synthetic aperture reflection imaging with correction for refraction and attenuation: Application of seismic techniques in medicine," presented at the San Diego Biomedical Symposium, San Diego, CA, 1978.
[Nor79a]	S. J. Norton and M. Linzer, "Ultrasonic reflectivity tomography: Reconstruction with circular transducer arrays," *Ultrason. Imaging,* vol. 1, no. 2, pp. 154–184, Apr. 1979.
[Nor79b]	——, "Ultrasonic reflectivity tomography in three dimensions: Reconstruction with spherical transducer arrays," *Ultrason. Imaging,* vol. 1, no. 2, pp. 210–231, 1979.
[Nor81]	——, "Ultrasonic reflectivity imaging in three dimensions: Exact inverse scattering solutions for plane, cylindrical and spherical apertures," *IEEE Trans. Biomed. Eng.,* vol. BME-28, pp. 202–220, 1981.
[Pap75]	A. Papoulis, "A new algorithm in spectral analysis and band limited extrapolation," *IEEE Trans. Circuits Syst.,* vol. CAS-22, pp. 735–742, Sept. 1975.
[Rob85]	B. A. Roberts and A. C. Kak, "Reflection mode diffraction tomography," *Ultrason. Imaging,* vol. 7, pp. 300–320, 1985.
[Wel77]	P. N. T. Wells, *Biomedical Ultrasonics.* London, England: Academic Press, 1977.

Index

Algebraic equations
  solution by Kaczmarz method, 278
Algebraic reconstruction techniques, 283–84
  sequential, 289, 293
  simultaneous, 285–92
Algebraic techniques
  reconstruction algorithms, 275–96
Algorithms
  cone beams, 104
  filtered backprojection, 60–63, 72, 104
  filtered backpropagation, 234–47
  Gerchberg–Papoulis, 313–14
  reconstruction, 49–112, 252–61, 275–96, 313–20
  re-sorting, 92–93
  SIRT, 295
  see also Reconstruction algorithms
Aliasing
  artifacts, 177–201
  bibliography, 200
  in 2-D images, 46
  properties, 177–86
Approximations
  Born, 212–14, 248–53
  comparison, 248–52
  Rytov, 214–18, 249–53
  to wave equation, 211–18
ART *see* Algebraic reconstruction techniques
Artifacts
  aliasing, 177–201
  beam hardening, 124
  bibliography, 200
  polychromaticity, 120–25
Attenuation compensation
  for positron tomography, 145–47
  for single photon emission CT, 137–42
Authors
  affiliations, 329
  Kak, Avinash C., 329
  Slaney, Malcolm, 329

Backprojection, 179
  filtered, 60–63, 65–72, 82, 84–85, 88, 104–7
  star-shaped pattern, 184
  weighted, 92, 106
  3-D, 104–7

Backpropagation algorithm, 242–47, 262
  filtered, 234–47
Bandlimited filter
  DFT, 74
Beam hardening, 118
  artifacts, 120, 124
Bibliographic notes
  algebraic reconstruction algorithms, 292–95
  algorithms for reconstructions with non-diffracting sources, 107–10
  aliasing artifacts and noise in CT images, 200
  measurement of projection data, nondiffracting case, 168–69
  reflection tomography, 321
  tomographic imaging with diffracting sources, 268–70
Bones, 122
Born approximation, 215–18, 249–53, 258
  evaluation, 248–49
  first, 212–14
Breasts
  mammograms, 159
  sonograms, 302
B-scan imaging, 297–303, 315
  commercial, 302

Cancer
  in breast, 159–60
Carcinoma
  sonogram, 302
Coincidence testing
  circuits, 143
  of positron emission, 143
Collinear detectors
  equally spaced, 86–92
Compton effect, 114–15, 119
Computed tomography *see* Computerized tomography
Computerized tomography
  applications, 132–33
  emission, 134–47, 275
  graduate courses, ix
  images, 177–201
  noise, 177–201
  scanners, 130
  ultrasonic, 147–58
  x-rays, 120–24

324 INDEX

Cone beams
    algorithms, 104, 108–9
    projection, 101
    reconstruction, 102, 108–9
Continuous signals
    Fourier analysis, 11
Convolution, 8–9, 31–32, 83
    aperiodic, 18
    calculation, 15
    circular, 18, 66
    Fourier transforms, 39
CT *see* Computerized tomography

Data collection process, 228–34
Data definition
    negative time, 25–26
    positive time, 26
Data sequences, 26
    padding, 23–25
    resolution, 23
Data truncation
    effects, 27–28
Delta functions, 28–30
    see also Dirac delta
Detectors, 75, 101, 127, 192
    arrays, 188
    collinear, 86–92
    equal spacing, 86–92
    ray paths, 190
    spacing, 78, 188
    xenon gas, 128
DFT *see* Fourier transforms—discrete
Diffracting sources
    filtered backpropagation algorithm, 234–47
    interpolation, 234–47
    tomographic imaging, 203–73
Diffraction tomography reconstructions
    limitations, 247–51
Dirac delta, 5–7, 12, 30, 32, 222
    see also Delta functions
Display resolution
    in frequency domain, 22–27
Distortions
    aliasing, 177–201
Dogs
    heart, 154, 156–57

Education
    graduate, ix
Emission computer tomography, 134–47
Equiangular rays, 77–86
Equispaced detectors
    collinear, 86–92
    reconstruction algorithms, 87
Evanescent waves, 261
    ignoring, 266

Fan beam reconstruction
    from limited number of views, 93–99

Fan beams, 78, 85
    projections, 97
    reconstruction, 93–99
    re-sorting, 92
    rotation, 126
    scanners, 188
    tilted, 105
Fan projections
    reconstruction, 75–93
FFT (Fast Fourier Transforms)
    inverse, 42, 240
    1-D, 45
    2-D, 45–47
FFT output
    interpretation, 20–22
Filters and filtering, 7
    backprojection, 60–63, 65, 68, 72, 82, 84–85, 88, 104–7
    backpropagation, 234–47
    bandlimited, 74
    ideal, 72
    low pass, 40–41, 266
    shift invariant, 8
    Wiener, 306
Finite receiver length
    effects, 263–66
    experiments, 266
    reconstruction, 266
Forward projection process
    modeling, 286–88
Fourier analysis
    of function, 9–13, 33–35
Fourier diffraction theorem, 218–34, 253–54, 259
    short wavelength limit, 227–28
Fourier series, 10–13
    triangle wave, 12
Fourier slice theorem, 228, 260, 307
    tomographic imaging, 49, 56–61
Fourier transforms
    diffraction, 219, 223–27
    discrete, 10, 13–15
    fast, 16, 18, 20–26
    finite, 10, 16–18, 42–45
    generalized, 13
    inverse, 13, 17, 34–35, 42, 226
    line integrals, 318
    Parseval's theorem, 39, 44
    properties, 35–41
    seismic profiling, 233
    1-D, 44–45, 56
    2-D, 34–35, 42–45, 222, 226–27, 229, 308
Frequency-shift method, 156–58
Functions
    continuous, 5–7
    discrete, 5–7
    Fourier representation, 9–13
    Green's, 220–23
    Hankel, 220

linear operations, 7-9
point spread, 29, 32
1-D, 5-7

Gibbs phenomenon, 178
Green's function
  decomposition, 220-23
Grids
  representation, 277
  square, 276
  superimposition, 276

Haunsfield, G. N., 1-2, 107
Head phantom
  of Shepp and Logan, 51-53, 69, 103, 198, 255, 259, 285
Helmholtz equation, 224
Hilbert transforms, 68
Homogeneous wave equation, 204-8
  acoustic pressure field, 204
  electromagnetic field, 204
Human body
  x-ray propagation, 116, 195
Hyperplanes, 279

Ideal filter, 72
  DFT, 74
Image processing, 28-47
  Fourier analysis, 33-35
  graduate courses, ix
Images and imaging, 276-83
  B-scan, 297-303, 315
  CT, 177-201
  magnetic resonance, 158-68
  noise, 177-201
  radar, 298-99
  reconstructed, 190-94, 281
  sagittal, 137
  SPECT, 136
Impulse response
  convolution, 9
  of ideal filter, 73
  of shift invariant filter, 8-9
Inhomogeneous wave equation, 208-11
  acoustics, 209
  electromagnetic case, 208
Interpolation
  diffracting sources, 234-47
  frequency domain, 236-42

Kaczmarz method
  for solving algebraic equations, 278
Kak, Avinash C. (Author)
  affiliations, 329

Limitations
  diffraction tomography reconstruction, 247-52
  experimental, 261-68
  mathematical, 247-48

receivers, 268-70
reflection tomography, 309-13
Line integrals, 49-56
  Fourier transforms, 318

Magnetic moments, 163
Magnetic resonance imaging, 158-68
Mammograms
  of female breasts, 159
Medical industry
  use of x-ray tomography, 132, 168
Modeling
  forward projection process, 286-88
Moiré effect, 46, 178
MRI see Magnetic resonance imaging

Negative time
  of data, 25-26
Noise
  in CT images, 177-201
  in reconstructed images, 190-99
Nondestructive testing
  use of CT, 133
Nondiffracting sources
  measurement of projection data, 113-74
  reconstruction, 49-112
Nyquist rate, 19-20, 180

Objects
  blurring, 192
  broadband illumination, 235
  Fourier transforms, 166, 235, 239
  illumination, 300, 304
  projections, 50, 59, 165, 182, 239
  reflectivity, 300
Operators and operations
  linear, 7-9, 30-32
  shift invariant, 8, 30-32

Parallel projections
  reconstruction algorithms, 60-75
Parseval's theorem
  Fourier transforms, 39, 44
Pencil beam
  of energy, 299
Phantoms, 122
  reconstruction, 198, 262
  x-rays, 127
Photoelectric effect, 114, 119
Photons
  emission, 146
  emission tomography, 135-37
  gamma-rays, 135, 138
Plane waves
  propagation, 207
Point sources, 28-30
Polychromaticity artifacts
  in x-ray CT, 120-25
Polychromatic sources
  for measuring projection data, 117-20

INDEX 325

Positron emission tomography, 142-45
Positron tomography
  attenuation compensation, 145-47
Projection data
  measurement, 113-74
  sound waves, 113
  ultrasound, 113
  x-rays, 113
Projections, 49-56
  backpropagation, 245
  cone beam, 101
  curved lines, 95
  diffracted, 204-11
  fan beams, 75-93, 97, 192
  forward, 286-88
  of cylinders, 2
  of ellipse, 54, 62
  of objects, 50, 59, 165, 182, 239
  parallel, 51, 60-75, 77, 100, 185
  representation, 276-83
  uniform sampling, 238
  x-ray, 114-16
  3-D, 100-104, 165

Radar
  imaging, 298-99
Radioactive isotopes
  use in emission CT, 134-35
Radon transforms, 50, 52, 93-97
Received waves
  sampling, 261-62
Receivers
  effect of finite length, 263-66
  limited views, 268-70
Reconstructed images
  continuous case, 190-94
  discrete case, 194-99
  noise, 190-99
Reconstruction
  algebraic, 280, 283-92
  algorithms, 49-112
  bones, 122
  circular, 287
  cone beams, 102
  cylinders, 256, 310
  diffraction tomography, 247
  dog's heart, 154, 156-57
  errors, 177-201
  fan beams, 93-99
  from fan projections, 75-93
  iterative, 284, 289-90
  large-sized, 282
  limitations, 261-68
  of ellipse, 178, 181
  of images, 83, 122, 198, 281
  of Shepp and Logan phantom, 70
  phantom, 198
  plane wave reflection, 310
  refractive index, 154
  simultaneous, 284-92

  tumors, 290, 294
  with nondiffracting sources, 49-112
  2-D, 100
  3-D, 99-107
Reconstruction algorithms, 313-20
  algebraic, 275-96
  cone beams, 103, 108-9
  evaluation, 252-61
  for equispaced detectors, 87
  for parallel projections, 60-75
  implementation, 288-92
Rectangle function
  limit, 29
  2-D Fourier transform, 34
Reflection tomography, 297-322
  experimental results, 320-21
  limits, 309-13
  of needles, 320
  transducers, 307
  vs. diffraction tomography, 307-9
  with basic aim, 297
  with point transmitter/receivers, 313-21
Refractive index tomography
  ultrasonic, 151-53
Re-sorting
  algorithm, 92-93
  of fan beams, 92
Rocket motors
  nondestructive testing, 133-34
Rytov approximation, 249-53, 258
  evaluation, 249
  first, 214-18

Sampling
  in real system, 186-89
  of data, 19-20
  of projection, 238
  received waves, 261-62
SART *see* Simultaneous algebraic reconstruction technique
Scanning and scanners
  B-scan imaging, 297-303
  CT, 130
  different methods, 126-32
  fan beams, 188
  fourth generation, 129
Scattering
  x-rays, 125-26
Seismic profiling
  experiment, 232
  Fourier transforms, 233
Shift invariant operations
  linear, 30-32
Short wavelength limit
  of Fourier diffraction theorem, 227-28
Signal processing
  fundamentals, 5
  graduate courses, ix
  one-dimensional, 5
Simultaneous algebraic reconstruction tech-

nique, 285-92
  implementation, 288
Simultaneous iterative reconstructive technique, 284
  algorithm, 295
Single photon emission tomography, 135-37
  attenuation compensation, 137-42
Sinograms, 94
SIRT *see* Simultaneous iterative reconstructive technique
Skull
  simulated, 121
Slaney, Malcolm (Author)
  affiliations, 329
Sonograms
  of breast, 302
  of carcinoma, 302
Sound waves
  projection data, 113
SPECT images, 136
Synthetic aperture
  tomography, 230-31

Tomography
  applications, 1
  definition, 1
  diffraction, 203, 221, 247, 307-9
  emission computed, 134-47, 275
  Fourier slice theorem, 49, 56-61
  imaging with diffracting sources, 203-73
  positron, 145-47
  positron emission, 142-45
  reflection, 297-322
  simulations, 55
  synthetic aperture, 230-31
  ultrasonic, 147-58, 205
  x-ray, 1-3, 114-33
  x-ray scanner, 1, 107
  3-D simulations, 102
  see also Computerized tomography, Reflection tomography, Single photon emission tomography, Ultrasonic computed tomography

Transducers
  plane wave, 303-7
  pulse illumination, 312
  reflection, 303-7
  rotation, 316
  ultrasonic, 149
Transforms *see* Fourier transforms, Hilbert transforms, Radon transforms
Transmitter/receivers
  point, 313-21
  reflection tomography, 313-21
Tumors
  reconstruction, 290-94

Ultrasonic beams
  propagation, 149, 153
Ultrasonic computed tomography, 147-58
  applications, 157-58
  attenuation, 153-57
  fundamentals, 148-51
  refractive index, 151-53
Ultrasonic signals, 152-53

Wave equation
  approximations, 211-18
  homogeneous, 204-8
  inhomogeneous, 208-11
Weighting functions, 99
  backprojection, 92
Windows
  Hamming, 291, 293-94
  smooth, 98

X-rays
  CT, 120-25
  in human body, 195
  monochromatic, 114-16
  parallel beams, 116
  phantoms, 127
  photons, 128
  projection data, 113
  scatter, 125-26
  sources, 129
  tomography, 114-33
  tubes, 115